Family-Centered Maternity Care

CELESTE R. PHILLIPS, RN, EdD

JONES AND BARTLETT PUBLISHERS

Sudbury, Massachusetts

BOSTON   TORONTO   LONDON   SINGAPORE

World Headquarters

Jones and Bartlett Publishers
40 Tall Pine Drive
Sudbury, MA 01776
978-443-5000
info@jbpub.com
www.jbpub.com

Jones and Bartlett Publishers Canada
2406 Nikanna Road
Mississauga, ON L5C 2WG
CANADA

Jones and Bartlett Publishers International
Barb House, Barb Mews
London W6 7PA
UK

Library of Congress Cataloging-in-Publication Data

Phillips, Celeste R., 1933–
    Family-centered maternity care / Celeste R. Phillips
        p. cm.
    Includes bibliographical references and index.
    ISBN 0-7637-2360-6
        1. Maternal health services.   2. Pregnant women—Family relationships.   3. Childbirth.   4.
    Family.   I. Title.

RG940.P494 2003
362.1'982—dc21   2002043337

Acquisitions Editor: Penny M. Glynn
Production Manager: Amy Rose
Associate Production Editor: Karen C. Ferreira
Associate Editor: Karen Zuck
Production Assistant: Jenny L. McIsaac
Senior Marketing Manager: Alisha Weisman
Associate Marketing Manager: Joy Stark-Vancs
Manufacturing and Inventory Coordinator: Amy Bacus
Cover Design: Kristin E. Ohlin
Interior Design: Anne's Books
Composition: Jackie Davies
Printing and Binding: Courier Stoughton
Cover Printing: Courier Stoughton

Printed in the United States of America
07   06   05   04   03   10 9 8 7 6 5 4 3 2 1

The family is one of nature's masterpieces.

—George Santayana, *The Life of Reason,* 1905

This book is dedicated to:

- ➤ my lifetime friend, companion, and husband, Roger Phillips

- ➤ my son, J. Duncan Phillips, his wife, Curlee-lyn Phillips, and their children, my grandchildren, Tyler and Lauren Phillips

- ➤ my daughter, Catherine Way, her husband, Lawrence Way, and their children, my grandchildren, Elizabeth and Caroline Way

- ➤ my step-grandsons, Stewart and Spencer Way

All together we compose a family.

Acknowledgments

In the course of visits to family-centered maternity programs, research, writing, and seeing this manuscript to publication, I have incurred many debts. During my travels I met wonderful, inspiring caregivers who graciously shared their experiences and materials used in providing family-centered maternity care. I would especially like to thank Melanie Dossey of Nativiti Women's Health and Birth Center, Houston, Texas; Karen Geiser and Vivian Houghton of The Good Samaritan Hospital, Lebanon, Pennsylvania; Barbara Pascoe of Boston Medical Center, Boston, Massachusetts; Urban Midwife Associates of Dorchester, Massachusetts; Jeanette Schwartz of Woodwinds Health Campus, Woodbury, Minnesota; Michelle Young, Cathy Lane, and Anne Maguire of Lawrence General Hospital, Lawrence, Massachusetts; Sister Jean Orsuto of Mercy Health Partners, Cincinnati, Ohio; Leslie Blasewitz of Mad River Community Hospital, Arcata, California; Emily Ousley and Linda Swift of Catawba Memorial Hospital, Hickory, North Carolina; Judy Roudebush and Debbie Brown of Evergreen Healthcare, Kirkland, Washington; Kathleen Besson and Montrice Chapman of Gaston Memorial Hospital, Gastonia, North Carolina; Kathleen Hale of Concord Hospital, Concord, New Hampshire; Beth Lavely of Moses Taylor Hospital, Scranton, Pennsylvania; Cynthia Eckert of Northeast Medical Center, Concord, North Carolina; Janet Bergdoll and Sarah Koontz of Rockingham Memorial Hospital, Harrisonburg, Virginia; and Sharon Schindler Rising of the Centering Pregnancy Program.

Emily Pascoe, a gifted young photographer, generously gave of her time to take numerous photos of childbearing families at Boston Medical Center because she believed in my work. I am grateful for her photos and for knowing her.

I owe a special debt to Rose Michelle Nagel who typed this manuscript one section at a time while taking care of my very active and bright nephew, Jeffrey Christian. I also appreciate the detail work Shirley Coe did to get the final manuscript ready for Jones and Bartlett.

Elizabeth Hamilton did a fine job on Chapter 6, and I thank her for contributing her knowledge about marketing. Barbara Ford contributed a wealth of information on breastfeeding, and I appreciate those contributions very much.

For publication itself, special thanks go to Penny M. Glynn, Nursing Acquisitions Editor of Jones and Bartlett, for believing in the value of my work and helping me to get this book published. Also, I want to thank Amy Rose, Production Manager, and Karen Zuck, Associate Editor, for their good work and all their help.

Of course, this book couldn't have been written at all without all the childbearing families and family-centered maternity care program staffs and leaders with whom I have worked over the years.

Closer to home, and close to my heart, I want to thank my family for their encouragement, love, and support. ∎

—C. P.

Introduction

Perhaps the greatest service that can be rendered by anybody to the country and to mankind is to bring up a family.

—George Bernard Shaw

It has been 42 years and 40 years since my own babies were born in a hospital delivery room. I was a young nurse then and had been socialized to believe that the American hospital way of birth was far superior to any other system in the world. After all, we had improved dramatically on the maternal and infant morbidity and mortality statistics of my mother's generation. In the process, we had mechanized and modernized birth to the point of making us all proud.

MY STORY

It took my own birth experiences to make me realize how much was missing from hospital birth. Knowing that I did not want a narcotized baby who would have to be stimulated to breathe, I had read and prepared for the births of my babies by studying the book *Childbirth without Pain* by Dr. Grantley Dick-Read and practicing relaxation and breathing techniques faithfully.

Although it was unusual to have fathers in the labor rooms in the early '60s, our situation was a bit different because of my nursing background and familiarity with the hospital nurses. It also helped to have a good friend, who was a nurse in the hospital, help me during these labors and smooth the way for my husband, Roger, to participate. Roger and I labored well together. He rubbed my back with each contraction, brought me cold cloths for my forehead, helped me to breathe and relax, and told me that he loved me.

But each time I was ready to deliver, my husband was sent to the fathers' waiting room located at the end of a long corridor distant from the delivery room. Our requests for his presence in the delivery room fell on deaf ears, and the response was, "It's against hospital policy. Fathers cannot come into the delivery room. If we allow one person to violate policy, we will have to allow others. You know this."

Immediately after their birth, each baby was alert, pink and had an APGAR score of 9 at one minute and 10 at five minutes. But each baby was placed in an infant warming bed where the nurse proceeded to weigh and bathe them on the other side of the room, where it was impossible for me to see what she was doing to my babies. On leaving the delivery room each time, I was handed my baby wrapped tightly in a blanket and admonished not to unwrap the blanket.

I was grateful for the safe passage for my babies and myself and for all the help that I had received from the doctors and nurses in the hospital, but it was clear to me that something had been missing. The births of my children were medical/surgical experiences, and those experiences belonged to the hospital. The most important person in my life was prohibited from sharing the births of our children. The feelings of joy that I experienced at the births were my own, and although I could describe the events to Roger, he could not experience them. I felt that a piece of our shared lives was missing.

In the years that have passed since those birth days, our family has grown close and our marriage has developed into a lifelong strong relationship. As a family, we experienced and survived all the passages through the toddler years. As a family, we experienced all the adjustments that have to be made as babies become children and children become adults. Sickness and death touched our family over the years as our parents died and Roger and I became the senior generation. The day also came when we became in-laws and then grandparents. And it all began more than forty years ago in a hospital delivery room.

I realize that there has been significant change in hospital births over the past 40 years. Delivery rooms have become birthing rooms or Labor-Delivery-Recovery (LDR) or Labor-Delivery-Recovery-Postpartum (LDRP) rooms, and fathers are active participants in the birth of their babies. Hospital visitation policies have been liberalized, and in some hospitals mothers and babies are not routinely separated. However, family-centered maternity care is still not standard practice, and in many instances birth is still a medical event that belongs to the hospital and not to the woman and her family.

I have told my story to help explain that birth is not a medical event. Birth is the beginning of a family.

FAMILIES

Families begin with a relationship between two people. It is often a complex relationship forged out of strong bonds of commitment and attachment and built on love. As a couple's relationship grows from being lovers and partners to being parents, their roles become even more complex. We often speak of pregnancy as "being in a family way"; a new person is added to the nucleus of two people as they become parents.

We all seek the ideal family. However, for many of us that perfect family will always be a dream and never a reality. We yearn for connection, trust, appreciation, support, respect, concern, and unconditional love to feel complete. Everyone needs someone to count on, no matter what. Whoever that is, they are our family.

As a family grows, the complexity of family relationships increases. Father, sister, grandparents, cousins, and a community of friends bind us to each other and define who we are. Each person plays many roles. An endless cycle shapes the family from generation to generation.

For many of us, the biggest fear in becoming parents was the fear of failure. Sometimes lacking positive role models, we did not learn how to relate to our children from our parents. Stressed by an increasingly complex world, we have to struggle to develop our own unique approaches to our new roles as parents.

FAMILY-CENTERED MATERNITY CARE

Childbearing couples need help as they become families. I believe family-centered maternity care (FCMC) can provide this help. Sharing information and collaborating between childbearing women, their families, and healthcare providers are the cornerstones of FCMC. Birth is viewed as a normal life event rather than a medical procedure, and women and their families are helped to make the transition to parenthood.

Defining quality maternity care has been the focus of debate and effort by healthcare practitioners, researchers, and consumer advocacy groups for years. Morbidity, mortality, costs, readmission rates, hospital length of stay, and consumer satisfaction are some of the ways that have been proposed to measure quality of care. But what if quality could be measured by childbearing families and healthcare providers together so that it focuses on what childbearing women and their families need in order to have safe, satisfying childbirth experiences and healthy, strong families?

Family-centered maternity care is timeless and should be universal. In writing this book, it is my hope that my grandchildren and their generation will all experience true family-centered maternity care.

ABOUT THIS BOOK

This book is concerned with the childbearing experience—one short but vitally important period of time in the life of a family. This book offers "how to" strategies and methods to translate the philosophy of family-centered maternity care into maternity services operations in hospitals. There are examples of innovative healthcare providers developing family-centered maternity programs in their respective facilities. There are samples of forms, policies, procedures, standards, and other program implementation tools that were contributed by centers of excellence in FCMC. Appendix H provides assessment criteria for self-assessing an existing maternity program in order to determine its level of compliance with the principles of family-centered maternity care. This book contains a wealth of information to help make family-centered maternity care a reality in your institution.

FCMC has the potential to re-energize providers who value quality care for families. There are suggestions throughout this book for ways to help physicians and nurses rediscover the joy of their work as they implement family-centered maternity care.

Family-centered maternity care is not pretty rooms and attractive surroundings. It is an attitude and a philosophy that supports and underpins the whole birth experience.

The doctors and nurses at the Mad River Birth Center in Arcata, California, have captured the essence of family-centered maternity care in their belief statement and welcoming message to new families. Read their statement, think about its meaning, and marvel in their sensitivity.

BEING BORN IS IMPORTANT

We *believe* that birth is:

- Normal
- A life-changing experience
- The beginning of a family
- A celebration

We *believe* we are here to meet the emotional and spiritual as well as physical needs of mother, father, and child.

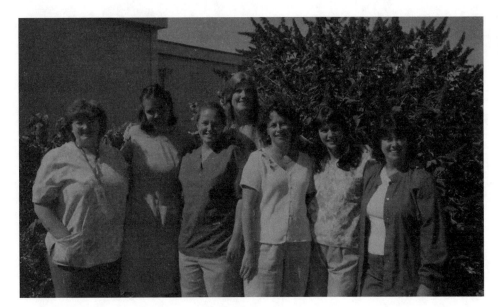

The Birth Center Nursing Team at Mad River Community Hospital, Arcata, California.

We *believe* in working as a team to provide family-centered care that promotes:

- Choices
- Nonseparation of mother and baby
- Breastfeeding
- Responsiveness
- Support and care
- Individualized, customized care
- Education and support of parenting

We *believe* that as caregivers we:

- Are sensitive and caring
- Recognize the need for support and nurturing
- Continually strive for excellence in professional responsibility and accountability
- Must be fiscally responsible

We *believe* that childbearing happens safely when it is a collaborative process between caregivers, women, and their families.

We *believe* that childbearing families are our honored guests.

Contents

CHAPTER THREE

Family-Centered Intrapartum Care   53

CHAPTER FOUR

Family-Centered Care for Pregnancy, Labor, Birth, and Babies at Risk   75

CHAPTER FIVE

Family-Centered Mother–Baby Care 101

CHAPTER SIX

Marketing Family-Centered Maternity Care 145

by Elizabeth Hamilton, PhD

EPILOGUE

Family-Centered Hospital Care: The Core Concepts   161

APPENDICES

INDEX   267

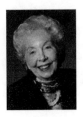

About the Author

Dr. Celeste Phillips, an internationally recognized expert and leader in Family-Centered Maternity Care, has pioneered efforts to improve maternity care through family-centered practice for more than 40 years. She is currently president of Phillips+Fenwick, a women's healthcare company. Founded in 1988, Phillips+Fenwick is located in Santa Cruz, California. Over the past 14 years, the firm has helped hundreds of hospitals throughout the U.S. and Canada to develop high quality, efficiently operated family-centered maternity programs and facilities.

A graduate of Hollywood Presbyterian Hospital, San Jose State University, and the University of Southern California, Dr. Phillips has an extensive clinical and educational background in maternal-child nursing, including staff, management, and educator roles. She has authored numerous books, monographs, and journal articles. Two of her books received the *American Journal of Nursing*'s Book of the Year Award. A prolific speaker on maternity care, she has served as keynote speaker and faculty member for 60 national conferences and symposiums. She has served two terms on the board of directors of the Association of Women's Health, Obstetrics and Neonatal Nursing (AWHONN) and one term on the board of the International Childbirth Education Association (ICEA). Dr. Phillips's work is well recognized, and she has received the Distinguished Professional Service Award from AWHONN and the Lifetime Achievement Award from the National Association of Women's Health (NAWH).

Information about Dr. Phillips's work can be obtained by viewing the Phillips+Fenwick website:

www.pandf.com

by calling her:

831-457-5640

or by writing her:

Celeste R. Phillips, RN, EdD
Phillips+Fenwick
343 Soquel Avenue, Suite 273
Santa Cruz, CA 95062

Family-Centered Maternity Care

INTRODUCTION

The family is the oldest human institution, and in many ways it is the most important. Families have survived as the basic unit of society because they serve vital human needs for nurture and emotional sustenance. The family shares a common culture, and each is unique.

The central purpose of a family is to create, maintain, and promote the social, mental, physical, and emotional development of each and all of its members (Taylor, 2000). This is becoming increasingly difficult. Data from a variety of sources describe a rise in the number of troubled families (Teachman, Tedrow and Crowder, 2000), and some researchers argue that the family is in decline (Popenoe, 1988, 1993; Skolnick, 1991; Munhall and Fitzsimons, 2001; Bennett, 2001).

Although the family has changed constantly throughout time, today the family is in the midst of a profound historical transformation. Older assumptions—such as the idea that marriage is a lifetime commitment, or even necessary—have eroded (Forste, 2002). We live in an era of transition in which families have grown less stable and uniform, and traditional family role definitions and expectations have been thrown into question (Mintz and Kellogg, 1988; Munhall and Fitzsimons, 2001; Bennett, 2001).

Today there are many family forms, including two-parent families, one-parent families, nuclear families, extended families, blended families, cohabiting couples, gay and lesbian families, skip-generation families, and people bonded together in a family through a loving relationship nurtured by proximity and mutual chemistry (Teachman et al., 2000). We become part of a family by birth, adoption, marriage, or from a desire for mutual support.

Increasingly, the childbearing population is becoming more diverse in terms of culture, ethnicity, race, socioeconomic status, and age. Over time, the racial/ethnic diversity will increase, with African-Americans, Hispanics, and Asians representing a greater proportion of the general population (Cox, 1997; Salimbene, 1999). In this extremely diverse environment, the intrinsic "rules" upon which the United States health system and approach to caregiving are based may no longer be valid (Salimbene, 1999).

The Challenge

The challenge today and in the years to come is not to hope nostalgically for a return to the "ideal" of the 1950s family—characterized by high rates of marriage, high fertility, and stable rates of divorce. Instead, the challenge is to help families adapt to the unique demographic and economic conditions of this time, and in so doing become strong families built on love, trust, respect, responsibility, and mutual obligation. This is extremely important because strong families form the foundation of a healthy, productive society.

The childbearing experience—pregnancy, birth, and the first year of life—can have a significant impact on the way parents relate to each other and to their infants and children. With the birth of her baby, the woman experiences one of the most profound life changes she will ever undergo (Simkin, 1991, 1992, 1996). When a woman becomes a mother, she is no longer a separate person. Instead she is intimately interwoven with her child. Neither one exists as totally separate from the other. The mother–child relationship begins with a look of love that can last a lifetime.

When a baby is born, a woman and her partner become parents, and their changing roles require new skills that demand hard work and commitment. Each member of the family is affected by the baby's birth, often in unexpected ways. Parents interpret the larger world for their children and model strategies for dealing with it, some more successfully than others (Munhall and Fitzsimons, 2001).

The Opportunity

Pregnancy and birth present an opportunity for the child-bearing family to develop confidence and mastery in their new roles. Intervention for positive parenting must begin prenatally and continue through the newborn and infancy periods. The way women are treated during their pregnancies and early months of mothering has a profound effect on their self-esteem and ability to parent. Quality educational programs and support for parenting and good health can have a lasting, positive impact on parents' confidence and competence in caring for their children.

Healthcare professionals are able to play a unique role in helping develop strong families through family-centered maternity care (FCMC) programs that support current changes in the structure and functioning of families. Because families are the experts on what family means to them, their active participation in FCMC program development is essential.

FAMILY-CENTERED MATERNITY CARE—WHAT IT IS

Maintaining normalcy in childbirth is a priority in a family-centered maternity program.

Definition of FCMC

Family-centered maternity care is a way of providing care for women and their families that integrates pregnancy, childbirth, postpartum, and infant care into the continuum of the family life cycle as a normal, healthy life event. The care provided is individualized and recognizes the importance of family support, participation, and choice. FCMC is a dynamic process based on a philosophy of care that empowers women and families and guides policy and program development, facility design, decision-making, and daily interactions. Healthcare professionals practicing FCMC recognize that the great majority of childbearing women are healthy and can birth their babies using normal physiological processes. Providing family-centered maternity care, based on the belief that birth is a natural process requiring minimal and selective intervention, in general results in the highest quality low-cost care (Simpson and Knox, 1999).

Family-centered maternity care is characterized by ten principles. These principles are shown in Exhibit 1–1.

Family-centered maternity care requires a fundamental shift from a professionally centered view of health care to a collaborative model (Ahmann, 1994; Phillips, 1996). Attitude about care shifts from control to collaborative decision-making, with the woman and her family as active partners in their health care during the childbearing experience. Services revolve around the needs and expectations of women and their families rather than those of the hospital staff.

EXHIBIT 1–1   Principles of Family-Centered Maternity Care

The following ten principles of operation summarize the philosophy of family-centered maternity care (FCMC):

FCMC Principle 1: Childbirth is seen as wellness, not illness. Care is directed to maintaining labor, birth, postpartum, and newborn care as a normal life event involving dynamic emotional, social, and physical change.

FCMC Principle 2: Prenatal care is personalized according to the individual psychosocial, educational, physical, spiritual, and cultural needs of each woman and her family.

FCMC Principle 3: A comprehensive program of perinatal education prepares families for active participation throughout the evolving process of preconception, pregnancy, childbirth, and parenting.

FCMC Principle 4: The hospital team assists the family in making informed choices for their care during pregnancy, labor, birth, postpartum, and newborn care, and strives to provide them with the experience they desire.

FCMC Principle 5: The father and/or other supportive person(s) of the mother's choice are actively involved in the educational process, labor, birth, postpartum, and newborn care.

FCMC Principle 6: Whenever the mother wishes, family and friends are encouraged to be present during the entire hospital stay including labor and birth.

FCMC Principle 7: Each woman's labor and birth care are provided in the same location unless a cesarean birth is necessary. When possible, postpartum and newborn care are also given in the same location and by the same caregivers.

FCMC Principle 8: Mothers are the preferred care providers for their infants. When mothers are caring for their babies, the nursing role changes from performing direct patient care to facilitating the provision of care by the mother or family.

FCMC Principle 9: When mother–baby care is implemented, the same person cares for the mother and baby couplet as a single family unit, even when they are briefly separated.

FCMC Principle 10: Parents have access to their high-risk newborns at all times and are included in the care of their infants to the extent possible given the newborn's condition.

Source: Phillips, C. R. (1994). Family-Centered Maternity Care. Minneapolis: ICEA.

The point-by-point comparison in Exhibit 1–2 illustrates the differences between many traditional or professionally centered models of maternity care and the family-centered model.

Actual day-to-day practice and attitude in the two care models is illustrated in Exhibit 1–3. In family-centered maternity care processes change from fragmented, compartmentalized experiences to ones that are integrated and seamless.

Advocates for FCMC

For more than thirty years individuals and organizations have been advocating for family-centered maternity care.

EXHIBIT 1–2   Traditional Care versus Family-Centered Maternity Care

Aspect of Care	Traditional Care	Family-Centered Maternity Care
Basic Philosophy	Labor and birth are potentially high-risk medical events that frequently or routinely require invasive procedures, drugs, and restrictions to prevent damage to the mother and/or fetus.	Labor and birth are normal physiologic events involving emotional, social, and physical change and stress, which in most cases require nothing more than close observation and support by medical and nursing staff.
Staff Attitudes	Staff attitude is based on their perception that their role requires them to implement hospital-based rules and regulations.	Staff attitude is based on an understanding of and sensitivity to the important role that childbirth plays in the lives of women and their families.
Policies and Procedures	Policies and procedures are rigid and are designed around hospital and staff needs. No provision is made to meet the needs of diverse populations.	Policies and procedures are individualized and flexible, balancing patient wishes with medical and nursing staff professional judgment. Policies and procedures accommodate all populations the institution serves.
Treatment Decisions	Staff makes treatment decisions, without consulting or collaborating with the family.	Staff uses their expertise to help the family make informed choices; the family and staff collaborate.
Childbirth Education	The primary goal of childbirth education is to instruct couples on the hospital program's policies and practices.	Childbirth education focuses on health promotion, making informed decisions, and self-efficacy strategies. Programs are designed to accommodate the education needs of all the populations that the hospital serves.
Facility	Labor, delivery, recovery, postpartum, and newborn care occur in different locations.	Labor, delivery, recovery, postpartum, and newborn care occur in one location, the LDRP room, or in two locations, the LDR room and a mother–baby room.
Environment	The environment is institutional; it is often unattractive and noisy.	Surroundings are comfortable, with a home–like environment, peaceful and quiet.
Efficiency of Care	Maternity care is fragmented and centered around the caregivers' task-oriented needs. Fragmentation leads to breakdowns in communication and often to longer-than-necessary hospitalization.	Maternity care is centered on case management, which ensures an integrated, cost-effective approach.
Patient Care	Mother and baby are considered separate patients, even when cared for by the same nurse.	Mother and baby are cared for together by the same nurse in mother–baby or couplet care.
Privacy	It is assumed that hospitalization and childbirth require the relinquishment of privacy.	Patients enjoy private room settings with private toileting and bathing facilities; all staff respect family privacy to the extent possible.
Labor Support	Labor support is limited to one person who is not allowed to remain during procedures such as epidural induction or cesarean section.	The mother determines how many and which people will be with her in labor, including children. At least one person may attend her during cesarean birth. Professional labor support (e.g., doulas) is encouraged.
Infant Care	The infant is primarily cared for in the nursery, with nursing staff providing basic infant care.	The infant is primarily cared for in the mother's room, with nurses teaching and modeling infant care and behaviors, and mothers and families taking an active learning role in the infant's care.
Visiting	Visiting hours are restricted for fathers and others in the mother's support network.	Family and friends, including children, are encouraged to be present at the mother's discretion, within safety and health parameters as required by the mother's physical condition.
Consumer Loyalty	Consumer satisfaction is not measured regularly or objectively, so there is little evaluation of or feedback on program components.	Frequent formal, comprehensive consumer evaluations ensure consumer feedback.

EXHIBIT 1–3   Traditional Care versus Family-Centered Maternity Care Behaviors

Aspect of Care	Traditional Maternity Care	Family-Centered Maternity Care
Patient Care	Registration (completion of admission and financial forms) must be done at the time of arrival. The father is asked to register while the mother goes alone to L&D.	Registration is done well in advance of labor and hospitalization. The father and laboring woman are not separated for admission.
Patient Care	The anesthesiologist interviews all women shortly after admission. The interview cannot be waived.	The anesthesiologist sees mothers only upon request.
Patient Care	The staff are brisk and "all business."	The staff are warm and encouraging.
Patient Care	Staff dislike patient "birth plans."	Women are encouraged to submit a "birth plan" prior to hospitalization, and the plan is honored.
Labor Support	The approach to care for the laboring woman emphasizes at-risk, high-tech, or ill aspects of care, such as: • Confinement to bed • Continuous fetal monitoring • Continuous IV infusions • Supine positions for labor and delivery	Care is individualized according to a physiologic approach to childbirth and is delivered in a high-touch, personalized environment.
Labor Support	The nurses prefer laboring women to remain in their room and in bed.	The nurses encourage ambulating and frequent position changes in labor.
Labor Support	Nurses prefer laboring women to have epidurals.	Nurses assist women with nonpharmacologic pain management strategies. Showers and deep hydro-jet tubs are available.
Labor Support	Professional labor assistants (doulas) are not allowed. Having more than one labor support person is discouraged.	Professional labor assistants (doulas) are welcome. Support people are encouraged to be present during labor.
Infant Care	Routine neonatal procedures are done in the nursery while the mother is still in labor and delivery.	Routine neonatal procedures are done at the mother's bedside.
Infant Care	Physicians examine babies in the well-newborn nursery, where they are lined up in cribs.	Physicians examine babies at the mother's bedside.
Education	Postpartum staff teach a class in mother care, and nursery staff teach infant care.	Mother–baby nurses teach both mother and infant care.

They have defined FCMC, developed guiding principles, identified core concepts, made recommendations, published position papers, developed initiatives, and incorporated FCMC principles into professional guidelines.[1]

---

[1] Interprofessional Task Force, 1978; International Childbirth Education Association (ICEA), 1975, 1978, 1986; Health Canada, 1968, 1974, 1987, 2000; Institute for Family-Centered Care, 1998; World Health Organization (WHO), 1996; The Cybele Society, 1980; Maternity Center Association (MCA) 1998, 1999; American Academy of Pediatrics (AAP) and American College of Obstetricians and Gynecologists (ACOG), 1997; Association of Women's Health, Obstetric and Neonatal Nurses (AWHONN), 1998; Coalition for Improving Maternity Services (CIMS), 1996.

The predominant theme in these publications is the goal of improving the overall health status of childbearing families. The focus is on health enhancement and disease prevention. In addition to physical care, social, emotional, and psychological aspects of childbirth and parenting are emphasized. Pregnancy and birth are considered normal life events. The woman is informed so that she can make choices and have a central role in all aspects of her care. Common concepts include: individualized care, respect for each woman's definition of family, empowerment of women and families, choice about care and care providers, information, education, support and follow-up, and partnerships with childbearing families and healthcare professionals.

Evidence-Based Practice

The most recent of these publications (Maternity Center Association, 1999; WHO, 1996; Health Canada, 2000;

AWHONN, 1998) address the issue of closing the gap between evidence and practice in order to make maternity care safer and more cost effective. The emphasis is on providing care that is consistent with the best scientific studies about safe and effective maternity care practices. The phrase "evidence-based" has become synonymous with quality health care.

In practical terms, evidence-based practice (EBP) means basing patient care on more than just tradition; i.e., avoiding a "We've always done it that way" mentality (Simpson, 1999; DeGeorges, 1999). At the same time, few providers change their knowledge, attitudes, and behaviors when new evidence is presented. This is because evidence threatens to end conventional practices, which can be very disturbing to all those who are comfortable with the status quo. The bottom line is that it is difficult to change knowledge, attitude, and behaviors. It is a constant struggle to improve practice (Goer, 1995). For example, research indicates that breastfeeding failure is more common when infants and mothers are separated, when first feedings at the breast are delayed, and when duration of breastfeeding is limited (Gennaro, 1994). However, hospital nursing models of care that support nonseparation of mothers and babies have not been uniformly instituted (Gennaro, 1994). In many hospitals mothers are still separated from their babies during the first hours of life when babies are "transitioned" in newborn nurseries. In addition, many hospitals keep babies in newborn nurseries and bring them to their mothers only for feedings at scheduled times.

Evidence from numerous sources supports many FCMC practices. Clinical practice guidelines, based on evidence, now proliferate in the fields of medicine, nursing, and midwifery. Little evidence has been found to support the use of many care practices previously deemed necessary, such as the use of intravenous fluids in labor and restrictions on positioning and movement (Lothian, 2001).

A valuable source of information about maternity practices is The Cochrane Pregnancy and Childbirth database. It is an ongoing meta-analysis of evidence documenting effective health practices for childbearing women and their babies (Callister and Hobbins–Garbett, 2000). Collaborative reviews from the Cochrane database are based on hand searches of the literature, searches of journals (including MEDLINE), and unpublished data where it is possible to include it. The Cochrane Database of Systemic Reviews (CDSR) is available in printed form, as a CD-ROM subscription, and on the Internet (see Appendix A). The CDSR summarizes the prenatal healthcare practices likely to be ineffective or harmful compared to those likely to be beneficial. Topics can be searched and abstracts accessed without subscribing to the database (www.update-software.com/cochrane/cochrane-frame.html). The family-centered practices discussed in this text are found by the CDSR to be beneficial (see Appendix B).

BENEFITS OF FCMC

The benefits of implementing FCMC are many. The following represent only the tip of the iceberg.

Reduced Healthcare Costs

Studies have documented the cost-effectiveness of family-centered practices. Specifically, these studies have found that family-centered practices lead to reduced use of emergency departments and fewer readmissions to the hospital (Forsythe, 1995; Solberg, 1996; Talbert-May, 1995).

The research of Als and colleagues on family-centered developmental neonatal care documented better medical and developmental outcomes, shorter stays in neonatal intensive care units, and cost savings (Als et al., 1994; Buehler et al., 1995).

When FCMC is practiced, the efficient use of staff, facilities, and supplies reduces costs for hospitals (American Academy of Pediatrics and American College of Obstetricians and Gynecologists, 1997).

Improved Medical and Developmental Outcomes

A 1995 study compared maternal behaviors of 31 young, unmarried, predominantly black, low socioeconomic level mothers who had extended and early contact (rooming-in) with their infants with peers who had contact only during feedings. The findings suggested that increased contact with infants not only led to more interaction between the mother and infant, but also to more touching, including touching in more intimate places, such as the infant's face and head (Prodromidis et al., 1995).

Numerous studies reveal that when a mother wants to breastfeed, has early contact with her infant with an opportunity for suckling in the first hours of life, and is rooming-in with her infant, she is far more successful with breastfeeding than mothers who do not have such experiences (Klaus and Kennell, 1982).

Review of infant feeding policies presented strong evidence that rooming-in and breastfeeding guidance in a rooming-in context has a beneficial impact on breastfeeding among primiparae. Breastfeeding on demand was positively associated with lactation success (Perez–Escamilla et al., 1994).

In caring for mothers and infants after birth, the standard hospital setting, with its orientation toward illness protocols and procedures, is not conducive to helping new parents develop the skills needed to be successful caregivers. It is recommended that when in the hospital setting new parents be treated as responsible adults and be given accurate and consistent information in order to make their own decisions. The parents' decisions should then be supported within the realm of proven good medical care (Enkin et al., 2000).

Evidence from randomized controlled trials conducted throughout the world shows that labor support provides relief of pain, and leads to a decrease in the need for operative vaginal delivery or cesarean section and a slight decrease in the length of labor (Brown et al., 2000; Kennell et al., 1991). Labor support also leads to an improved sense of maternal satisfaction with labor and decreases the incidence of postnatal depression (Hodnett, 1999). Positive effects of continuous labor support by a trained lay person are greater for low-income women who do not have a supportive companion in labor than for middle-class women who do (Simkin and O'Hara, 2002).

Enhanced Satisfaction of Childbearing Women and Their Families

A study examining differences in women's perceptions of quality and benefits of postpartum care in traditional postpartum care versus family-centered postpartum care (FCPPC) revealed that women receiving FCPPC had higher satisfaction with the quality and the benefits of postpartum care than women receiving traditional postpartum care (Hunter and Larrabee, 1998).

Informal evaluations of FCMC programs indicate that the programs are popular with parents. There is little to lose by promoting maternity practices that enhance parents' feelings of satisfaction with their birth experiences.

Personnel expectations, the amount of support from caregivers, the quality of the caregiver–patient relationship, and involvement in decision making are the most important determinants of a woman's satisfaction with her birth experience (Hodnett, 2002).

Enhanced Staff Satisfaction

In a separate study, data were collected both before and after mother–infant care (couplet care) was implemented. Benefits of the new system included increased maternal competence and satisfaction with parent education, parent–infant contact, and the nurse–client relationship, as well as increased staff satisfaction—all with no increase in operational expenses (Watters and Kristiansen, 1995).

A perinatal cross-training program to prepare mother–baby nurses at one hospital demonstrated increased flexibility and efficiency of staffing. This led to improvements in the hospital's finances and employee morale, as well as increasing the skills and marketability of the nursing staff (Altimier et al., 1995).

Janssen and colleagues found that obstetrical nurses experienced improved overall satisfaction with the work environment when they transitioned to family-centered single-room maternity care (Janssen et. al., 2001).

More Effective Positioning of the Organization in the Marketplace

Hospitals also benefit from implementing a maternity program that focuses on the needs of childbearing women and their families. Patient satisfaction is high in FCMC pro-

grams (Janssen et al., 2000). As a result, FCMC hospitals achieve a high level of awareness as the "best place" to have a baby.

FAMILY-CENTERED MATERNITY CARE—WHAT IT IS *NOT*

Despite consumer and professional support for the belief that "birth is not an illness," and that care can be delivered with women and families being full participants in the decision making, there is still a long way to go in completely implementing FCMC.

A Marketing Slogan

In some communities, the term "FCMC" has become a cliché or a marketing slogan employed by hospitals eager to increase their market share of educated, discriminating consumers. A hospital's marketing brochures, newspaper and television ads, and Web site describe beautiful private rooms, décor, and furnishings as being "family-centered," but there is no reference to the actual care provided in those rooms.

Lack of Understanding

In other communities, staff perceive that they practice FCMC by "allowing" fathers to be present in the maternity service at all times. Another belief is that FCMC is practiced when mothers "may have" their babies with them whenever they request. These practices comprise only a small part of an FCMC program, and are not in themselves FCMC.

Inconsistency in Practice

Many healthcare professionals respect and support the idea of family-centered care, but some of their practices suggest otherwise (Rothman, 1996). For example, it is not uncommon to hear nursing staff speak of the importance of nonseparation of new mothers and babies in order to enhance bonding and attachment and facilitate breastfeeding. However, some of these nurses are reluctant or actually refuse to expand their knowledge and skills to provide care for mothers and babies together, as couplets. Instead, they fragment the family unit and provide care for either mothers or babies in the separate postpartum and nursery model. This fragmented care model does not allow the nurse to view and interact with the family as a unit, with each member affecting the other.

Pediatricians recognize the importance of nonseparation of new mothers and their babies. However, they often insist on examining newborns in the well-baby nursery instead of at the mother's bedside. Doing so requires that the baby be separated from the mother, and thus an opportunity to teach the mother about her baby while doing the exam is lost. In family-centered maternity care, the family is regarded as a unit, not as separate, individual patients. Mothers and babies are cared for as a family to facilitate the teaching of newborn and parenting skills and to promote family attachment. This is operationalized in *mother–baby nursing*, in which mother and baby remain, and are cared for, in the same room by the same nurse.

Physicians and nurses may espouse the value of offering women options for managing the pain of labor, but may then insist on women laboring in bed while attached to an electronic fetal monitor. This continuous monitoring preempts the woman's options to ambulate, find her own positions of comfort, or use hydrotherapy while in labor. These methods of pain relief may have been discussed with the woman in prenatal classes, though, and may be among the options she selected to include in her "birth plan." When this happens, the mother's birth plan is of little use to her and she feels disappointed and powerless.

In other cases, FCMC is said to be an important goal in providing care, but the maternity unit doctors and nurses define the family as a nuclear family of mother and child with her choice of one significant other person (Rouse, 2000). Restrictive visitor policies are in place and perceived as necessary in order to protect against infant abduction, conserve patient privacy, and facilitate safe unit operations (Rouse, 2000).

Dysfunctional Operations

The routine practice of separating well mothers and babies, restrictive visitation policies, and the refusal to provide options for labor are often conducted in a well-meaning manner by people who are truly caring, nurturing, and protective. In some cases, though, the hospital policies, schedules, and routines block the practice of FCMC. In fact, the maternity program itself may be lacking in organization and leadership.

As a result, nursing staff may be frustrated by poor communication from management, inadequate orientation or in-service education, and unnecessary or redundant tasks and documentation. When the staff does not feel valued and validated, teamwork suffers.

All the family-centered philosophies in the world will be difficult to implement if the maternity program lacks leadership and its operations are chaotic. A family-centered care initiative that addresses the needs of patients and their families but neglects the needs of the staff will not succeed. In these situations, existing maternity program operations must be improved before FCMC can be implemented. Failure is inevitable if the organization does not spend time developing the basics before introducing a full FCMC initiative.

In other cases, there is no clear direction for care and thus "modified" FCMC is practiced by "exception." For example, family-centered care is given "except" at night, "except" when a staff member does not believe in it, "except" when the census has peaked, "except" when there is not enough staff, and so on.

Medicalization of Birth

It is easy to get caught up in the day-to-day tasks and routine of a busy hospital. There are many people with whom to interact and numerous written and unwritten rules to follow each day. Sometimes coping mechanisms include tightening already rigid rules and regulations to "control the traffic," or simply going about one's tasks "on auto-pilot," oblivious to the hustle and bustle of the system. There is often comfort in the perception that "the way we've always done it" is the only choice.

For the past 30 years, paralleling the movement to FCMC, there has been a proliferation of technologies for use in maternity care. Recent years have witnessed an intensified medicalization of the labor and birth process. In many maternity services, the use of ultrasound, oxytocin (to induce and augment labor), continuous electronic fetal monitoring (EFM), IVs, and epidurals has become routine (Rooks, 1999; Simpson, 2000). Some critics believe that this approach to labor and birth disempowers childbearing women. The concern is that eventually all pregnancies and births will be seen as "high–risk conditions," i.e., potential illnesses needing to be controlled with drugs and technology by physicians in hospitals. If this happens, choice by women would become severely restricted. On the other side of the argument, there are interesting studies demonstrating that some women today deliberately opt for a medicalized birth as a way of exercising control over the unruly process of reproduction, while at the same time gaining "convenience" to select the time and day of birth (Zadoroznyj, 1999).

It is the trend today for couples to accept this purely medicalized labor and birth with little understanding of the impact of the "convenience" approach—almost as if the last four decades of humanizing hospital maternity practices never happened. But these practices did happen, and the advances made in family-centered practice that today's families accept as "standard of care" were hard-won. To understand, it is necessary to take a brief look at the significant changes in the practice of maternity care over the past eighty or so years and then place today's practices within the context of that history.

THE HISTORY AND EVOLUTION OF FCMC

At the beginning of the twentieth century, most women gave birth at home, generally attended by midwives or physicians. Anesthesia and pain medications were not standard practices. Childbirth was accepted as part of the life cycle, and the woman and her family controlled the event (Wertz and Wertz, 1989).

1920–1940

In the third decade of the twentieth century, however, the hospital came to be known as the "modern" place of birth.

It offered women a medical specialist attendant and obstetric analgesia in the form of diethyl ether, or repeated injections of morphine and scopolamine, known as "twilight sleep" (Gogarten and Van Aken, 2000). Upper middle-class women in America formed "twilight sleep societies" and advocated its use for labor, and obstetric analgesia became a symbol of the progress possible through medicine. The twilight sleep movement helped change the definition of birthing from a natural home event to an illness requiring hospitalization. Due to scopolamine's amnesiatic effect, few women remembered their labor and birth experiences.

Childbirth As a Pathologic Process   In the first volume of the *American Journal of Obstetrics and Gynecology* (published in 1929), Joseph De Lee, MD, described childbirth as a "pathologic process" from which few escaped "damage," and urged routine use of forceps, episiotomy, and anesthesia (Speert, 1980). Dr. De Lee believed that childbirth was not a normal function, and that midwives had no place at a birth. He proposed a program of active control over labor and birth, attempting to prevent problems through a routine of intervention that included sedation for labor, anesthesia for birth, episiotomies, forceps deliveries, placental extraction, and oxytocics to help the uterus contract (De Lee, 1927; Leavitt, 1988). All of these interventions became routine for hospital births. The training of obstetricians emphasized the worst-case scenarios possible, and the task of delivery rather than the process of supporting a woman through normal labor and birth.

By 1936, approximately one-third of all live births occurred in hospitals (*American Journal of Public Health*, 1983). Within minutes after birth, babies were transported to large, central newborn nurseries and brought to their mothers in assembly-line fashion for twenty-minute feeding periods scheduled every three to four hours. Mothers commonly bottle-fed their babies with modern "scientific" formula (Apple, 1987).

Restrictive Visitation Policies   The expectant father was relegated to the waiting room for labor and birth to spare him from the "woman's work" of childbirth. Hospital policies restricted his visitation and participation in the infant's care because he was viewed as a source of infection. Of course, other family members and friends were also seen as sources of infection and rigid visitation policies ensured that they had limited access to mother and baby (Leavitt, 1989; Simpson, 2000).

Women remained in the hospital in postpartum wards for seven to ten days where, separated from their families, they often felt lonely and isolated (Leavitt, 1989). Impersonal bureaucracy, efficiency, and medical professionalism dominated the hospital birth experience in the first two decades of the advent of hospital birthing and laid the foundation for years to come.

1940–1960

By the late 1940s, a few women had begun to perceive and regret the costs—many of them psychological—of what they had gained in pain control and convenience. At the same time, several small groups of psychologically oriented, hospital-based academic pediatricians, obstetricians, and child psychiatrists became advocates of early contact between infants and their mothers and the restoration of "family-centered" birth and care of infants.

Rooming-In   Dr. Gisell and his colleague, Dr. Frances Ilg, coined the term "rooming-in," referring to a hospital arrangement of keeping the newborn infant at the mother's beside and allowing the mother to take as much care of the baby as she wished (Gisell and Ilg, 1943). Dr. Edith Jackson directed an experimental rooming-in project at the Grace–New Haven Community Hospital from 1946 to 1952, where rooming-in was practiced in two four-bed units. Rooming-in, under Dr. Jackson's leadership, effectively eased the tensions of new motherhood by allowing the mother to become familiar with her infant before leaving the hospital (Klaus and Kennell, 1976).

Prepared Childbirth   At about the same time, in England, Dr. Grantly Dick-Read began to advocate natural childbirth. Dick-Read had started as a physician who supported the use of anesthesia during childbirth. After assisting at a natural childbirth, he became a supporter of drug-free delivery. Coining the term "childbirth without fear," Dick-Read emphasized relaxation techniques and prenatal education (Dick-Read, 1953).

In France, Dr. Ferdinand Lamaze developed "childbirth without pain," the *Lamaze* method. Dr. Lamaze observed women in the Soviet Union give birth without anesthesia. The women had been trained to use specific breathing patterns and relaxation techniques with the assistance of a trained woman, called a "monitrice." The Russian childbirth system was based on Pavlovian conditioning. Dr. Lamaze borrowed from this technique. In addition, he developed a series of breathing patterns and nonpharmacologic techniques women could use to cope with the pain of labor. The Lamaze method gained popularity in the United States after Marjorie Karmel wrote of her childbirth experience using the Lamaze method in the 1957 book, *Thank You, Dr. Lamaze.* Women began preparing themselves for birth using both Dick-Read's method and the Lamaze method and found that their pain was relieved and their birth experiences were rewarding. They felt a sense of control again.

FCMC   In the 1950s, Sister Marie Stella, CNM, introduced the concept of "family-centered maternity care" at St. Mary's Hospital in Evansville, Indiana (Young, 1987). Later in the decade, Ernestine Wiedenbach, a certified nurse–midwife, authored a nursing classic, *Family-Centered Maternity Nursing*. In this book, she challenged conventional nursing practices by encouraging nurses to provide supportive maternity nursing care based on recognizing the needs of each mother, father, infant, and family (Wiedenbach, 1959).

La Leche League   Seven suburban women eager to promote the "womanly art of breastfeeding" founded the La Leche League in 1956. At the time, only about 20 percent of American women breastfed their babies, but many were learning about the benefits of breastfeeding and were eager to try it. These women welcomed breastfeeding assistance from the La Leche League (Leavitt, 1989).

Women Speak   By the late 1950s, articles appeared in the popular literature denouncing American hospital practices for birth. In May 1958, *The Ladies' Home Journal* published letters from American women in an article titled "Mothers Report on Cruelty in Maternity Wards" (Shultz, 1958).Women reported being strapped down on delivery tables or being left alone for long periods of time while in labor. One woman wrote: "Our biggest enemy is smugness and indifference" (Schultz, 1958).

The Social Movement of FCMC   By 1960, 97 percent of births occurred in hospitals and the stage was set for the social movement of family-centered maternity care. Throughout history, most social movements have begun in reaction to situations that people perceive to be intolerable. Many women and their families and a small group of professionals, unwilling to tolerate the obstetric practices of the time, began the revolution to FCMC (Zwelling and Phillips, 2001).

1960–1980

In the 1960s consumer organizations formed and advocated for FCMC.

Consumer Organizations   The International Childbirth Education Association (ICEA) was founded in 1960 at its first convention, in Milwaukee, Wisconsin, under the motto, "Freedom of choice based on knowledge of alternatives." In New York in 1960, the American Society for Psychoprophylaxis in Obstetrics (ASPO) was founded to promote the Lamaze method and educate Lamaze teachers (Phillips, 1996).

In the early 1950s, Dr. Robert Bradley, an American obstetrician, became familiar with the work of Dr. Grantly Dick-Read. He believed women should be awake during childbirth, and because of this became an advocate of natural childbirth. Whereas most practitioners left men in the waiting room, Bradley felt that husbands should be included in the birth experience. He focused on educating the pregnant couple so that the husband could serve as "coach" during labor. The Bradley Method®, also known as Husband-Coached Childbirth, emphasized education, controlled breathing and relaxation, breastfeeding, and maternal nutrition and exercise. The American Academy of Husband-Coached Childbirth (AAHC) was founded in 1970 to promote Dr. Bradley's methods and train teachers (Wallace, 2000).

The National Association of Parents and Professionals for Safe Alternatives in Childbirth (NAPSAC) was also influential at this time. NAPSAC emphasized a strong commitment to family values and responsibility in childbearing.

Grassroots leaders evolved out of these organizations. Numerous childbirth educators were prepared, and all taught choice and alternatives and diligently searched for the truth about childbearing. As expectant couples became better informed they asked more questions. Couples flocked to childbirth classes. By the 1970s, "natural childbirth" was the vogue.

Women's Self-Help Movement   In the 1970s, the women's self-help movement emerged. *Our Bodies, Ourselves* was published, epitomizing the movement. Women consumers and women health professionals openly challenged many assumptions of the obstetrical system and demanded new models of care delivery. Women complained bitterly about their babies being taken away from them after birth and their husbands being separated from them.

Articles appeared in popular magazines—*McCalls* (1976), *Good Housekeeping* (1974), and *People Weekly* (1975)—about the new concept: family-centered childbirth and husbands delivering their own babies. The emphasis was on birth as a joyful celebration and not a disease to be cured.

The 1970s was also a turbulent decade that brought an end to many traditional values and beliefs. As educated childbearing couples became more and more unhappy with the rigid obstetrical practices of hospitals, some turned to home birth as the preferred alternative. Although the American College of Obstetricians and Gynecologists (ACOG) actively discouraged home births, some physicians attended women birthing at home, CNMs attended more, and lay midwives attended many. Despite a lot of divisiveness, consumer demand for changes began to result in changes in hospital practices.

Alternative Birth Centers   Alternative birth centers (ABCs), also called "birthing rooms," were opened in many hospitals. These more attractive "homelike" settings offered an alternative to the conventional labor and delivery rooms. The birthing rooms were often located adjacent to or near existing labor wards, and were intended for the care of women whose pregnancies were considered low-risk and who both desired and required little or no medical intervention during labor and birth.

The policies and procedures in the ABCs encouraged family participation and nonseparation of well mothers and babies. Obstetric interventions typically were not permitted and thus any maternal or fetal deviations from a normal labor required transfer out of the ABC to conventional labor and delivery units (Hodnett, 1998). As a result, many women were "risked out" of the birthing room when they needed intravenous fluids, oxytocin, labor augmentation, electronic fetal monitoring, analgesia, forceps delivery, and induction of labor (Hodnett, 1998). However, despite these reasons for transfer, many women who might have chosen home birth instead came to hospitals because of the birthing room option (Tegmeier and Elsea, 1984; May and Ditolla, 1984).

Freestanding Childbearing Centers   Freestanding childbearing centers were developed in 1976, with the Maternity Center Association (MCA) in New York City leading the way. The MCA demonstrated that the New York Maternity Center could provide high-quality, homelike birthing experiences at costs less than hospital deliveries. Using nurse–midwives to provide most of the care was an important factor in savings (Lubic, 1983).

As the 1970s came to a close, the hospital birth experience was changing again. The natural childbirth movement remained active, but many women chose medications and epidurals to cope with the pain of labor. The hard-fought battle for consumer choice, father participation in labor and birth, and the liberalization of rigid rules and regulations for hospital maternity care had been won. But most women were still separated from their babies within one to two hours after birth, and were moved through the assembly line of labor to delivery to recovery and then to postpartum. Electronic fetal monitoring was standard of practice and the cesarean birth rate increased from 5.5 per 100 births in 1970 to 14.7 percent in 1978 (Taffel, et al., 1987). Questions began to arise about the association between electronic fetal monitoring and the increasing cesarean birth rate (Schmidt and McCarthey, 2000).

1980–2000

Access to Care   During the 1980s there was a widening and deepening sense of crisis regarding the country's ability to provide adequate and effective maternity and other reproductive health care to all of its women. Racial and ethnic minority women, rural women, and women living with poverty and social distress were particularly likely to have limited access to effective care.

During the late 1980s, Congress enacted legislation to make Medicaid available to more women and also required states to make Medicaid-eligible women's access to obstetric care equal to that of other women. Also, most state governments began to contribute more for maternity care.

In the early 1990s, some physicians who were once disinterested in taking care of poor, pregnant women became more willing to do so as Medicaid increased its fees paid for services and made it easier to obtain these fees. This provided an opportunity for disadvantaged women to have more choices in care providers and places for birth. However, these same women now found themselves in healthcare environments that often were not cognizant of and prepared to deal with their unique social situations and family needs.

Also during the 1980s, the hospital setting for birth was dramatically changing. Responding to a need to reduce costs as well as attract insured patients and improve their payer mix, many hospitals converted to more functional and homelike obstetrical designs through the 1980s and into the early 1990s (Nathanson, 1985).

LDRs and LDRPs   New hospital facility designs were developed that allowed for the replacement of multitransfer OB units with labor/delivery/recovery rooms (LDRs), and postpartum units with separate central nurseries. Some hospitals went a step further and converted to one room for labor/delivery/postpartum and well-newborn care (LDRP rooms) and did not build central nurseries. Instead, these hospitals designed small "baby holding or respite areas" where well babies could be cared for while out of their mother's rooms for short periods of time. The goal in these hospitals was nonseparation of well mothers and babies. To accomplish this goal, postpartum and nursery nurses were cross-trained to function as mother–baby, or couplet, nurses.

Focus on Facility   The new facility designs of LDRs and LDRPs do *not* in themselves provide FCMC. LDRs and LDRPs are only rooms. It is the program that must change. Unfortunately for many families, the program of care offered in many new LDR and LDRP units maintains a philosophical orientation to high-tech care in labor and birth management (Midmer, 1992). Mothers and babies are often separated for the first few hours of life and postpartum nurses provide care for the mother while nursery nurses care for the baby (Zwelling and Phillips, 2001).

Many physicians and nurses are torn between their belief in FCMC and their desire to hold onto the old clinical practices into which they were socialized. Changing to FCMC requires a change in attitude that must start at the top of the organization, with its administration.

REACHING CONSENSUS ON FCMC

FCMC is not practiced in a vacuum. The hospital culture must support the care practices and the caregivers. For FCMC to succeed, the hospital must prioritize the creation of a culture that supports and prepares providers and staff to practice FCMC. The hospital maternity service must exist for the families it serves. Whenever a change in policy or procedure is being considered, the first question to answer must be: "What is best for the patient and her family?"

It is possible to create a new future for an organization—to break down outmoded structures and create organizations that can thrive. The process is grounded in values, shaped by vision, guided by strategy, and focused on deliberate day-to-day actions. Values and vision provide a basis for change to FCMC.

Purpose, Values, and Mission

A hospital revolves around people: providers, nursing staff, support staff, all the workers, and the families these people serve. The hospital literally exists for the patients. Without them, there is no need for a hospital. This may sound simplistic and foolish, but it is essential to the practice of FCMC.

When nurses say, "I don't want to take care of mothers, I only want to take care of babies," and physicians say, "I don't want to examine babies in front of their mothers," the question is not about what the physicians and nurses want. The question is always: What is best for the mothers and babies? We must keep going back to the purpose and values that provide the foundation for the sense of professionalism that defines each job in the hospital (Gerteis et al., 1993).

Purpose   Inside each healthcare professional is a person with ideals who entered the caring profession because of a belief in the importance of the work. That person inside is often waiting to be drawn out, recognized, and given a purpose with which to identify. People aspire to identify with organizations that can respect and perform work that contributes value in ways they can understand (Sullivan and Harper, 1996). Doing what is best for mothers and babies must always come first. Doing that work better than anyone else can be a powerful, uniting purpose.

Values   Core values guide and shape the way the people who provide FCMC fulfill their purpose or mission. Values align people and get them committed to working together for common goals. FCMC begins by clarifying the maternity service purpose: the vision, mission, and values.

FCMC Task Force   The process used to arrive at a mission and values begins with the formation of a multidisciplinary FCMC task force, or planning work group, to serve as a leadership team for achieving FCMC. Members of this group should include top management and key stakeholders, including childbearing families. The team members become informed on FCMC through reading the research, studying the evidence, making site visits to benchmark FCMC programs, reviewing information on local consumer preferences and patient satisfaction data, and meeting with childbearing families that serve in an advisory capacity. After completing the initial study and data gathering, the FCMC task force agrees on a draft mission and a set of prioritized values for the maternity service. FCMC core values are listed in Exhibit 1–4.

Mission   The mission focuses on the present and provides a sense of purpose for everyone who provides care for childbearing families. The mission explains what the maternity program is all about. It should remain constant, providing meaning for generations of employees (Buckingham and Coffman, 1999). The mission of the Birthplace at Gaston

EXHIBIT 1–4   FCMC Core Values

- Mutual respect and trust
- Informed choice
- Empowerment
- Collaboration
- Flexibility
- Quality
- Individualized care

Memorial Hospital in Gastonia, North Carolina, sets the foundation for quality FCMC programming at that hospital. The mission is as follows:

Mission
- We value the knowledge that promotes women's health and wellness and strive to continually educate ourselves and our patients on these issues.

- We respect the importance of the family and encourage family involvement and support in our patients' lives.

- We recognize birth to be a unique, individual, and natural process and provide competent and caring staff to support mother, child, and family during this joyful event.

Before completing the mission and values draft, it is important to discuss actual implementation of the mission and determine how current practice will have to change so that the mission can become reality. This exercise is essential in order to answer staff questions when the draft is circulated.

When the FCMC task force has agreed upon the draft mission, a set of prioritized values, input, and feedback are gathered from providers, staff, board members, and childbearing families. This process occurs over several months and involves unit-based groups consisting of staff from each shift and a family advisory group. Unless employees can link the mission and values to their actual work lives, the mission and values will be meaningless (Blanchard and O'Connor, 1997). Thus, effective communication is essential. Everyone involved must understand the mission and core values and "buy into" them.

Vision

Grounded in purpose, values, and mission, the leadership team next creates a vision, a context within which the maternity program's future can be created. The vision must *pull* the maternity program into the future. In developing the vision statement, the following questions must be answered: What is the situation now? Who is served? What do they receive? What are the main issues and opportunities we face? What will make the difference between success and failure? Where should we be going in the future? What changes would we like to make? Is our mission statement congruent with where we are going? How committed is the group to new possibilities? What activities will help us accomplish our goals?

What resources do we need to accomplish our goals? How will we know when we have accomplished our goals?

A forum for developing the vision is often a planning and consensus building retreat attended by the FCMC leadership team. The planning process consists of presentations on FCMC and the work completed to date as well as large and small group activities and discussions. Childbearing families participate in the retreat and are active members of the FCMC leadership team.

The vision statement that is developed should describe an achievable future, such as the vision statement that follows, from The Family Place at Concord Hospital, Concord, New Hampshire. Note that it forms the basis for looking ahead, not for affirming the past or the status quo:

Vision

- The Family Place at Concord Hospital will be a center of excellence in family-centered obstetric, gynecologic, and pediatric services across the continuum of care.

- The emphasis in all programs will be on offering excellent, safe, accessible, and cost-effective health care.

- The environment will promote collaboration between families and staff to be working partners in designing and building positive health care experiences.

- These services will be a model of developmental, holistic, age-appropriate care delivered in an atraumatic environment.

- The maternity services will be provided in an innovative single-room maternity model.

Vision and Critical Mass   Once the leadership team has reached consensus on the maternity program's purpose, values, and vision, the vision must be communicated and understood in a way that empowers people to seek to achieve it (Sullivan and Harper, 1996). Staff must be infused with a sense of enduring purpose in order to provide day-to-day care in these difficult times. The vision must describe the future in a way that gives meaning to the work of patient care. A shared vision that has been developed by hospital planning teams using a consensus process can serve as the driving force for change to FCMC. It takes time for a vision to become embedded in an organization; sometimes it may take years.

Philosophy

A philosophy for a maternity program is a "belief" statement that directs caregivers in the achievement of their mission. The philosophy provides the basis for decision making about care provided for families in the childbearing year. All policies, procedures, protocols, standards of care, position descriptions, and staff selection and evaluation methods are based on this philosophy. The written FCMC policy is publicly displayed, reviewed, and reaffirmed annually.

A philosophy for an FCMC program should be a thoughtful expression of group values, such as this statement of philosophy from Evergreen Family Maternity Center in Kirkland, Washington:

Our Philosophy

We believe that:

- Birth is one of life's most special events.

- Birth and parenting occur with greater ease, comfort, and joy when parents assume their role with knowledge.

- Birth is a natural, physiological process that can be a positive time of growth.

- Parents can make decisions and accept responsibility for their own health care.

- Family, visitors, nurses, physicians, midwives, and all hospital personnel are regarded with dignity and respect.

Another thoughtful philosophy statement is the one developed for the Birth Place at Boston Medical Center. It is a philosophy that emphasizes the provider's beliefs when caring for a very diverse urban population:

- The Birth Place at Boston Medical Center promotes and supports family-centered care.

- The Birth Place recognizes the importance of the family unit and strives to enhance family cohesion. This is accomplished using a family systems approach and through the use of advocacy. Family values and priorities as well as cultural mores are used as a basis for establishing a plan of care.

At the Birth Place we strive to:

- Facilitate collaboration between parents and healthcare team.

- Honor the racial, ethnic, cultural, and socioeconomic diversity of families.

- Recognize family strengths and individuality.

- Encourage and facilitate family-to-family support and networking.

- Incorporate the developmental needs of infants and their families into the healthcare delivery system.

- Implement comprehensive policies and programs to meet the needs of the families.

Figure 1–1 illustrates a multidisciplinary team working on policies at Boston Medical Center. Representatives from midwifery, nursing management, nursing education, and the medical staff are present at this meeting.

Another approach to philosophy emphasizes "team" provision of family-centered care at Mad River Community Hospital in northern California:

Philosophy

We believe in working as a team to provide family-centered care that promotes:

- choices

- responsiveness

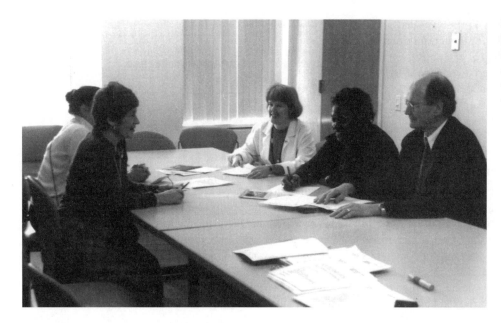

FIGURE 1–1 Multidisciplinary team, The Birth Place at Boston Medical Center. *Source: Photo by Emily Pascoe. Photo courtesy of Boston Medical Center, Boston, Massachusetts.*

- support and comfort
- individualized, customized care
- education and support for parenting
- nonseparation of mother and baby
- breastfeeding

Strategies for Change

As important as values, mission, vision, and philosophy are, they must be joined by a strategy—a set of concepts for action—before positive change can result (Sullivan and Harper, 1996). Strategies outline how the vision will be achieved within the context of the mission and values. Strategies change as the program changes. Managers may need to develop strategies to deal head-on with stubborn pockets of resistance (Gerteis et al., 1993). Developing a family-centered mission and building the organizational culture to sustain that mission will take considerable effort over time.

Goals It is at this point that goals can be set. Goals are broad and general statements about ways to make the mission and the philosophy functional. They are part of the overall plan for an FCMC program. Once again, the goal development can originate with the FCMC leadership team and then be reviewed and perhaps revised by the unit-based teams and the family advisory members. Examples of goals that, when achieved, contribute to the practice of FCMC are to:

- Facilitate the bonding process between parents and infants.
- Provide an environment in which the family unit is minimally disrupted.
- Promote family growth and education.
- Assist the expectant family to identify, determine, and meet their own health goals.

- Assist the expectant family to understand and cope with the impact of pregnancy and parenthood.
- Assist individuals and family to prepare for healthy and wanted pregnancies through family planning education.
- Prepare the expectant family to achieve a satisfying labor and delivery experience.
- Teach and promote appropriate parenting skills.

It is essential that the first strategic goal selected be achievable and capable of yielding immediate benefits. One step at a time, success in implementing one new family-centered policy or procedure leads to the next success.

Objectives Unlike goals, objectives are specific, measurable, and observable. Objectives are behavioral expectations that can be expressed in definite, tangible, quantitative terms. Every objective should:

1. Be written.
2. Be clear.
3. Outline the method by which it is to be achieved.
4. Indicate the reason that it was developed.
5. Set the time by which it is to be achieved.
6. Enclude a method of evaluation.

In order to be useful, an objective must be stated in terms of the results to be achieved, instead of the method to be used. For example, the objective "mothers will be taught about breastfeeding" focuses on the activities of the nurse rather than on the resulting benefits to the new mother. In contrast, a measurable objective would be stated as, "by the second day postpartum, each new mother will demonstrate on her own breasts the correct method of hand expression of breast milk." With this objective the focus is on outcome.

As is true in the development of philosophy and goals, the development of objectives calls for thoughtful examination of the reasons for them. Each goal and objective needs to be consistent with available research ("evidence-based") and/or established standards and guidelines from professional organizations. Objectives that are written in terms of outcomes to be achieved and behaviors to be observed can be useful tools for the evaluation of care provided.

Culture Change and Development

When benchmarking against successful FCMC programs, it is easy to identify some commonalities. These are: a genuine passion for FCMC; a sense of being part of a work in process; always striving to improve the FCMC program; an openness of vision grounded in values; a zest for continuous learning; and a deep, abiding belief in people. In the final analysis, everything comes back to people. People are the FCMC program. The bricks and mortar and equipment are only there to provide a functional environment in which the people can achieve the goals of FCMC. Success in implementing FCMC is 80 percent people and processes and 20 percent facility design (see Exhibit 1–5).

The excellent family-centered program at Gaston Memorial Hospital is an example of success being 80 percent people and processes. Figure 1–2 presents some of the nursing staff responsible for that family-centered program. Note how happy they are.

Family Involvement   As recipients of care, families bring expertise to the planning and operations of FCMC programs. Successful FCMC programs are based on patient and family identified needs rather than professional assumptions. Family members can be included as members of leadership teams, task forces, and advisory boards. They can

EXHIBIT 1–5   Success

> Success =
> 80% people and processes
> 20% facility

participate in focus groups, conferences and work meetings, fundraisers, and committees hiring new staff. Family members can be involved as program evaluators, paid program staff, grant reviewers, or mentors for other families (Institute for Family-Centered Care, 1994).

At Markham Stouffville Hospital in Markham, Ontario, Canada, community members sit on the maternal–child System Advisory Committee. Other committee members include the system director, chief, physician coordinators, clincial managers, professional representatives, a midwife, and the chief of anesthesia. The committee meets quarterly, and membership is renewed annually.

Leadership   The process of cultural change is most successful when the hospital's top leaders "walk the talk" of FCMC. Walking the talk means that leaders' attitudes and actions are consistent with their words. There is power in personal example. Physician champions who believe in the practice of family-centered obstetrics, pediatrics, and also in utilization of multidisciplinary care teams and collaborative practice are essential to gain the support of their colleagues for FCMC program goals.

Because nurses provide most of the day-to-day patient care, nursing leaders are pivotal to the successful implementation of the FCMC program. Effective nursing leadership requires very special qualities. First and foremost is the ability to inspire others with the leader's personal vision and commitment to the values, mission, vision, and philosophy

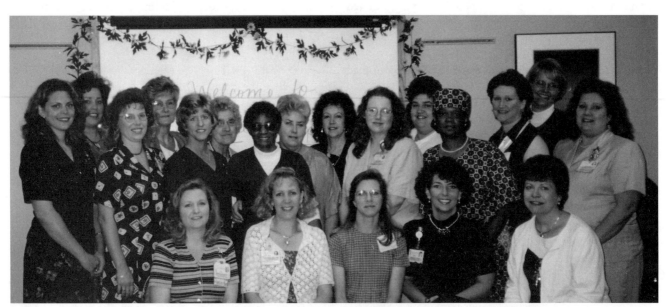

FIGURE 1–2 Nursing staff dedicated to the practice of FCMC at Gaston Memorial Hospital, Gastonia, North Carolina.

of FCMC as exemplified through daily actions and behaviors—again, walking the talk. However, physicians or nurses alone will not achieve FCMC. Respectful collaborative practice is required, and not separate nurse and physician committee structures.

The authors of the book *Managing from the Heart* have identified the essence of successful management in the following five principles, or requests, employees make of their managers (Bracey et al., 1990). They are:

1. Please don't make me wrong, even if you disagree.
2. Hear and understand me.
3. Tell me the truth with compassion.
4. Remember to look for my loving intentions.
5. Acknowledge the greatness in me.

When these fundamental requests of employees are fulfilled, the skilled nurse leader demonstrates caring.

People asked to make a change are really being asked to take a risk. They're thinking, "Will I still have a job? Will it be a job I can do? Will I look stupid? Will I be trained for the new job?" In hospitals characterized by high levels of caring, employees are more willing to take this leap of faith. It's basic: A staff must feel cared for before they themselves can provide care to families. It is a functional family of care providers that provides quality family-centered care.

Standards of Family-Centered Maternity Care Standards describe a competent level of performance in the professional nursing role. These standards include activities related to nursing practice, competencies, ethics, family health education and counseling, collaboration, and professional responsibility and accountability. See Appendix C for six standards of family-centered maternity care.

Select for Talent The front-line manager is key to attracting and retaining talented employees. The best managers select employees for talent rather than for skills or experience. Everyone has talents—recurring patterns of thought, feelings, and behavior that can be applied productively (Buckingham and Coffman, 1999). The trick in hiring staff for FCMC is to discover the talent inside a person that demonstrates caring. It is important, of course, to also screen applicants for technical and clinical skills. But it is critical to screen for those who have the "talent" to be happy and successful in an FCMC environment. An overview of a family-centered maternity nursing screening tool can be found in Appendix D.

Invest in People When a staff with desirable talents is in place, continuous support for that staff is needed. Orientation, in–service, team building, respect, praise, and rewards for family-centered practice become part of the culture. Supporting staff through change to FCMC means understanding that resistance is personal. According to Kriegel and Brandt (1996), the personal motives that drive resistance are fear, feeling powerless, inertia, and absence of self-interest. Each one is powerful and must be addressed.

Negative staff members can quickly poison their coworkers by complaining nonstop from the start to the end of the work day. Anger from staff who are resistant to FCMC can be destructive. It must be dealt with quickly and effectively.

People can be motivated to change through rewards and recognition, empowering with information, responsibility and accountability, support for ongoing learning, enthusiasm for FCMC, and inspiration around the mission and vision.

Physicians and nurses are inspired when they feel they are making their community a better place by supporting family beginnings. However, if all efforts to empower staff and assist them in the practice of FCMC fail, nurse leadership must have the authority and ability to transfer or remove staff. When such a decision has been made, it is important to take action as soon as possible.

Nurses staffing the Mother–Infant and Women's Care Unit at Northeast Medical Center in Concord, North Carolina, are evidence of a dedicated and inspired family-centered staff. Figure 1–3 illustrates a small group of these excellent nurses in Concord, North Carolina.

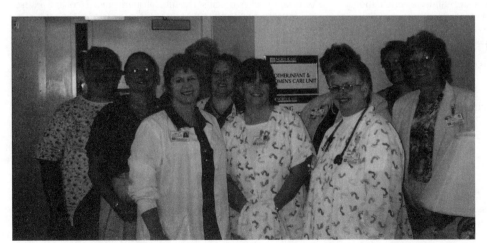

FIGURE 1–3 Family-Centered Maternity Care nurses at Northeast Medical Center, Concord, North Carolina.

CHAPTER SUMMARY

Family-centered maternity care supports the family as a unit. Family-centered care is based on the premise that the family is the constant, providing the ongoing care and support for one another well beyond the health care provider's brief time with them. Family-centered maternity care views birth as a normal life event rather than a medical procedure, and is the optimal model of care for all women and their families.

Developing successful FCMC programs means changing the institutional culture into one in which families come first. A vision about what the maternity service wishes to become is the next step in transforming the maternity service to family-centered care. A mission statement and a philosophy are developed to describe the core ideology or values of the maternity program and explain why it exists. Throughout this process, childbearing families are involved, included in relevant task forces, committees, advisory boards, work groups, and discussion groups.

The hospital family must be a functional family in order to provide FCMC. Superimposing FCMC on a dysfunctional operating system is not possible. Success = 80 percent people and processes and 20 percent facility.

Components of Family-Centered Maternity Care

Values and Mission
- The mission for maternity services reflects the basic values and defines the services for the maternity program.
- The mission reflects the principles of family-centered care.
- Community and hospital-based providers, staff, administration, and families are all actively involved in developing the mission.

Vision
- The maternity program is directed by a vision for the service.
- The vision is the focus of action.
- Providers, staff, administration, and families are all involved in the vision's development.

Philosophy
- A written philosophy statement defines how the mission will be accomplished.
- The philosophy statement reflects the principles of family-centered care.
- Community and hospital-based providers, staff, administration, and families are all involved in developing the FCMC philosophy.

Strategies
- Specific evidence-based goals and objectives with accompanying timelines and responsibilities have been developed for implementing the mission and philosophy of care.

Program Leadership
- A qualified leader oversees the maternity program.
- The maternity nurse leader is paired in the leadership role with a strong physician who champions FCMC.

Value Sharing
- There is evidence that values embodied in the vision, mission, and philosophy statements are reflected in communication, treatment of employees, policies, and decision making.

BIBLIOGRAPHY

Ahmann, E. 1994. Family-centered care: Shifting orientation. *Pediatric Nursing* 20, no. 2: 113–117.

Als, H., Lawhon, G., Duffy, F. H., McAnulty, G. B., Gibes-Grossman, R., and Blickman, G. 1994. Individualized developmental care for the very low-weight preterm infant: Medical and neurofunctional effects. *Journal of the American Medical Association*, 272, 853–858.

Altimier, L., et al. 1995. Aotearoa International Paediatric Nursing Conference, Auckland, September 27–29, 343.

American Academy of Pediatrics and American College of Obstetricians and Gynecologists. 1997. *Guidelines for Perinatal Care*, 4th ed. Elk Grove, IL: American Academy of Pediatrics.

American Journal of Public Health. 1983. The valley of the shadow of birth. T3 (6): 635–638.

Apple, R. 1987. *Mothers and Medicine: A Social History of Infant Feeding, 1890–1950.* Madison: University of Wisconsin Press.

Association of Women's Health, Obstetric and Neonatal Nurses (AWHONN). 1998. *Standards and Guidelines for Professional Nursing Practice in the Care of Women and Newborns*, 5th ed. Washington, DC: Author.

Bennett, W. 2001. *The Broken Hearth: Reversing the Moral Collapse of the American Family.* New York: Doubleday.

Blanchard, K., and O'Connor, M. 1997. *Managing by Values.* San Francisco, CA: Berrett-Koehler Publishers, Inc.

The Boston Women's Health Book Collective. 1971. *Our Bodies, Ourselves: A Book By and For Women.* New York: Simon and Schuster.

Bracey, H., et al. 1990. *Managing from the Heart.* New York: Dell Publishing.

Brown, H., et al. 2000. Evidence-based maternity care and labor support. *International Journal of Childbirth Education* 15, no. 4: 26–31.

Buckingham, M., and Coffman, C. 1999. *First, Break All the Rules: What the World's Greatest Managers Do Differently.* New York: Simon and Schuster.

Buehler, D. M., Als, H., Duffy, F. H., McAnulty, G. B., and Liederman, J. 1995. Effectiveness of individualized developmental care for low-risk preterm infants: Behavioral and electrophysiologic evidence. *Pediatrics* 96, 923–932.

Callister, L., and Hobbins-Garbett, D. 2000. Cochrane Pregnancy and Childbirth Database: Resource for evidence-based practice. *Journal of Obstetric, Gynecologic, and Neonatal Nursing* 29, no. 2: 123–128.

Coalition for Improving Maternity Services (CIMS). 1996. *The Mother-Friendly Childbirth Initiative.* Available on the Internet at www.motherfriendly.org.

Cox, R. 1997. Family health care delivery for the 21st century. *Journal of Obstetric, Gynecologic, and Neonatal Nursing* 26, no. 1: 109–118.

The Cybele Society. 1980. Unpublished material describing a national demonstration unit. Spokane, WA: Author.

DeGeorges, K. 1999. Evidence! Show me the Evidence! Untangling the web of evidence-based health care. *AWHONN Lifelines* 3, no. 3: 47–48.

De Lee, J. B. 1927a. How should the maternity ward be isolated? *Modern Hospital*, 29(3), 65–72.

———. 1927b. What are the special needs of modern maternity? *Modern Hospital*, 27(8), 59–69.

Dick-Read, G. 1953. *Childbirth Without Fear.* New York: Harper and Row.

Enkin, M., Keirse, M., Renfrew, M., and Neilsen, J. 1995. *A Guide to Effective Care in Pregnancy and Childbirth*, 2nd ed. New York: Oxford University Press.

———. 2000. *A Guide to Effective Care in Pregnancy and Childbirth*, 3rd ed. New York: Oxford University Press.

Family-Centered Maternity and Newborn Care: National Guidelines is available on the Internet at www.hc-sc.gc.ca.

Forste, R. 2002. Where are all the men? A conceptual analysis of the role of men in family formation. *Journal of Family Issues* 23, no. 5: 579–600.

Forsythe, P. 1995. Changing the ecology of the NICU. *Designing for Child Health* 3: 11–14.

Gennaro, S. 1994. Research utilization: An overview. *Journal of Obstetric, Gynecologic, and Neonatal Nursing* 23: 313–319.

Gerteis, M., et al. 1993. *Through the Patient's Eyes: Understanding and Promoting Patient-Centered Care.* San Francisco: Jossey-Bass.

Gisell, A., and Ilg, F. 1943. *Infant and Child in the Culture of Today.* New York: Harper and Brothers.

Goer, H. 1995. *Obstetric Myths versus Research Realities: A Guide to the Medical Literature.* Westport, CT: Bergin and Garvey.

Gogarten, W., and Van Aken, H. 2000. A century of regional analgesia in obstetrics. *Anesthesia Analog* 91: 773–775.

Health Canada. 2000. *Family-Centered Maternity and Newborn Care: National Guidelines.* Ottawa: Minister of Public Works and Government Services.

Hodnett, E. D. 1998. Home-like versus conventional birth settings. (Cochrane Review). *The Cochrane Library*, Issue 4, Oxford: Update Software.

———. 1999. Caregiver support for women during childbirth. (Cochrane Review). *The Cochrane Library*, Issue 1, Oxford: Update Software.

———. 2002. Pain and women's satisfaction with the experience of childbirth: A systematic review. *American Journal of Obstetrics and Gynecology* 186, S1: 60–72.

Hunter, M. A., and Larrabee, J. H. (1988). Women's perceptions of quality and benefits of postpartum care. *Journal of Nursing Care Quality* 13, no. 2: 21–30.

Institute for Family-Centered Care. 1994. Essential allies: Families and professionals working together to improve quality of care. *Advances in Family-Centered Care* 1, no. 2: 1–6.

———. 1998. Core principles of family-centered health care. *Advances in Family-Centered Care* 4, No. 1: 2–4.

International Childbirth Education Association, Inc. 1975. *The Pregnant Patient's Bill of Rights: The Pregnant Patient's Responsibilities.* Minneapolis: Author.

———. 1978. *ICEA Position Paper on Planning Comprehensive Maternal and Newborn Services.* Minneapolis: Author.

———. 1986. *ICEA Position Paper on the Role of the Childbirth Educator and the Scope of Childbirth Education.* Minneapolis: Author.

Interprofessional Task Force on Health Care of Women and Children. 1978. *Joint position statement on the development of family-centered maternity/newborn care in hospitals.* Chicago, Author.

Janssen, P., Klein, M., Harris, S., Soolsma, J., and Seymour, L. 2000. Single room maternity care and client satisfaction. *Birth* 27, no. 4: 235–243.

———. 2001. Single room maternity care: The nursing response. *Birth* 28, no. 3: 173–179.

Kennell, J., Klaus, M., McGrath, S., Robertson, S., and Hinkley, C. 1991. Continuous emotional support during labor in U.S. hospitals: A randomized controlled trial. *Journal of the American Medical Association* 265: 2197–2201.

Klaus, M. H., and Kennell, J. H. 1976. *Maternal–Infant Bonding.* St. Louis: C. V. Mosby.

———. 1982. *Parent–Infant Bonding*, 2nd ed. St. Louis: C. V. Mosby.

Kriegel, R., and Brandt, D. 1996. *Sacred Cows Make the Best Burgers.* New York: Warner Books, Inc.

Lake, A. 1976. Childbirth in America. *McCalls* 83: 128–130, 142.

Leavitt, J. W. 1988. Joseph B. De Lee and the practice of preventive obstetrics. *American Journal of Public Health* 76: 1353.

———. 1989. Joseph B. De Lee and the practice of preventative obstetrics. *Obstetrical and Gynecological Survey* 44, no. 9: 682–683.

Lothian, J. A. 2001. Back to the future: Trusting birth. *Journal of Perinatal Neonatal Nursing* 15, no. 3: 13–22.

Lubic, R. 1983. Childbirthing centers: Delivering more with less. *American Journal of Nursing* 83, no. 7: 1053-1056.

Marshall, M. 1974. My husband delivered our baby. *Good Housekeeping.* 78–82.

Maternity Center Association. 1998. A new definition of family-centered maternity care. *Birth*, 25, no. 4: 270–271.

———. 1999. *Your Guide to Safe and Effective Care During Labor and Birth.* New York.

May, K., and Ditolla, K. 1984. In-hospital alternative birth centers: Where do we go from here? *Maternal Child Nursing* 9: 48-51.

Midmer, D. 1992. Does family-centered maternity care empower women? The development of the woman-centered childbirth model. *Family Medicine* 24, no. 3: 216–221.

Mintz, S., and Kellogg, S. 1988. *Domestic Revolutions: A Social History of American Family Life.* New York: The Free Press, a division of Macmillan, Inc.

Mother-Friendly Childbirth Initiative. 1996. *The Coalition for Improving Maternity Services (CIMS)*. Washington, DC.

Munhall, P., and Fitzsimons, V. 2001. *The Emergence of Family into the 21st Century*. Sudbury, MA: Jones and Bartlett.

Nathanson, M. 1985. Single-room maternity care seen as a way to attract patients, cut costs. *Modern Healthcare* 15, no. 7: 72, 74.

Obstetrician teaches dad to deliver his baby himself. 1975. *People Weekly*, 20 January.

Perez-Escamilla, R., et al. 1994. Infant feeding policies in maternity wards and their effect on breastfeeding success: An analytic overview. *American Journal of Public Health* 84, no. 1: 89–95.

Phillips, C. R. 1996. *Family-Centered Maternity and Newborn Care: A Basic Text,* 4th ed. St. Louis: C.V. Mosby.

Popenoe, D. 1988. *Disturbing the Nest: Family Change and Decline in Modern Society*. New York: Aldine de Gruyter.

———. 1993. American family decline, 1960–1990: A review and appraisal. *Journal of Marriage and the Family* 55: 527–542.

Prodromidis, M., et al. 1995. A comparison of rooming-in versus minimal contact. *Birth* 22, 196–200.

Rooks, J. 1999. Evidence-based practice and its application to childbirth care for low-risk women. *Journal of Nurse-Midwifery* 44, no. 4: 355–369.

Rothman, B. 1996. Women, providers, and control. *Journal of Obstetric, Gynecologic, and Neonatal Nursing* 25, no. 3: 253–256.

Rouse, C. 2000. Should there be policies to restrict visitors during labor and birth? *Maternal Child Nursing* 25, no. 1: 8.

Salimbene, S. 1999. Cultural competence: A priority for performance improvement action. *Journal of Nursing Care Quality* 13, no. 3: 23–35.

Schmidt, J., and McCarthey, P. 2000. History and development of fetal heart assessment: A composite. *Journal of Obstetric, Gynecologic, and Neonatal Nursing* 29, no. 3: 295–305.

Schultz, D. G. 1958. Cruelty in the maternity wards. *Ladies Home Journal*, May: 44–45, 152–155.

Simkin, P. 1991. Just another day in a woman's life? Part 1. Women's long-term perceptions of their first birth experience. *Birth: Issues in Prenatal Care*, 18: 203–210.

———. 1992. Just another day in a woman's life? Part 2. Nature and consistency of women's long-term memories of their first birth experiences. *Birth: Issues in Prenatal Care* 19: 64–81.

———. 1996. The experience of maternity in a woman's life. *Journal of Obstetric, Gynecologic, and Neonatal Nursing* 25, no. 3: 247–252.

Simkin, P., and O'Hara, M. A. 2002. Nonpharmocologic relief of pain during labor: Systematic reviews of five methods. *American Journal of Obstetrics and Gynecology*, 186, S1: 31–59.

Simpson, K. 1999. Strategies for developing an evidence-based approach to perinatal care. *American Journal of Maternal Child Nursing* 24, no. 3: 122–131.

Simpson, K., and Knox, E. 1999. Perinatal teamwork: Turning rhetoric into reality. Chapter 3 in Simpson and Creehan.

Perinatal Nursing, 2nd ed. Philadelphia: Lippincott Williams and Wilkins.

———. 2000. A critical evaluation of the past 25 years of perinatal nursing practice: Opportunities for improvement. *American Journal of Maternal Child Nursing* 25, no. 6: 300–304.

Skolnick, A. 1991. *Embattled Paradise: The American Family in an Age of Uncertainty*. New York: Basic Books.

Solberg, B. 1996. Wisconsin prenatal care coordination proves its worth: Case management becomes Medicaid benefit. *Inside Preventive Care* 2, no. 3: 1, 5–6.

Speert, H. 1980. *Obstetrics and Gynecology in America: A History*. Chicago: American College of Obstetricians and Gynecologists.

Sullivan, G., and Harper, M. 1996. *Hope Is Not a Method*. New York: Random House.

Taffel, S. M., et al. 1987. Trends in the United States cesarean section rate and reasons for the 1980–1985 rise. *American Journal of Public Health* 77: 955–956.

Talbert-May, A. 1995. The effects of a non-traditional hospital environment for premature infant care on maternal state anxiety. Unpublished master's thesis, Case Western Reserve, Cleveland, OH.

Taylor, S. 2000. Orem's general theory of nursing and families. *Nursing Science Quarterly* 13, no. 4: 7–9.

Teachman, J., et al. 2000. The changing demography of America's families. *Journal of Marriage and the Family* 62: 1234–1246.

Tegmeier, D., and Elsea. S. 1984. Wellness throughout the maternity cycle. *Nursing Clinics of North America* 19, no. 2: 219–227.

Wallace, K. 2000. The Bradley method. *International Journal of Childbirth Education* 15, no. 1: 9–10.

Watters, N. E., and Kristiansen, C. M. 1995. Two evaluations of combined mother–infant versus separate postnatal nursing care. *Research in Nursing and Health* 18, no. 1: 17–26.

Wertz, R. W., and Wertz, D. C. 1989. *Lying-In: A History of Childbirth in America* (expanded edition). New Haven: Yale University Press.

Wiedenbach, E. 1959. *Family-Centered Maternity Nursing*. New York: G. P. Putnam.

World Health Organization. 1996. *Care in Normal Birth: A Practical Guide*. Report of a Technical Working Group. Publication no. WHO/FRH/MSM/96.24. Geneva: WHO. To order write: Documentation Centre, Family and Reproductive Health, World Health Organization, CH-1211 Geneva 27, Switzerland.

Young, D. 1987. Family-centered maternity care: Yesterday and today. *International Journal of Childbirth Education*, 5–7.

Zadoroznyj, M. 1999. Social class, social selves and social control in childbirth. *Sociology of Health and Illness* 21, no. 3: 267–289.

Zwelling, E., and Phillips, C. 2001. Family-centered maternity care in the new millennium: Is it real or is it imagined? *Journal of Perinatal and Neonatal Nursing* 15, No. 3: 1–15.

Family-Centered Antepartum Care

INTRODUCTION

Family-centered antepartum care addresses all aspects of pregnancy, childbirth, and parenting—emotional, psychosocial, biological, and medical—for all childbearing women and their families. Family advocacy in FCMC requires efforts to keep normal pregnancies normal and to provide the best healthcare services possible for all pregnant women. Those providing family-centered antepartum care for women and families practice according to the fundamental principles of family-centered maternity care: informed choice, continuity of care, evidence-based care, and respect for individuality (Health Canada, 2000). Emphasis is on providing care that promotes family unity while reaching or maintaining a high level of wellness during and after pregnancy (Ramer and Frank, 2001).

As discussed in Chapter 1, families come from a wide range of age, economic, social, ethnic, and cultural backgrounds. The family is no longer defined by blood ties, such as in a biological family, but is becoming instead a psychological family. However, regardless of the diversity of today's families, each and every pregnant woman wants a healthy baby, and a supportive and safe birth.

Although only the woman is physically pregnant, family members are also experiencing the shifts and changes in feelings, relationships, and lifestyle that are associated with pregnancy. To care for the woman without considering her family members is to ignore her most important support system.

The stress that pregnancy exerts on each family member is caused in large part by developmental tasks and adaptational demands that can be puzzling and anxiety-producing. If the family is highly functional and able to be mutually supportive, psychological adjustment is smoother as pregnancy proceeds. Social support and communication within the family are key buffers of stress (Health Canada, 2000).

GOALS OF PRENATAL CARE

- Improve and maintain the health and well-being of the mother, her unborn child, and her family.
- Prevent preterm delivery and low birth weight. (U.S. Department of Health and Human Services, 2000)

PRECONCEPTION CARE

Ideally, prenatal care should begin with preconception care that includes an assessment not only of health, but also of risk (Maloni et al., 1996). Healthy pregnancies begin well in advance of conception. A woman's behavior before and during pregnancy can have a profound impact on her health and the health of her baby (Center for the Advancement of Health, 2001).

In FCMC there is education and care for women and men of childbearing age before they are pregnant. Thus, interventions can be designed to reduce risks and promote general health and well-being. These interventions help improve pregnancy outcomes.

Preconception care focuses on promotion of healthful behaviors and education that provides general knowledge of pregnancy and parenting, and imparts information on personal care and community resources. Information is given regarding family planning and genetic counseling. Opportunities for rubella immunization, counseling about smoking, substance abuse, teratogens, and sexually transmitted diseases all help to ensure healthy conception. In addition, information about breastfeeding is presented during preconception care because most women decide whether to breastfeed by early pregnancy. Therefore, educators and healthcare providers should explore breastfeeding attitudes and knowledge with potential parents (AAP, 1997). The preconception period is an ideal time to correct myths and give women and their partners information that will help them make an informed decision about breastfeeding.

Whether a woman has a healthy pregnancy depends largely on her success in taking good care of herself. This includes proper exercise, nutrition, and other preventive measures such as avoiding sources of infections like toxoplasmosis or listeria. Taking good care of herself may include smoking cessation, reduction in stress, and elimination of substance and alcohol abuse. All these factors not only improve health, but also can substantially reduce costs of medical care.

Preconception evaluation of family issues includes assessment of family function. Assessment of social supports available, child or spouse abuse, economic hardships, and other stressors that can affect the pregnancy needs to be done so that assistance can be initiated as early as possible (Scherger et al., 1992).

Once pregnancy is suspected, immediate contact with a prenatal care provider is necessary for assessment of health and risk.

PRENATAL CARE

Early entry into care, health promotion, risk screening for specific fetal and maternal problems, and medical and psychosocial interventions and follow-up are important aspects of prenatal care (Fiscella, 1995; American College of Obstetricians and Gynecologists, 1995). According to priorities established in *Healthy People 2010,* prenatal care should be initiated during the first trimester of pregnancy and include early and continued risk assessment, health promotion, and medical, nutritional, and psychosocial interventions and follow-up (USDHHS, 2000). Prenatal care not only must begin early, but also should continue regularly (March of Dimes, 2001). Unfortunately, some women do not come for prenatal care in the first trimester, and still others seek care that is sporadic, if at all (Beckmann et al., 2000).

Timing of entry into prenatal care often reflects factors associated with low birth weight, such as poverty, maternal age, and other barriers to care. Adequacy of prenatal care varies by race and ethnicity. Native-American, African-American, and Hispanic women were most likely to receive inadequate prenatal care (March of Dimes, 2001). Negative attitudes toward pregnancy and unwanted pregnancies are also associated with inadequate and absent prenatal care (Hulsey, 2001).

Barriers

There are numerous barriers to obtaining early prenatal care. They include cost of care and transportation and lack of understanding about government programs that address cost issues, long waiting time in the pregnancy clinic, difficulty obtaining a provider and an appointment, and negative atti-

tudes toward the provider (Beckmann et al., 2000). Psychological stresses and the wantedness and planning of the pregnancy also contribute to a woman's decision to seek or avoid prenatal care (Meikle et al., 1995; Hulsey, 2001).

Omar and Schiffman used focus groups to determine women's perceptions of their expectations of and satisfaction with prenatal care. The attentiveness of the provider was the most commonly identified aspect on which the women focused their overall feelings of satisfaction or dissatisfaction (Omar and Schiffman, 1995). In other words, positive encounters with providers and staff can do much to encourage women to seek and continue prenatal care.

CNM Model

A real need exists to develop culturally meaningful and specific programs to motivate women to obtain early prenatal care, particularly those at risk for adverse outcomes.

An example of a culturally meaningful prenatal care program is found at Catawba Memorial Hospital in Hickory, North Carolina. At Catawba, certified nurse midwives (CNMs) provide care for approximately 55 percent of the birth population of 1,500 births per year. They offer CNM-managed prenatal clinics in outlying areas, provide flexible scheduling for appointments through after-hour and weekend appointments, and conduct prenatal groups for patient education and peer support. Some of the prenatal groups are held in a church, and others are held at Central Latino center, where the Latino community of Catawba Valley meets for educational and community support.

Figure 2-1 shows several proud expectant mothers in a prenatal group at Central Latino. Since this midwifery service began eight years ago, the number of births per year has not declined but the number of pregnant women without prenatal care *has* declined from an estimate of 120 per year to 6 per year. (Interview with Emily Ousley, CNM, and Linda Swift, Director MCH at Catawba Memorial Hospital, June 2001).

The CNMs at Catawba have found group teaching to be particularly meaningful for the community of Latina women. The group provides peer support that is lacking when families immigrate to an unfamiliar place from their native country and cannot speak the language of their new home.

The Centering Pregnancy Program is the interdisciplinary model utilized for group teaching by the midwives in Hickory, North Carolina. The Centering Pregnancy Program abolishes routine prenatal care by bringing women out of examination rooms and into groups for their care.

A prenatal group meeting in the Centering Pregnancy Program at Catawba Memorial Hospital is shown in Figure 2-2. The design incorporates the three components of prenatal care—risk assessment, education, and support—into one entity. Women are placed in groups of eight to twelve based on estimated dates of delivery, and meet for ten 90-minute prenatal or postpartum visits at regular intervals. During these visits, standard prenatal risk assessment is completed within the group setting, an educational format is followed

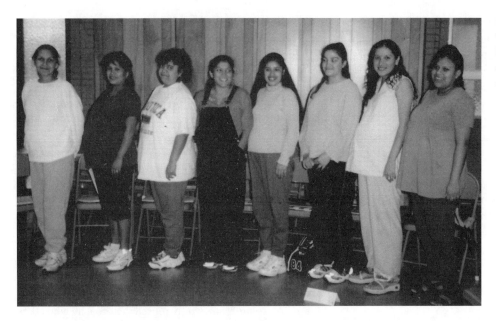

FIGURE 2–1 A prenatal group at the Central Latino center in Hickory, North Carolina. *Photo courtesy of Catawba Memorial Hospital.*

that uses a didactic discussion format, and time is provided for women to talk and share with one another. By incorporating these three components into a whole, emphasis is placed on their collective importance. Women are encouraged to take responsibility for themselves; this leads to a shift in the client–provider power base.

A sampling of comments from women who completed the program includes the following:

- "I liked everything about the group. The companions we had made us happy. All the people felt that the time was well spent. I am well pleased with the support of the nurses. I am happy."

- "Truly it felt good sharing with the other women. It was an agreeable time. I appreciate with all my heart the midwife, the nurse, and Maria, all the beautiful help that I was given. Thank you."

- "They gave us trust and support."

- "I got to know the other mothers, and I felt assisted and comforted in every moment. We set up friendships, and we hope to communicate in the future."

- "It seems to me an excellent program. It has helped me very much to know all the symptoms and stages of pregnancy as well as labor and the care of the baby. Furthermore in every moment we felt supported and encouraged, and I liked the company of the other mothers. I recommend it to all future mothers. The nurse and midwife are wonderful people."

Evaluative data demonstrated that 96 percent of the women preferred receiving their prenatal care in groups. This model is interdisciplinary in design and demonstrates provider satisfaction, as well as efficiency in delivery of

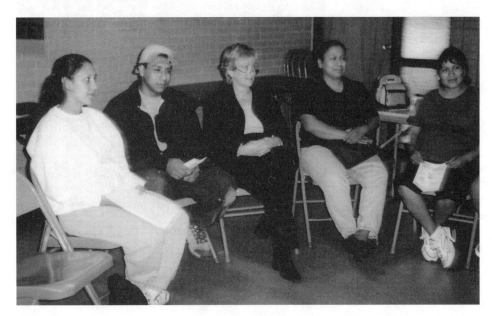

FIGURE 2–2 The Centering Pregnancy Program participants at Hickory, North Carolina. *Photo courtesy of Catawba Memorial Hospital.*

care. It is an excellent model for the care of teens, and for midwives and nurse practitioners to lead. The combination of satisfaction, good outcomes, and effective delivery of care makes this an attractive model for agencies to implement (Rising, 1998). For detailed information on The Centering Pregnancy Program see Appendix E. Also explore the Web site www.centeringpregnancy.com.

LIFE TRANSITIONS

Life transitions involve the human experience of moving from one phase of life to another. There is a sense of loss for the old ways, fear of the unknown, anxiety, and frustration with new ways. There is often expectant joy (Ramer and Frank, 2001).

The Expectant Mother

Each pregnancy involves preparation for becoming the psychosocial mother to the new child (Rubin, 1984). With any pregnancy, whether planned or unplanned, a woman has many new and different feelings, including ambivalence toward the pregnancy (Rubin, 1970). As the pregnancy progresses, the fetal presence becomes obvious on ultrasound and as fetal movement is felt, any uncertainty about really being pregnant is gone. If women have accepted the pregnancy and moved through the ambivalence of the first trimester, the focus is now on the baby. Feeling the baby move for the first time is a profound experience for men, and they begin thinking seriously about becoming fathers.

Rubin (1970) described the last trimester as a period of "watchful waiting" for women; it can be a period of anxious concern and waiting for the father. The father is often very concerned about his partner's physical safety as the time for birth approaches. Attachment with their unborn baby begins as both the man and the woman move through these emotional phases of pregnancy on their way to successful role changes.

Men's reactions to becoming a father are numerous and diverse.

The Expectant Father

Many expectant fathers have a joyful reaction to impending fatherhood, whereas others may react with depression, fear, anger, or jealousy. How a man reacts may depend on his childhood memories of his own father, his culture, his concerns over increasing financial responsibilities, anxiety about the potential loss of a partner or child, and concerns about the man–woman relationship (Phillips, 1996).

Pregnancy can be a crisis time for men as well as women. During pregnancy a man must adapt to the change in his partner's role to mother while he is becoming a father. In addition, he may become concerned when his partner begins to

evaluate him in terms of what kind of father he will be, because he may be wondering that himself.

Pregnancy can be an ideal time for a man to become aware of his own health and lifestyle and their potential effects on his growing family. As fatherhood approaches, a man may see his partner's pregnancy as an opportunity to improve his own health by modifying his lifestyle, for the benefit of both himself and his family.

Most people view the father's presence during labor and birth as important. For some men, witnessing the birth of his child can actually help him begin to accept the reality of fatherhood (Jordan, 1990). However, the role of active participant and labor coach may not be consistent with all women's expectations of the father's role (Raines and Morgan, 2000), or with all cultures. It is not unusual for expectant fathers to feel anxiety about their ability to perform as labor coaches.

Lamaze International's position paper in 2002, *Lamaze for the 21st Century*, officially retired the "coach" who takes charge of the birth, calling the plays and instructing the mother. The emphasis is now on the fathers, family members, and other supporters of the laboring woman learning how to provide quiet, gentle, encouraging support and comfort measures.

Throughout the pregnancy it is essential to include the father by encouraging him to assume the role that is most comfortable for him (White, 2000). Also, inclusion of the father in developmental assessment and intervention is very important for family maturation (Malnory, 1996). The Centering Pregnancy Program at Catawba Memorial Hospital encourages father participation throughout his partner's pregnancy. (See Figure 2-3.)

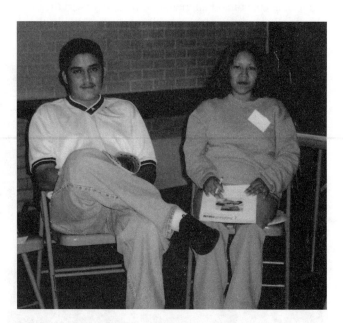

FIGURE 2–3 The Centering Pregnancy Program includes fathers. *Photo courtesy of Catawba Memorial Hospital.*

FAMILY ATTACHMENT

Attachment is the process of forming an enduring bond between parents and babies (Klaus and Kennell, 1982; Todd, 1998). This life long love relationship between parents and child does not occur magically at the time of birth, but instead progresses throughout pregnancy. As a sensitive receiver of family messages, the fetus is thought to be influenced not only by the mother's responses, but also by those of the father. For example, there is evidence that hearing the father's voice has a profound effect on the fetus. Studies have shown that newborn babies who heard their fathers' voices during pregnancy were able to pick out and respond to their fathers' voices even in the first one or two hours of life. As knowledge of fetal responsiveness expands, practices in antepartum care will be oriented toward facilitating the family–infant attachment process during pregnancy. This care will be especially beneficial beginning with the sixth month of pregnancy (and perhaps earlier), when the fetus is capable of seeing, hearing, tasting, responding, and primitive learning.

Examples follow that demonstrate how caregivers can facilitate attachment during the antenatal period. The father is encouraged to attend the first antepartum visit. He is included as an integral part of the care process and encouraged to show continued interest. Care providers can encourage other family members to accompany the woman on antepartum visits. Children in the family can assist with care procedures, feel fetal movements, listen to the fetal heartbeat, and learn about pregnancy and the birth process, all of which can help them form a bond with their unborn sibling (Fortier et al., 1991). As you can see from Figure 2-4, children are welcome in prenatal care at Catawba Memorial Hospital.

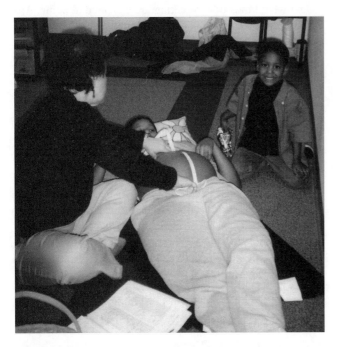

FIGURE 2–4 Family-centered antepartum care. *Photo courtesy of Catawba Memorial Hospital.*

It may be necessary to schedule appointments on weekend days and evenings to provide times when family members can be present, but the benefits to the family are well worth the inconvenience to the providers.

Care providers can also educate families about fetal growth and development. Most families are fascinated to know that, as mentioned earlier, from the sixth month of pregnancy (and perhaps earlier) the fetus is capable of experiencing sight, sound, taste, and touch. Families are encouraged to talk and sing to the baby, and to play with the baby by patting or gently palpating the mother's belly. Family members can be supported in playing music for the baby and calling the baby by a pet name (Booth, 2001).

CULTURALLY COMPETENT CARE

Culture is a set of behaviors, beliefs, and practices that can be passed from one woman in a group to another (Simpson and Creehan, 2001). Different cultures focus on different aspects of the childbirth experience according to their view of the world, and according to the meanings given to events such as birth and death. The high rate of immigration today means that more women from a variety of cultural and ethnic backgrounds are giving birth in hospital maternity programs that are based on the traditional western model of practice. This may be in conflict with the woman's cultural beliefs and expectations (Raines and Morgan, 2000). Thus, women may be unwilling to use existing healthcare services or may use the services but continue with their own cultural patterns and not comply with physicians' recommendations for diet, medication, or treatment protocol.

Cultural Competence

Cultural competence is not just understanding other cultures but embracing diversity. Cultural competence is a combination of knowledge, attitudes, and clinical skills and is a dynamic process that occurs over time (Callister, 2001). It is essential that all providers of FCMC become culturally competent.

Cultural competence begins with healthcare providers knowing their own cultural heritage and how their own cultures affect their views of what is important. This basic understanding of self is followed by wanting to know the view of the families for whom care is provided (Mattson, 2000). Education for providers about varied health beliefs, practices, and mores of specific ethnic and cultural groups is required in order to practice family-centered care. However, because there is considerable heterogeneity within cultural groups (Callister, 2001), care is always individualized rather than standardized for each culture studied.

Cultural Assessment

Cultural assessment includes learning about a woman's beliefs and values, health-related behaviors, and cultural rituals and practices (Mattson, 2000b). The following list[1] provides some critical questions for cultural assessment within the perinatal period:

Antepartum

- Society's acceptance of the pregnancy—age, marriage requirement.
- Consideration of pregnancy as a state of illness or health.
- *Dietary prescriptions or restrictions.* Adherence to the hot and cold theory of health and diet? What particular foods must she have or avoid?
- *Activity restrictions or prescriptions, including the use of massage.* What is a "good" environment for the expectant mother?
- *Expression of emotions, including what sexual activity is permitted.* What emotions may be expressed and what should be restrained?
- *Modesty and its influence on seeking care.* Who may be present during an examination?

Intrapartum

- *What is the appropriate setting for labor and delivery.* Home, hospital, special birth center? This information will tell you what dangers are anticipated and how they will be handled. What is an acceptable length for labor? What are acceptable interventions to assist the child during birth?
- *Who are appropriate birth attendants.* Most non-western cultures consider childbearing as being within the woman's domain, and don't necessarily expect or want male support. Male practitioners may be refused.
- *Activity expectations.* Is walking permitted? Can massage be used for discomfort? What position is ideal for delivery?
- *Dietary expectations.* Should food intake be permitted? Are herbal teas used (for pain relief and to "hasten birth")?
- *Expression of emotions.* What is acceptable for relief of discomfort? What expressions of discomfort are allowed?
- What is expected in terms of disposition of placenta and/or umbilical cord?

Postpartum

- *Determine when it begins and ends.* Western culture says it is 6 weeks, other cultures believe it lasts 30 days, still others believe it lasts longer. It may be different for primiparas versus multiparas.
- *Activity restrictions/prescriptions.* This period is viewed by many as one that is fraught with dangers for both

mother and infant, and may include restrictions on ambulating, bathing, and infant care-taking. In some cultures, women are also considered to be in a state of impurity during the puerperium, which results in seclusion and avoidance of contact with others as well as avoidance of sexual relations during the time of lochial flow.

- *Dietary expectations.* Many of the same requirements that are based on a theory of hot and cold also affect postpartum rules. The puerperium is a "cold" time (heat has been lost at delivery from the pregnancy that was a "hot" time), so foods should be "hot" in nature.
- *Use of therapeutic heat and cold.* The use of cold packs or sitz baths for perineal comfort and healing may not be acceptable to women from many cultures, because cold air and water are believed to be harmful and the cause of uterine problems.

Newborn

- *Feeding of the infant, including best method and timing of the first feed.* A culture's advocacy of breastfeeding varies and many influences must be taken into consideration. Hispanic women and some Asian women believe that colostrum is bad for the baby (or is dirty) and prefer to bottle feed until the milk comes in. In cultures that restrict the mother's activity, this may be the only care-taking permitted, or it may be curtailed. In this situation another person would need to bottle feed the baby.
- *Bathing, including the time of the first bath and the appropriate person to bathe the infant.* Certain measures may be required to protect the baby during this activity.
- *Activity expectations.* These include swaddling practices, and what kinds of care-taking are expected at home. Are babies allowed to cry or be comforted immediately? Are there ritual beautification practices? Where does the baby sleep? How is the umbilical stump cared for?
- *Circumcision.* Cultures vary greatly in their beliefs about this practice; ritual circumcision is frequently practiced in traditional Judaism.
- *Expression of emotions.* When is the infant recognized and accepted by society? Because of traditionally high infant mortality rates, some cultures don't recognize the baby, even with a name, until some time after its birth. Attachment behaviors differ, at times because of the fear of losing the child. Some Asian women maintain a distance and do not praise their infants because of fear of evil influences; they may be erroneously assessed as demonstrating maladaptive behaviors.

---

[1] From Mattson, S. (2000). Working toward cultural competence: Making the first steps through cultural assessment. *AWHONN Lifelines* 4(4), 42. ©2000 by the Association of Women's Health, Obstetric and Neonatal Nurses. All rights reserved.

SOCIAL SUPPORT DURING PREGANCY

A woman needs social support during pregnancy. Social support reflects a woman's sense of belonging and safety with respect to a caring partner, family, or community (Health Canada, 2000). Lack of social support has been associated with abuse of the child and/or woman and postpartum depression (Midmer et al., 1996).

Most pregnant women receive their primary social support from their spouse or partner and their mothers (Logsdon, 2001). Well over a quarter of a century ago, it was recognized that there is a strong relationship between a woman's feelings toward her mother and the course of her pregnancy.

Partner Support

Researchers have found that women in good marital relationships are less likely to be depressed and anxious during pregnancy than women in unhappy marriages (Newton, 1963). Rubin (1975) explained the importance of a woman having the acceptance of her baby by the persons with whom she is intimately involved. In her estimation, this one task of security in acceptance seemed to be the keystone to a successful pregnancy.

Although families have changed over the past three decades, this basic need for the support and concern of a partner during pregnancy has not changed. In a recent study (Kroelinger and Oths, 2000), a partner's stability, status, feelings toward the pregnancy, and level of dependability and support all influence whether a woman experienced her pregnancy as "wanted" or "unwanted." Women whose partners were unhappy about the pregnancy were more likely to experience their pregnancies as unwanted. In other words, the father of a baby has a notable impact on pregnancy wantedness. This is significant because women who experience unwanted pregnancy are at a greater risk of complicated pregnancy outcomes. In addition, their children are more likely to experience physical or psychological problems in infancy when compared with those women with wanted pregnancies.

Before the use of the term social support, research on stress and its effects on pregnancy outcome (Nuckolls, Laplan, and Cassel, 1972) investigated the relationship between attitudes toward pregnancy, personality characteristics, and social support (known as psychosocial assets) and health in pregnancy. It was found that women with high life stress and low psychosocial assets had pregnancy complication rates three times higher than those women with high life stress and high psychosocial assets (Logsdon, 2001).

Single Mothers

Achieving emotional well-being during the transition to parenthood is extremely important. Developing a strong support system is essential for healthy adaptation to the new roles of father and mother. For women who will be parent-

ing alone, social support is critical. Being able to confide in someone and having a support network can help the single mother emotionally (Bianchi, 2000).

Violence in Pregnancy

Pregnant women commonly encounter violence in intimate relationships. Domestic abuse crosses all ethnic, racial, age, national origin, and socioeconomic levels (McFarlane, Parker, and Cross, 2001). Although the relationship before the pregnancy may have been satisfactory, it has been documented that many of the assaults within a relationship begin with the first pregnancy (Polomeno, 2000). Pregnancy is a time of increased risk for abuse because of ambivalent feelings about the pregnancy, decreased sexual availability, increasing financial pressures, and increased vulnerability of the woman (Health Canada, 2000).

A pregnant woman's sense of loneliness and social isolation can be profound if she is in a relationship filled with physical and psychological violence. There may be hesitancy on the part of the woman and the care provider to broach the issue of violence. However, hesitancy or reluctance is never an excuse. Because domestic abuse increases during pregnancy, affecting up to 30 percent of pregnant women (Canterino et al., 1999), screening methods are needed to identify women at risk for domestic abuse.

ASSESSMENT TOOLS

Women who have a greater than normal amount of stress or who live in nonsupportive or abusive family situations should be identified early in pregnancy, so that appropriate intervention plans can be developed and pregnancy outcome improved as a consequence. All assessment for abuse must be done in a private setting where the provider can assure confidentiality. Women must be assessed for abuse at each visit (McFarlane, Parker, and Cross, 2001).

Canterino et al. (1999) discovered a standardized domestic abuse questionnaire to be superior to a direct interview in identifying self-reported domestic abuse in pregnancy. However, when a directed interview was used along with the standardized domestic abuse questionnaire, a greater number of patients with domestic abuse were identified. The efficient and simple screening tool they used asked the following questions:

1. Have you ever been emotionally or physically abused by your partner or someone important to you?

2. Within the last year, have you been hit, slapped, kicked, or otherwise physically hurt by someone?

3. Since your pregnancy began, have you been hit, slapped, kicked, or otherwise physically hurt by someone?

4. Within the last year, has anyone forced you to have sexual activities?

5. Are you afraid of your partner or anyone else?

Some healthcare providers, themselves, may be victims of abuse. This makes it very difficult for them to approach women in their care with questions about violence. It is very important for healthcare providers involved in abusive relationships to seek help and support (Health Canada, 2000).

Maternity Social Support Scale

A maternity social support scale has been incorporated into prenatal assessment and documentation at the Royal Women's Hospital in Brisbane, Australia (Webster et al., 2000). This assessment tool helps identify at-risk women during the prenatal period so that appropriate referrals, counseling, monitoring, and crisis interventions can be provided. (See Exhibit 2-1.) With the woman's consent, the caregiver can share the information with appropriate professional(s) in order to provide necessary care and support to the woman.

DEVELOPMENTAL–PSYCHOLOGICAL ASSESSMENT TOOL

Malnory (1996) has developed a tool—the MPDP-2—that identifies the developmental tasks of pregnancy (Rubin, 1984), as well as expected behaviors and appropriate nursing interventions for each parent and each stage of pregnancy. This tool can become a permanent part of the prenatal/perinatal record. (See Exhibit 2-2.) Inpatient nursing staff and home-care nurses can review a summary of the MPDP-2 and have valuable information to help in their care of the family. In this way continuity of care and teaching is enhanced because the documentation provides effective communication between providers.

Ideally, the first interview and observation is conducted at the first prenatal visit. The second assessment occurs at 24–26 weeks into the pregnancy, and the third assessment takes place at 34–36 weeks into the pregnancy.

The MPDP–2 report includes the father's adaptational changes in the assessment process. Taking time to elicit and understand some of the father's concerns and their changes as pregnancy advances, and planning for the father's role in

EXHIBIT 2–1   Maternity Social Support Scale (MSSS)

The Royal Women's Hospital, Brisbane

MATERNITY SOCIAL SUPPORT SCALE (MSSS)

For each of the following statements, please tick one box

which shows how you feel about the support you have

right now.

	Always	Most of The time	Some of the time	Rarely	Never
A. I have good friends who support me	5	4	3	2	1
B. My family is always there for me	5	4	3	2	1
C. My husband/partner helps me a lot	5	4	3	2	1
D. There is conflict with my husband/partner	1	2	3	4	5
E. I feel controlled by my husband/partner	1	2	3	4	5
F. I feel loved by my husband/partner	1	2	3	4	5

Source: Webster et al., 2000. Measuring Social Support in Pregnancy. Can It Be Simple and Meaningful? Birth, 27, No. 2: 98. Reproduced with permission.

EXHIBIT 2–2   Maternal–Paternal Developmental–Psychological Assessment Tool

	Task	*Expected Behavior (+) (−)*	*Intervention*
Maternal Trimester 1	Seeking safe passage: Assessment of changes related to pregnancy	Demands nurturance and protection, worried about oneself	Instruct woman about most worrisome aspects of pregnancy. Let woman drive direction of instruction.
	Integration and incorporation of fetus as an important part of woman	Ambivalence	Help her to understand that ambivalence is the first emotion of pregnancy, explore her desire for the pregnancy and motherhood, let her "tell her story."
	Binding-in: being pregnant	Changing self-image, mood swings, introversion, passivity, narcissism	Discuss hormonal influence, self-limiting nature of symptoms. Remember that discomforts that are overemphasized may be continuing sign of ambivalence.
	Acceptance by others	Shares news with partner, family, and friends	Encourage sharing of information if no past history precludes this.
	Giving of oneself: Reality testing about pregnancy	Seeks clues, signs, and symptoms of pregnancy, change in sexual activity	Heighten her awareness to early pregnancy changes through anticipatory guidance and education, especially fetal development.
		May experience unusual dreams or fantasies about self	Stress normalcy of these dreams and fantasies; encourage her to talk about them.
	Expected outcome	Resolution of ambivalence, trusting relationship developed with caregiver	Education source: *Women's Health Patient Education Resource Manual*, Aspen Publishers, Inc., 1994.
Paternal Trimester 1	Seeking safe passage: Realization or confirmation of pregnancy	Ambivalence, potential guilt or pride in ability to impregnate woman	Help him to understand that ambivalence is the first emotion of pregnancy, and guilt or pride are normal reactions.
	Binding-in: Couvade syndrome	Increasing physical symptoms such as nausea, unexplained weight gain: guilt or pride regarding woman's pregnancy	Minor physical discomforts and symptoms are normal and may be his way of becoming involved with the pregnancy. Explore feelings and encourage him that either feeling is normal.
	Increased need to protect and control	Encourage nurturing feelings and discuss need to control with woman	Discuss changes he can expect in partner and encourage expressions of his feelings.
	Identity formation of new role	Financial worries, may take on extra work, home improvements	Provide sounding board for him to balance perceived financial worries with real financial worries.
		Possible decrease in communication, may also have fantasies, begin role playing and mimicry	Encourage couple to talk frequently; dreams also help person to test out ideas and strategies.
	Acceptance by others		May not occur in the first trimester for man.
	Giving of oneself: Inadequacy, helplessness, and anxiety	May feel left out, unable to verify pregnancy by physical symptoms	Encourage him to get involved with the pregnancy by encouraging woman to incorporate healthful behaviors and help her with duties, discuss fetal development.
	Expected outcome	Trust relationship between partners and care provider	Education source: *Women's Health Patient Education Resource Manual*, Aspen Publishers, Inc., 1994.

EXHIBIT 2–2   Maternal–Paternal Developmental–Psychological Assessment Tool, *continued*

	Task	Expected Behavior (+) (−)	Intervention
Maternal Trimester 2	Seeking safe passage	Protective avoidance behaviors	Discuss patient's perceived need to avoid perceived dangerous situations.
		Possible decrease in sexual activity	Initiate discussion with the couple to explore alternate positions; encourage mutual nurturing.
		Decrease in other physical activities	Encourage the continuation of usual physical activities, encourage walking.
		Increased information seeking	Center guidance and education around the growing child. Include her when performing routine assessments.
	Binding-in: Realization that child is a separate entity	Quickening is an important event	Alert her to early fetal movement feelings such as butterflies or gas bubbles.
		Interactions with fetus (naming, patting, talking to, singing to)	Reinforce interactions; educate about fetal capabilities.
		Feeling of wellness	Hormonal changes result in feelings of wellness.
		Change in body image; wearing of maternity clothes	Explore feelings about changing body image, effect on partner and sexuality.
	Acceptance by others	Fantasies and dreams about own relationship with mother and new child and her relationship	Continue opening avenues for discussion between couple and among family members, dreams allow the trying out of ideas and strategies; mother is most important role model.
		Relationship with mother becomes important	Need to resolve old conflicts with mother; encourage her to do so.
	Binding in	Increase in role playing and mimicry; identification with mothering role	Explore cultural influences on mothering role, role models also will be found throughout the media and Internet.
		Reality testing and learning about her child; nesting begins	Encourage abdominal palpation, counting fetal movements, naming, or nicknaming: encourage mother to pick song or rhyme to repeat to fetus daily.
		Changing role may cause feelings of loss and grief	Discuss process of role change: Who am I, What will I be. Anticipate life changes.
	Giving of oneself	Preparations begin for labor, delivery, and infant care	Help mother to enroll in classes for labor, delivery, parenting, infant care, and feeding; discuss with her.
	Expected outcome	Couple begins to prepare for role change; beginning attachment evident	

EXHIBIT 2–2   Maternal–Paternal Developmental–Psychological Assessment Tool, *continued*

	Task	Expected Behavior (+) (−)	Intervention
Paternal Trimester 2	Seeking safe passage	Anxiety about labor and delivery	Encourage networking with other expectant men or new fathers; discuss realistic expectations for the birth.
	Binding-in	Fears about mutilation or death of mother or child Increased irritability, anxiety, decreased physical symptoms, nesting behaviors, fantasies, and dreams about fatherhood, may buy items for child Dreams assist role development	Encourage communication between partners about fears. Encourage couple to work together; dreams continue to allow working through of fathering role conflicts; educate about fetal capabilities (hearing, dreaming, memory).
	Acceptance by others	Announcement made to coworkers, friends, and buddies; ambivalence resolving	
	Giving of oneself	Protective of partner	May enroll in fathering course.
	Expected outcome	Father announces role change to others: couple begins attachment with child	
Maternal Trimester 3	Seeking safe passage	Introjection-projection-rejection (looking into herself, trying on roles and deciding)	May experience decreasing memory (pregnancy amnesia).
		Safety has heightened importance, increased vulnerability	Discuss nutrition, exercise, and self-protective behaviors.
		Anxiousness to end pregnancy	Discuss cultural influences that are important for a positive labor and delivery experience.
		Fantasies/dreams continue but decrease; may include stressful dreams of death and infant intactness	Encourage open discussion and reassurance of normalcy.
		Possible continuation of decrease in sexual activity	Explore alternate mechanisms for maintaining intimacy.
	Anxiousness to deliver	Mother should be prepared for labor, delivery, and infant care and knows signs and symptoms	Review signs and symptoms with her; review breathing techniques and relaxation techniques.
			Discuss change in body after birth.
		Has plans for postpartum period	Use anticipatory guidance to help prepare for common postpartum situations.
	Acceptance by others	Increased sensitivity to rejection and need for acceptance by family and friends, especially mother; increased need for acceptance	Social support is very important; other women used as confidantes; may be provider if social network is small or not helpful.
	Binding-in: separating from pregnancy	Binding-in endures; she may be irritable and susceptible to insults	Compliment mother about appearance and positive actions she is taking.
	Giving of oneself	Feels overwhelmed with demands; less confident, nesting behaviors continue	Needs constant reassurance and social support; new role relationships become more defined.
	Expected outcome	Confidence with upcoming labor and delivery, beginning interest in infant care	

EXHIBIT 2–2   Maternal–Paternal Developmental–Psychological Assessment Tool, *continued*

	Task	*Expected Behavior (+) (−)*	*Intervention*
Paternal Trimester 3	Seeking safe passage: Awareness of mother's size	Excitement about fetal movements	Let him listen to fetal heart tones and feel fetal parts through abdomen.
		Some anxiety about woman's changing body	Encourage him to express feelings about partner's changing body.
	Anxiousness to deliver	Father should be prepared for labor, delivery, the postpartum period, and infant care	Review signs and symptoms of labor, comfort measures, and coaching techniques with him.
		Plans for getting to hospital	Begin to anticipate with him his postpartum needs.
		Decreased sexual activity	Initiate discussion with couple; discuss alternatives to traditional position and intercourse; encouraging nurturing; reassure partner of his love for her.
	Binding-in	Couvade continues: Increased physical symptoms	Empathize with continuation of couvades, explore feelings with father.
	Giving of oneself	Introspection may increase	Encourage open communication about changing roles and needs between couple.
		Increase mimicry and role playing	Discuss with him his concept of fatherhood and how involved he plans on becoming; include him in decision about feeling.
		Increase in dreams and fantasies	Encourage him to talk about them with you and partner.
	Acceptance by others	Relationship with own father becomes important	Needs to resolve old conflicts with father; encourage him to do so by talking with father or by working through reasons within himself.
		Role of being provider increases in importance	Anticipate this with him.
		May become irritated with job	
	Expected outcome	Comfort with upcoming labor, delivery, and fathering role	

Source: Malnory, M., 1996. Developmental Care of the Pregnant Couple. Journal of Obstetric, Gynecologic and Neonatal Nursing, *vol. 25, no. 6: 527–530. Reproduced with permission.*

the care process, are all part of family-centered maternity care.

CONTINUITY OF CARE

During pregnancy and childbirth, continuity of care is very important. Every effort should be made to provide women with care from the same healthcare provider, or from a familiar group, with a shared philosophy of care. Documentation systems can be used to provide effective communication between providers (Health Canada, 2000).

Care Coordinators

In an effort to provide comprehensive, nonfragmented care some hospitals have developed care coordination programs. In these programs, perinatal care coordinators follow each patient throughout pregnancy and provide a link between patient, hospital, and physician (Ashe, 2000). The care coordinators see the expectant mother at specific intervals at the hospital where she plans to give birth. Assessment, problem identification, patient and family education, and appropriate referrals to community resources are all part of the program.

A needs assessment is performed early in the pregnancy to identify any high-risk problems and address them promptly. The number of visits and interventions are determined according to whether the woman is low, moderate, or high risk. The care coordinator collaborates with the physician or midwife on all aspects of the patient's care and coordinates all referrals.

At Catawba Memorial Hospital, patient care coordinators identify high-risk mothers and families and establish a plan for their care throughout the childbearing year. This plan is developed collaboratively with certified nurse midwives, physicians, dieticians, public health nurses, clinic maternal–child nurses, social workers, and the care coordinator.

There are multidisciplinary team meetings where the team members discuss each high-risk mother's needs for care and progress along the care path and appropriate referrals are made. Care coordinators at Catawba Memorial Hospital make antepartum home visits if needed as determined by the multidisciplinary team.

Saint Luke's–Shawnee Mission Health System in the Kansas City area uses maternity care coordinators to help coordinate the women's childbirth care and hospital stays. The maternity care coordinators are registered nurses with a variety of experience in maternal/child care. Their role is to prepare the expectant mother and her family for the birth experience, answer their questions, and identify any special needs the woman or her family might have.

In one-on-one sessions in the last trimester of pregnancy, the care coordinators give the family a chance to discuss their family's healthcare and educational needs, hospital admission, discharge planning, and services available. The woman has an opportunity to discuss her concerns and preferences for labor and birth and this information is relayed to the hospital nursing staff by the care coordinator.

Pregnancy Guides

A book that serves as a pregnancy guide is distributed to all pregnant women planning to birth in the Saint Luke's–Shawnee Mission Health System. Women are encouraged to take their book to appointments with their healthcare provider so that they can record important information. Also, they are asked to take their book to their childbirth and parenting classes, to their maternity care coordinator visit, and to their hospital stay.

The 130-page softcover book is a comprehensive overview of what to expect during the childbearing year. Helpful phone numbers, community resources, parent and family education offerings, and class enrollment forms are included. It is an easy-to-read, well-illustrated, and thorough road map for expectant families.

At Evergreen Family Maternity Services in Kirkland, Washington, at the first pregnancy visit, all families receive a book as a guide for use durng pregnancy, a text for prenatal classes, and an aid to parenting. At 12 weeks of pregnancy, families receive a stylized binder, "The Maternity Patient Information Guide," which contains information about their healthcare provider, the maternity education program, what to expect in the hospital, and an overview of all the programs designed to support them as they become parents (Keppler and Roudebush, 1999).

The content of the "Maternity Patient Information Guide," used at Evergreen Family Maternity Services is outlined below:

The Maternal Patient Information Guide

Chapters 1 and 2: Information about the care provider's office and a "Pregnancy, Having a Baby, and Parenting Pathway" designed to help families know what to expect during each phase of pregnancy and during their hospital stay.

Chapters 3 and 4: Information on Evergreen's childbirth and parenting education program. Contains handouts and evaluation forms for each seminar and course.

Chapter 5: Infant care; information about choosing a physician for the baby, car seat safety, and immunizations.

Chapter 6: Infant feeding; health benefits of breastfeeding.

Chapter 7: Information a family needs for an inpatient stay, including the hospital's philosophy, a sample consent form, a discussion about the expected length of the hospital stay, instructions for obtaining a social security number and birth certificate, how to register a baby online with us, and how to have photographs of the baby taken.

Chapter 8: Description of the hospital's postpartum follow-up appointment procedure for mother and baby.

Chapter 9: Information on the hospital's baby beeper rental program, health resource line, and information about domestic violence.

Chapter 10: Provides the family with a place to store other important papers they acquire.

Adapted from The Evergreen Story—Moving toward Family-Centered Care (Roudebush, *J. Advances in Family-Centered Care*, p. 11. Summer 2000).

Clinical Pathway

At Gaston Memorial Hospital, expectant mothers are given maternal and newborn clinical pathways during prenatal classes. The clinical pathways are discussed with the woman and her family during the classes so that they are informed of the plan of care for hospitalization. This is a detailed account of what the woman can expect for herself and her infant and helps the mother work with the nurse toward mutually planned goals. These clinical pathways are reproduced in Exhibits 2-3 and 2-4.

EXHIBIT 2–3   Newborn Clinical Pathway. *Courtesy of The Birthplace, Gaston Memorial Hospital, Gastonia, North Carolina. Reproduced with permission.*

The Birthplace
Gaston Memorial Hospital

Newborn Clinical Pathway

label

Name:_____

Date/time of birth_____

☐SVD ☐VAC ☐FORCEP ☐ C/S (reason:_____)

Mother's blood type:_____ Infant's MD_____ Feeding: ☐Breast ☐Formula type:_____

Expected Patient Outcomes	Birth to 4hours of Age (Time_____ to _____)
Physiological ❖ Infant will establish and maintain stable respiratory rate and lung sounds.(RR 30-60) ❖ Infant will establish and maintain stable heart rate and rhythm; skin will be well perfused, pink centrally.(HR 120-160) ❖ Thermoregulation will be established and bath given. (Temp 97.6-98.9 axillary)	**Time/Initials** _____VS and assessment at admission _____ _____VS and assessment Q 30minutes x 4 *if unstable _____ consult with nursery _____VS and assessment 2hrs after last 30min check _____ _____Thermoregulation: skin to skin_____; warmer _____ _____Admission assessment within 60 minutes of birth_____ _____Admission bath_____
Nutrition ❖ Infant will breastfeed within 1st hour. ❖ Breastfeeding Assessment ❖ Formula feed infants will eat at least ½ oz. within the 1st 2 hours. ❖ Blood sugar levels will stabilize and be maintained, no signs of hypoglycemia.	_____Breastfeeding Assessment: _____ _____Breastfeeding (assist with positioning, latch-on) _____ _____Formula feeding education (positioning, amount, frequency and burping) _____
Hydration/Elimination ❖ Infant will void and stool at least once by 24hours of life	_____Void _____Stool
Labwork/Medications ❖ Infant will remain free of infection and electrolyte imbalances.	_____Erythromycin withheld until bonding process begun_____ _____Erythromycin Ointment OU within 1st hour_____ _____Aquamephyton 1mg IM within 1st hour (site)_____ _____Dextrostix if indicated (see assessment sheet) _____ _____Hepatitis B vaccine information given/ consent signed_____
Psychosocial and Bonding ❖ The bonding process will begin at birth. ❖ Mother and father/significant other will be allowed to hold infant within 1st 15 minutes. ❖ Skin to skin care will be encouraged.	_____Mother will hold infant_____ _____Skin to skin care_____ _____Age appropriate care_____
Security/Identification ❖ Infant security will be maintained throughout hospital stay.	_____Bracelets to baby, mother, father/s.o. within 15 minutes of birth_____ _____Security process explained to mother, father/s.o., family_____ _____Footprints to footprint identification sheet and souvenir birth certificate after feet have been washed_____ _____Mother's index fingerprint to footprint identification sheet_____
Discharge Planning/Education ❖ Mother will be able to independently perform all aspects of newborn care by the end of her hospital stay.	_____Mother informed of Baby Care Basics class/times_____

❖   If variance significantly alters plan of care, see nurses narrative.
     Revised 4/01

EXHIBIT 2–3   Newborn Clinical Pathway *(continued). Courtesy of The Birthplace, Gaston Memorial Hospital, Gastonia, North Carolina. Reproduced with permission.*

label

✚ The Birthplace
Gaston Memorial Hospital

Date/time of birth_____

☐NSD ☐ C/S (reason:_____)

Mother's blood type:_____ Infant's MD_____Feeding: ☐Breast ☐Formula type:_____

Expected LOS_____

Expected Patient Outcomes	**4hrs to 24hrs of Age (Date/Time_____ to _____)**
Physiological ❖ Infant will maintain normal parameter of vital signs throughout hospital stay.(HR 120-160, RR 30-60, T 97.6-98.9 Ax) ❖ Infant will remain free from infection processes ❖ Physical assessment will remain within defined limits as stated on Newborn Admission Record.	Time/initials _____ VSS done at 4hours of age or 2hours after stable then_____ _____ VSS done q 12hours 0800 and 2000, and PRN_____
Nutrition ❖ Infant will maintain adequate nutritional intake: - Breastfeeding on demand (at least 6-8 times per 24 hours) -Formula feeding every 3-4 hours on demand ❖ Blood sugar levels will stabilize and be maintained, no signs/symptoms of hypoglycemia. ❖ Infant will not have weight loss > 7% of birth weight.	_____ Observe a least one complete breastfeeding q 12hrs_____ _____ Dextrostix glucose with s/s hypoglycemia or with inadequate nutritional intake > 5 hours_____
Hydration/Elimination ❖ Infant will void and stool within 1st 24 hours. ❖ Infant will void after circumcision (if applicable)	_____ Void-notify MD if no void by 24 hours of age_____ _____ Stool-notify MD if no stool by 24 hours of age _____ _____ Circumcision permit if applicable_____ _____ Circumcision checks if applicable_____ _____ Void after circumcision_____
Labwork/Medications	_____ Hepatitis B vaccine given_____ _____ Vaccine card given to parents_____ _____ Assess coombs status _____ **(All OPos and Rh negative moms)**
Psychosocial / Bonding/ Developmental ❖ Infant/parents will demonstrate appropriate bonding process and attachment. ❖ Infant displays appropriate newborn behavior. ❖ Parents respond appropriately to newborn cues.	_____ Assess bonding process (eye contact, touch, verbal, enface response) _____ _____ Age appropriate care_____
Security/Identification ❖ Infant security will be maintained throughout hospital stay and at discharge.	_____ Identification band checked with each release of infant _____
Discharge Planning Education ❖ Infant's mother & father/s.o. will verbalize and demonstrate all aspects of appropriate caregiving by discharge.	_____ Mother attended Baby Care Basics class_____ _____ BCB teaching sheet signed by mother_____

❖ If variance significantly alters plan of care, see nurses narrative.

EXHIBIT 2–3   Newborn Clinical Pathway *(continued). Courtesy of The Birthplace, Gaston Memorial Hospital, Gastonia, North Carolina. Reproduced with permission.*

The Birthplace
Gaston Memorial Hospital

24 hrs to 48 hrs of age (Date/time_____ to_____)	48 hrs to Discharge (Date/time_____ to_____)
Time/initials _____ VSS done q 12hrs 0800 and 2000, & PRN_____ _____ Cord clamp removed_____	**Time/Initials** _____ VSS done q 12hrs 0800 and 2000, & PRN_____ _____ Cord clamp removed_____
_____ Observe two complete breastfeedings. _____ _____ D/S glucose with s/s of hypoglycemia or with adequate nutritional intake > 5 hours. _____ _____ Daily weight (Weight_____) _____ Less that 7% wt loss_____ _____ Greater that 7%wt loss ☞indicates variance_____	_____ Observe one complete breastfeeding_____ _____ Daily weight (weight_____)_____
_____ Circumcision checks if applicable. _____ _____ Voided after circumcision_____	_____ Circumcision checks if applicable_____ _____ Voided after circumcision_____
_____ PKU done > 24 hours after 1st feed (time_____) _____ Hearing screen	
_____ Assess bonding process (eye contact, verbal, interaction care) _____ _____ Age appropriate care_____	_____ Assess bonding process (eye contact, verbal, interaction care) _____ _____ Age appropriate care_____
_____ Identification band check with each release of infant_____	_____ Identification band check with each release of infant_____
_____ Mother attended Baby Care Basics class_____ _____ BCB teaching sheet signed by mother_____	_____ Mother & father/s.o. independently perform all aspects of infant care_____

❖   If variance significantly alters plan of care, see nurses narrative.

EXHIBIT 2–3   Newborn Clinical Pathway *(continued). Courtesy of The Birthplace, Gaston Memorial Hospital, Gastonia, North Carolina. Reproduced with permission.*

The Birthplace
Gaston Memorial Hospital

Label

Date of Discharge_____
Actual LOS_____

Discharge Criteria to be completed by 48 hours of age (Date/time_____)	Discharge Checklist
Date/initials _____ Vital signs stable x 24hours_____ _____ Adequate feeding after _____ hours_____ _____ Weight check done > 24hours of age_____ _____ PKU completed and documented_____ _____ Hearing screen done_____ _____ Cord clamp removed. Cord WNL_____ _____ Hepatitis B vaccine given and immunization card given _____ _____ Circ site without bleeding (if applicable) _____ _____ Infant pictures offered/ done_____ _____ Car seat available_____	**Date/initials** _____ Clinical path/ variances completed_____ _____ Discharge order received_____ _____ Infant discharge instruction sheet given, explained, signed_____ _____ Birth Certificate completed_____ _____ ID bracelet to footprint identification sheet and signed by mother_____
❖ **Variance Report**	❖ **Variance Report**
Date/time Variance and Reason	Date/time Variance and Reason

Initials	Signature/Title	Initials	Signature/Title

❖   If variance significantly alters plan of care, see nurse's notes.

EXHIBIT 2–4   Admission through Discharge Clinical Pathway. *Courtesy of The Birthplace, Gaston Memorial Hospital, Gastonia, North Carolina. Reproduced with permission.*

The Birthplace
Gaston Memorial Hospital

Admission through Discharge
Clinical Pathway

Age:_____ MD:_____

G:_____ P:_____ ρBreast ρFormula Type:_____

Blood Type:_____

Rubella ρImmune ρNon-Immune
ELOS

Expected Outcome	Delivery - 4hrs Date/Time to
Physiological: Pt. will maintain vitals throughout hospital stay (T <100.4, P- 60-110, BP 90/60, 140/90) Pt. will have minimal blood loss. (Lochia small, moderate; fundus firm) Dressing dry/intact/incision free of redness, drainage, infection	**Time/Initial** _____Assessment q 15 x 4_____,_____,_____,_____ _____Assessment q 30 x 2_____,_____ _____Assessment q 1 hr x 2_____,_____ _____Assessment q 6 hrs_____
Nutrition/Hydration: Pt tolerates regular diet as evidenced by the absence of nausea, vomiting, or anorexia.	_____Progression to regular diet: ____Clear liquids ____Regular _____IV fluid type:_____ rate:____ _____ _____D/C IV fluids/convert to prn adapter _____D/C IV_____
Elimination: Output will be > 30 ml/hr	_____Bladder non-palpable _____Voids without difficulty _____Foley cath
Labwork: Labs/tests will be WNL	_____H & H ordered for 1st PP day _____Fetaldex drawn if indicated
Medication: Medication will be given as ordered.	_____Rubella status assessed _____Antibiotics
Pain Management: *Maximum level of pain control will be achieved as per patients needs/expectations. Pain assessed minimum 1 time per shift (q12hrs)	_____Pain assessed a/p_____ _____Pain assessed p/a_____ _____Analgesics _____Epidural/PCA _____Ice pack for epis/hem/lac _____Tucks/Dermoplast _____Whirlpool
Activity: Activity will progress to ambulation	_____Up with assistance first time _____Ambulatory _____Bedrest
Psycho-Social: Patient/SO and family involvement will be evidenced by a demonstration of eye contact/holding/and participation of care. Transition to parenting will be demonstrated.	_____Bonding _____SO present _____Family present _____Care specific to patient age and needs _____High risk (reason: _____)
Teaching/Discharge Planning: Patient will be able to demonstrate required aspects of self care/infant care by discharge.	_____Breastfeeding education/breast care _____Care of perineum, involution/lochia _____Infant safety/security

*see nurses notes

EXHIBIT 2–4 Admission through Discharge Clinical Pathway *(continued). Courtesy of The Birthplace, Gaston Memorial Hospital, Gastonia, North Carolina. Reproduced with permission.*

4hrs – 24hrs Date/time _____ to	24hrs – 48hrs Date/time _____ to
Time/Initial _____ Assessment q 6hrs (0800,1400,2000,0200) _____ Incision check	Time/Initial _____ Assessment q 12hrs (0800,2000)vaginal _____ Assessment q 6hrs (0800,1400,2000,0200)C/S _____ Incision care _____ Remove/change post-op dressing
_____ Regular diet _____ Clear liquid diet _____ Encourage po fluids _____ IV fluid type:_____ rate:_____ _____ D/C IV fluids/convert to prn adapter _____ D/C IV	_____ Regular diet/encourage po fluids _____ PO intake _____ % _____ Dietary consult (po intake <75%)
_____ Voids without difficulty _____ Remove foley cath at _____ _____ 1st void amount _____	_____ Voids without difficulty _____ Passing flatus _____ Bowel movement _____ Fleets enema
_____ H&H reviewed (Level:_____)	_____ _____
_____ Rubella permit signed _____ Rubella given _____ Rhogam eligible ____ Given (site:_____) _____ Antibiotics	_____ Depo Provera given _____ _____
_____ Pain assessed a/p _____ _____ Pain assessed p/a _____ _____ Analgesics _____ Epidural/PCA _____ Ice pack for epis/hem/lac _____ Tucks/Dermoplast _____ Whirlpool	_____ Pain assessed a/p _____ _____ Pain assessed p/a _____ _____ Analgesics
_____ Ambulate with assistance _____ Ambulate ad lib _____ TCDB q 2hrs _____ Incentive spirometry q 2hrs	_____ Ambulate ad lib
_____ Bonding _____ SO present _____ Care specific to patient age and needs	_____ Assuming care of infant _____ Care specific to patient age and needs
_____ Informed of Baby Care Basics Class & times _____ Newborn Channel (English 39, /Spanish 49) _____ Discharge/Education Sheet Introduced	_____ Discharge/Education sheet signed by patient _____ Newborn picture information given _____ Attended Baby Care Basics class _____ BCB teaching sheet signed

*see nurses notes

EXHIBIT 2–4   Admission through Discharge Clinical Pathway
(continued). Courtesy of The Birthplace, Gaston Memorial Hospital, Gastonia, North Carolina. Reproduced with permission.

The Birthplace
Gaston Memorial Hospital

48hrs to D/C
Date/time   to

Physiological:
Time/Initial
_____Assessment q 12hrs (0800,2000) vaginal
_____Assessment q 6hrs (0800,1400,2000,0200) C/S
_____Incision site WNL
_____Staples removed/Steri strips applied

Nutrition:
_____PO Intake _____%
_____Dietary consult (PO intake <75%)

Elimination:
_____Voids without difficulty

Labwork:
_____ _____

Medication:
_____ _____

Pain Management:
_____Analgesics PRN

Activity:
_____Ambulate ad lib

Psycho-Social:
_____Assuming care of infant
_____Care specific to patient age and needs

Teaching/Discharge Planning:
_____Discharge education sheet completed

EXHIBIT 2–4   Admission through Discharge Clinical Pathway *(continued). Courtesy of The Birthplace, Gaston Memorial Hospital, Gastonia, North Carolina. Reproduced with permission.*

Actual LOS

To be completed by 0700 day of Discharge
Discharge Checklist

Date/Initial

_____Vital signs stable

_____Clinical path/Variances completed

_____Self care/infant care evident at discharge

_____BCB Teaching sheet signed by mother

_____Rubella given(if needed)

_____Rhogam given (if needed)

_____Depo Provera given (if ordered)

_____Rx with patient

_____Medication fact sheet(s) given

list:_____

_____

_____Diaper bag given

_____Other:_____

_____

_____

_____

_____

_____

_____

Date/Time	Variance and Reason

_____Isolation precautions (type:_____

See Isolation Flowsheet)

_____D/C to courtesy room_____

_____Infant in NICU_____

_____

_____

_____

_____

_____

_____

_____

Initials	Signature/Title	Initials	Signature/Title

INFORMED DECISION MAKING

A basic tenet of family-centered antepartum care is that decisions about care are made collaboratively. Some families prefer to leave all decisions up to their doctor or midwife; however, most welcome and appreciate the opportunity to explore the pros and cons of their various options under a trusted healthcare professional's guidance. Although this can be time consuming, good, open communication between care provider and family is the best way to develop a trusting relationship. The antepartum period offers many opportunities for providers to give parents the information they need to learn about the influence of the new family member on their lives.

This is the time for providers to educate couples about normal pregnancy, labor, birth, and parenting. Emphasis is on pregnancy not as a disease state but as a state of wellness, during which individuals move from the role of expectant parents to the role and responsibilities of parents of a new baby.

The Pregnant Patient's Bill of Rights and The Pregnant Patient's Responsibilities (Haire, 1975), published by the International Childbirth Education Association, can form the foundation from which healthcare providers inform families of their rights and responsibilities during the childbearing experience. The Bill of Rights and Responsibilities for a Pregnant Patient follow (see Exhibit 2-5). (See Appendix J for a full-page version of the exhibit.)

The Maternity Center Association (MCA, 1998) has developed the Statement of the Rights of Childbearing Women. Selected key points of the Statement of the Rights of Childbearing Women (MCA, 1998) are included in Exhibit 2-6.

All or part of MCA's Rights of Childbearing Women can be incorporated into FCMC policies and procedures.

Choosing a Pediatrician or Family Care Physician

During the pregnancy, families need to understand the importance of interviewing and selecting a pediatrician, family care physician, or nurse practitioner for newborn care before their baby's birth. As mentioned earlier, in almost all cases, data indicate that a mother's feeding decision is made early in pregnancy, or, in many cases, before she becomes pregnant (Hill, 2000). Thus, the family and infant care provider should share similar philosophies regarding decision making, breastfeeding, and parenting in general. Arranging for a meeting before the baby is born assures the opportunity to talk about feeding and parenting issues as well as to clarify the provider's availability and role.

Choosing a Hospital or Birthing Center

During the early stages of pregnancy families need to consider where the birth is going to take place. The hospital or birthing center chosen will depend on the insurance plan, healthcare provider, and maternity care program offered. It is important to understand the hospital's or birthing center's philosophy and policies about FCMC; options and resources available; the program's cesarean, induction, and epidural rates; and whether or not mother–baby nursing is practiced.

EXHIBIT 2–5   Bill of Rights and Responsibilities for a Pregnant Patient. Policy and Procedure.

BILL OF RIGHTS AND RESPONSIBILITIES FOR A PREGNANT PATIENT

Procedure

Provide care for all antepartum and postpartum patients according to The Pregnant Patient's Bill of Rights and The Pregnant Patient's Responsibilities.

Policy

Staff will ensure that all antepartum and postpartum patients are encouraged to participate in decisions affecting their well-being and that of their unborn children.

Equipment

1. The Pregnant Patient's Bill of Rights (attached).
2. The Pregnant Patient's Responsibilities (attached).

Implementation

I. Follow the guidelines of The Pregnant Patient's Bill of Rights and The Pregnant Patient's Responsibilities when providing care to the antepartum or postpartum patient.

II. Assist the mother in understanding her rights and responsibilities.

VP Nursing

Department Chair

EXHIBIT 2–5 Bill of Rights and Responsibilities for a Pregnant Patient *(continued)*. *Reproduced here with permission of the International Childbirth Education Association (ICEA).*

THE PREGNANT PATIENT'S BILL OF RIGHTS

I. The pregnant woman has the right to:

A. Be informed, prior to the administration of any drug or procedure, by the health professional caring for her of any potential direct or indirect effects, risks, or hazards to herself or her unborn or newborn infant that may result from the use of a drug or procedure prescribed for or administered to her during pregnancy, labor, birth, or lactation.

B. Be informed, prior to the proposed therapy, not only of the benefits, risks, and hazards of the proposed therapy, but also of known alternative therapy.

C. Be informed, prior to the administration of any drug, by the health professional who is prescribing or administering the drug to her that any drug which she receives during pregnancy, labor, or birth, no matter how or when the drug is taken or administered, may adversely affect her unborn baby, directly or indirectly, and that there is no drug or chemical that has been proven safe for the unborn child.

D. Be informed, if Cesarean section is anticipated, prior to the administration of any drug, and preferably prior to her hospitalization, that minimizing her intake and, in turn, her baby's intake of nonessential preoperative medication will benefit her baby.

E. Be informed, prior to the administration of a drug or procedure, if there is no properly controlled follow-up research that has established the safety of the drug or procedure regarding its direct and/or indirect effects on the physiologic, mental, and neurologic development of the child exposed, via the mother, to the drug or procedure during pregnancy, labor, birth, or lactation.

F. Be informed, prior to the administration of any drug, of the brand name and generic name of the drug so she may advise the health professional of any past adverse reaction to the drug.

G. Determine for herself, without pressure from her attendant, whether she will accept the risks inherent in the proposed therapy or refuse a drug or procedure.

H. Know the name and qualifications of the individual administering a medication or procedure to her during labor or birth.

I. Be informed, prior to the administration of any procedure, as to whether that procedure is being administered to her for her or her baby's benefit (medically indicated) or as an elective procedure (for convenience or teaching purposes).

J. Be accompanied during the stress of labor and birth by someone she cares for and to whom she looks for emotional comfort and encouragement.

K. Choose a position, after appropriate medical consultation, for labor and for birth which is least stressful to her baby and herself, and promotes her comfort and the physiologic progress of her labor.

II. The new mother has the right to:

A. Have her baby cared for at her bedside if her baby is normal, and to feed her baby according to her baby's needs rather than according to hospital regimen.

B. Be informed in writing of the name of the person who actually delivered her baby and that person's professional qualifications. This information should also be on the birth certificate.

C. Be informed if there is any known or indicated aspect of her or her baby's care or condition that may cause her or her baby later difficulty or problems.

D. Have her and her baby's hospital medical records complete, accurate, and legible, and to have the hospital retain these records, including nurses' notes, until the child reaches at least the age of majority or, alternatively, to have the records offered to her before they are destroyed.

E. Have access, both during and after her hospital stay, to her complete medical records, and to receive a copy upon payment of a reasonable fee and without incurring the expense of an attorney.

It is the obstetric patient and her baby, not the health professional, who must sustain any trauma or injury resulting from the use of a drug or obstetric procedure. Observing the rights listed above will not only permit the obstetric patient to participate in decisions involving her and her baby's health care, but will help to protect the health professional and the hospital against litigation arising from resentment or misunderstanding on the mother's part.

Prepared by: Doris Haire, Chair, Committee on Health Law and Regulation, International Childbirth Education Association.

THE PREGNANT PATIENT'S RESPONSIBILITIES

In addition to understanding her rights, the pregnant woman should also understand that she too has certain responsibilities.

I. The pregnant woman is responsible for:

A. Learning about the physical and psychological process of labor, birth, and postpartum recovery. The better informed expectant parents are, the better they will be able to participate in decisions concerning the planning of their care.

B. Learning what comprises good prenatal and intranatal care and for making an effort to obtain the best care possible.

C. Knowing about those hospital policies and regulations that will affect their birth and postpartum experience.

D. Arranging for a companion or support person (husband, mother, sister, friend, etc.) who will share in her plans for birth and who will accompany her during her labor and birth experience.

E. Making her preferences known clearly to the health professionals involved in her care in a courteous and cooperative manner and for making mutually agreed-upon arrangements regarding maternity care alternatives with her physician and hospital in advance of labor.

F. Listening to their chosen physician or midwife with an open mind, just as they expect him or her to listen openly to them.

G. Seeing, to the best of their ability, that their program, once the have agreed to a course of health care, is carried out in consultation with others with whom they have made the agreement.

H. Obtaining information in advance regarding the approximate cost of her obstetric and hospital care.

I. Notifying all concerned, when intending to change her physician or hospital, well in advance of the birth if possible, and for informing both of her reasons for changing.

J. Learning, during her hospital stay, about her baby's continuing care after discharge from the hospital.

II. The parents are responsible for:

A. Behaving toward those caring for them, in all their interactions with medical and nursing personnel, with the same respect and consideration they would like.

B. Writing, after birth, constructive comments and feelings of satisfaction and/or dissatisfaction with the care (nursing, medical, and personal) they received. Good service to families in the future will be facilitated by those parents who take the time and responsibility to write letters expressing their feelings about the maternity care they received.

All the previous statements assume a normal birth and postpartum experience. Expectant parents should realize that if complications develop in their cases, there will be an increased need to trust the expertise of the physician and hospital staff they have chosen. However, if problems occur, the childbearing woman still retains her responsibility for making informed decisions about her care or treatment and that of her baby. If she is incapable of assuming that responsibility because of her physical condition, her previously authorized companion or support person should assume responsibility for making informed decisions on her behalf.

Prepared by members of the International Childbirth Education Association.

EXHIBIT 2–6   Key Points of the Statement of Rights of Childbearing Women

- Every woman has the right to receive care that is consistent with the best available current scientific evidence on its effectiveness.

- Every woman has the right to be fully informed about the benefits, risks, and costs of the procedures, drugs, tests, and treatments considered for use during her pregnancy, labor, birth, and postpartum periods, or for use by her child, and the right to informed consent or refusal.

- Every woman has the right to maternity care that is appropriate to her cultural and religious background.

- Every woman has the right to maternity care that identifies and addresses social and behavioral factors that put her or her baby at increased risk of harm.

- Every woman has the right to receive continuous social, emotional, and physical support throughout labor and birth from a professional who has knowledge of labor support. She also has the right to have a companion or companions of her choice present throughout labor and birth.

- Every woman has the right to choose from a variety of natural and pharmacologic methods to control and relieve the pain of labor. She has the right to change her mind at any time during pregnancy and labor and to make new choices.

- Every woman has the right to decide collaboratively with her caregivers when she and her baby will leave the birth site for home, based on their individual conditions and circumstances.

Source: Maternity Center Association. (1998). Statement of the Rights of Childbearing Women. New York, NY: Author.

BIRTH PLANS

In addition to engaging in dialogue about diagnostic and treatment options for the intrapartum and postpartum periods, providers should also invite discussion of the woman's attitudes, fears, preferences, and desires about the birth experience. This process allows providers to present the pros and cons of medical and nursing procedures as they relate to maternal–infant bonding and attachment, family formation, and attaining parenting skills. Armed with this information, parents can put their preferences into a written birth plan and give that plan to the hospital staff so that all providers who come into contact with the family will know their preferences. Because birth plans encourage parent involvement in the decisions surrounding their baby's birth and early care, they are positive and practical tools for communication between healthcare providers and family members. The birth plan becomes a permanent part of the prenatal record and is sent from the provider's office to the birth facility along with the woman's history and copies of her physical forms. An example of a birth plan is shown in Exhibit 2-7.

EXHIBIT 2–7 Birth Plan, Gaston Memorial Hospital, Gastonia, North Carolina. *Reproduced with permission.*

The Birthplace
Gaston Memorial Hospital
<u>Birth Plan</u>

Welcome to The Birthplace! Our goal is to make your birth experience positive and unique, personal and private.

Name_____ **Date of Admission**_____

Support person(s)_____

Please check the options below <u>in the shaded boxes</u> which you would like to try (your nurse can describe them if needed):

Comfort Measures	Yes	No	Used by pt.	Stage of Labor/RN Comments
Jacuzzi				
Birthing Ball				
Walking				
Rocking Chair				
Labor Massage				
Relaxation/Breathing				
Visualization				
Position Changes				
Counter Pressure				
Knee Press				
Pain Medication				
Epidural				
Following Delivery:				
Labor partner to cut umbilical cord?				
Baby to be placed on Mom's abdomen?				
Pediatrician to check baby in Mom's room?				
I plan to: Breastfeed				
Bottle-feed				

Special Requests _____

_____

(See Appendix J for a full-page version of the exhibit.) This plan is specific to the birth experience itself.

EDUCATION FOR PREGNANCY, BIRTH, AND PARENTING

A major portion of family-centered and wellness health care for childbearing families is education and guidance (Ramer and Frank, 2001). Integrated throughout a FCMC program, childbirth and parent education are often anticipatory, informal, and focused on the expectant mother, a parent couple, or a small group. Complementing informal education is a family-centered, comprehensive education program for pregnancy, birth, and parenting. This program may be organized and offered by the birth facility staff, the physician's and midwife's offices, clinics or public health departments, or by community childbirth educators (ICEA, 1999). Sometimes the knowledge and skills of all groups are combined in a cooperative program of childbirth education.

When prenatal education is offered in hospitals, it may be tempting to promote a philosophy of care that reflects what is done rather than one that clearly presents options. It is important to recognize that there are distinct advantages to providing childbirth and parenting education programs that utilize the unique skills of both experienced staff from the birth facility and community childbirth educators.

Standards for Family-Centered Perinatal Education

A family-centered childbirth and parent education program emphasizes wellness, information for all family members, health enhancement, and family autonomy, which are all foundations of family-centered care (Westmoreland and Zwelling, 2000). Standards for a family-centered perinatal education program, based on experience and published recommendations, were identified by Westmoreland and Zwelling in 2000 and can be seen in Exhibit 2-8.

Education Course Guide

An exemplary comprehensive family-centered education program can be found at Concord Hospital in Concord, New Hampshire. The class offerings are described in the Childbirth and Parent Education Course Guide shown in Exhibit 2-9.

Parenting in Pregnancy Curriculum

Ann Corwin has developed a curriculum for integrating parenting information into an existing traditional child-

EXHIBIT 2–8   Standards for a Family-Centered Perinatal Education Program

- Courses offered encompass the entire childbearing year.

- In order to meet the changing needs of families during the childbearing year, education offerings include early pregnancy, mid-pregnancy, and late pregnancy classes, as well as postpartum and parenting information.

- The long-term emotional significance of the childbearing experience is addressed in all courses.

- Classes reflect the cultural needs of the participants.

- Class size facilitates the group process, with an ideal size of 6–10 couples and a maximum of 12 couples.

- Teachers utilize a variety of reaching strategies during each class to meet the needs of different types of learners.

- The Lamaze class series for first-time parents includes at least 12 hours of instruction with emphasis on skills practice (especially positioning and relaxation), comfort measures, and class discussion.

- Classes include discussion of consumer rights and responsibilities for making informed choices based on knowledge of alternatives.

- Family input and evaluation of class content and process is actively sought and used to improve classes.

- Childbirth instructors are certified.

(AWHONN, 1993, 2000; Haire, 1975; ICEA, 1999; Lamaze International, 2000; Phillips, 1994, 1996.)

Source: Westmoreland, M., and Zwelling, E. 2000. Developing a Family-Centered, Hospital-Based Prenatal Education Program. The Journal of Perinatal Education, *Vol. 9, No. 4. Reprinted with permission.*

birth education program. She emphasizes that parents spend an average of 10 hours preparing for a 10- to 16-hour labor and almost no time in childbirth classes preparing for 18 or more years of parenting (Corwin, 1998). A sample content outline of such an integrated curriculum is shown in Exhibit 2-10.

EXHIBIT 2–9   Childbirth and Parent Education

CHILDBIRTH AND PARENT EDUCATION
CONCORD HOSPITAL CENTER FOR HEALTH PROMOTION

Breastfeeding and Returning to Work

This open discussion addresses the rewards and challenges of breastfeeding and working outside the home. Topics include breast pumps, scheduling feedings and pumpings, storing breastmilk, and strategies for "keeping it all together." Babies are always welcome!

Parent Preview

An informational program designed to update you on maternity services and programs, what to expect during your hospital stay, and a guided tour of The Family Place, the maternity unit at Concord Hospital.

Sibling Preparation

Information, discussion, and activities aimed at increasing the sibling's sense of participation for the arrival of a new baby and for a new role as big brother or sister. Also included is a tour of The Family Place, the maternity unit at Concord Hospital.

Early Pregnancy Class

For women in their first four months or pregnancy and women thinking about getting pregnant. Led by a childbirth educator, registered dietician, and physical therapist, topics include nutrition, fitness, comfort measures, posture, fashion, and health tips to help make your pregnancy a safe and positive experience.

Expectations: Preparing for Your First Birth

This childbirth education program is devoted to preparing women and their support partners for labor, birth, and recovery during postpartum. Coping with the challenges of labor and birth will be discussed, including labor support, comfort measures, birthing positions, relaxation and breathing techniques, and pain control options. A newborn care class is also offered as part of this educational package.

Newborn Care

Learn the basics of newborn care from bathing, swaddling, and feeding to diapering, infant massage, and more! A "How to Be a Parent" manual does not exist, but you will get the "basic training" to get you started on your journey into parenthood!

Hypnobirthing

The Hypnobirthing childbirth method is as much a philosophy of birth as it is a technique for achieving a satisfying, relaxing, and stress-free birth. You will not be in a trance or a sleep state; you will be aware and fully in control, yet very relaxed throughout your birth. Hypnobirthing teaches you and your birth companion the art and job of experiencing birth in an easier, more comfortable way.

Infant and Child CPR

American Red Cross class for expectant and new parents.

Source: "Childbirth and Parent Education Course Guide," courtesy of Concord Hospital, Concord, New Hampshire.

EXHIBIT 2–9   Childbirth and Parent Education *(continued)*

One More Time: Preparing for Another Birth

This program is designed for women/partners who have experienced a previous childbirth. Includes review of the childbirth process and labor coping skills, including breathing and relaxation, labor support, pain control options, and update on hospital care policies.

Breastfeeding: Is It for Me?

Expectant mothers, fathers, and grandparents are all invited to join an open discussion on breastfeeding—the advantages, necessary preparation, and impact on the family. Participants will receive a copy of the book *Breastfeeding: A Parent's Guide*.

Vaginal Birth after Cesarean (VBAC)

This informational session is designed for pregnant women and their support partners who have experienced a prior Cesarean birth. Participants review the option of a VBAC delivery with an opportunity for questions and sharing of concerns.

Prenatal Fitness[*]

This fitness program combines exercise and discussion in sessions held twice a week. Emphasis is on improving muscle tone, strength, flexibility, and endurance during pregnancy.

Postpartum Fitness[*]

This exercise class for new moms emphasizes getting back to pre-pregnancy shape in a safe and healthy manner. Cardiovascular, toning, and stretching exercises will be incorporated into the class. Babies are welcome!

Baby Steps: Parent/Baby Group

Information and support for new parents regarding what's next in baby's steps toward growing and developing. Timely topics on caring for a new baby and dealing with the challenges and rewards of parenting will be presented, with ample time for friendly discussion. Babies are welcome!

Beyond Baby Steps

A parenting group for "graduates" of the Baby Steps program, or for parents and their 6- to 12-month-old babies.

"Just for Dads"

Led by experienced fathers, *Just For Dads* enables fathers-to-be to step up to the challenge of being a new dad and feel confident bringing the new baby home. A 3-hour class covering not only baby care and fatherhood, but also the needs of new mothers.

New Dads Discussion Group

This support group, facilitated by a "seasoned" Dad, meets monthly to discuss the challenges of living with a newborn, changes in relationship and roles, and resources available to the new dad.

---

[*]Indicates that a medical clearance is required before participating in class.

EXHIBIT 2–10 **Broad Concepts That Integrate Preparation for Birth and Preparation for Parenthood**

I. Building Support Systems

The necessity of a support system in order to cope with the important life transitions such as before and after birth include the following:

1. Other parents in similar transitions

2. Healthcare providers and caregivers

3. Identification of primary support person—just as the coach in labor provides dependability for labor and the postpartum

4. Use of support group(s)

5. Identification and locations of other resources as needed

II. Responding to Change in Normal Life Transitions

1. The body changes to accommodate the fetus, and the family must change to accommodate the infant.

2. Changes brought by life transitions require new coping techniques. In pregnancy, the challenge may be a sore back. Postnatally, the challenge may be sleep deprivation.

3. The need to cope and change should be viewed as a positive force in the transition to becoming a family.

4. The orderly sequential nature of labor phases, accompanied by the uniqueness of each labor, is similar to the expected stages and phases of infancy accompanied by the uniqueness of every child.

III. Specific Examples

1. Early labor parallels immediate postpartum (i.e., the infant is in a restful state, and the mother/caregiver is preparing for the job of caretaking).

2. Active labor parallels the first weeks postpartum as the caregiver's hard work has begun, accompanied by little sleep and the constant dependency needs of the infant.

3. Transition, which is the toughest part of labor, parallels the first 2 weeks to first 3 months as the mother/caregiver may think this phase will NEVER end and that she/he will NEVER get needed sleep. Just like transition, postpartum can be one of the hardest stages of parenting, but it is the shortest.

4. Similar parallels can be drawn through second stage (or pushing), as compared to the relief the mother/caregiver finally gets when reciprocal responses from the infant begin (i.e., smiling at 3 months). Delivery parallels the infant's first 6 months to first year of life as the road to autonomy and less dependency is begun.

Corwin, A. 1998. Perinatal Education, vol. 7, no. 4: 31. Reprinted with permission.

PARENT ADVISORY COUNCIL

FCMC programs involve families as advisors to the maternity services. In serving on a Parent Advisory Council (PAC), parents become part of the fabric of policy and program design.

A parent advisory council is a forum for ongoing discussion with families in the community. The membership consists of couples or single parents who became parents within three years of sitting on the advisory council. The parent members of the parent advisory council listen and provide input for maternity program development and implementation but have no decision-making authority. They offer suggestions, give feedback, and become involved in specific projects. There are quarterly meetings of one or two hours and members are reimbursed for childcare and transportation expenses (Jeppson and Thomas, 1994).

The range of advisory roles that families can play is almost limitless. Serving on a parent advisory council is just one role. Exhibit 2-11 identifies some of the advisory roles and functions that families can perform.

EXHIBIT 2–11 **Advisory Roles Patients and Families Can Play**

Members of task forces

Advisory board members

Program evaluators

Co-trainers for preservice of inservice sessions

Paid program staff

Paid program or policy consultants

Mentors for other families

Grant reviewers

Participants in needs assessment process

Reviewers of audiovisual and written materials

Group facilitators

Witnesses at hearings

Advocates

Participants in focus groups

Members of committees hiring new staff

Fundraisers

Members of boards of trustees

Participants at conferences and working meetings

Participants in quality improvement initiatives

Source: Adapted from Jeppson, E., and Tomas, J. (1994). Essential Allies: Families As Advisors. Bethesda, MD: Institute for Family-Centered Care.

FAMILIARIZATION WITH THE PLACE OF BIRTH

To help families prepare for the actual labor and birth and become more comfortable with the maternity care unit, FCMC programs invite small groups of expectant families to visit the childbirth facility. For their convenience, hospitals schedule tours at a variety of times, including evenings and weekends. The purpose of this tour is not to acquaint family members with policies, rules, and regulations, but to introduce families to staff members, to the system of care, and to resources. Further, family members become familiar with the facility, its physical layout, and features such as the patient/family resource library. A guide can explain the maternity program's components and provide information on the FCMC philosophy, present media materials, and explain consent procedures. The orientation tour also offers hospital staff and visiting families an opportunity to discuss birth options and resources available both through the hospital and in the wider community. Families are given a copy of the hospital's maternity care philosophy. This is also the appropriate time for consultation with hospital business staff about financial arrangements, prepayment options, and insurance requirements.

CHAPTER SUMMARY

Prenatal care begins with preconception care that includes not only an assessment of health, but also of risk. Early entry into care, health promotion, continued risk assessment, cultural assessment, and medical, nutritional, and psychosocial interventions are all important components of prenatal care.

Social support during pregnancy is extremely important and a woman especially needs the support and care of her partner. Assessment of social support and the presence of excessive stress and/or violence in pregnancy is necessary so that appropriate intervention plans can be developed and pregnancy outcome improved. There are numerous tools for providers to use in this assessment, a few of which can be found in this chapter. (See questions from Canterino et al. [1999], the maternity social support scale from Webster et al. in Exhibit 2-1, and the maternal–paternal developmental–psychological assessment tool from Malnery [1996] in Exhibit 2-2.)

Throughout pregnancy continuity of care is essential and again, care practices and useful tools to establish that continuity are included in this chapter. A major portion of family-centered and wellness health care for childbearing families is education and guidance integrated throughout the FCMC program.

Families are an integral part of planning and implementing FCMC programs. They can serve as active members of task forces, advisory boards, and even as paid program staff. The variety of options for inclusion of childbearing families in the development of FCMC is limited only by one's imagination.

FACILITY FEATURES FOR FAMILY-CENTERED ANTEPARTUM CARE

Facility Design

The following facility design features provide a physical environment that supports the practice of FCMC:

- A contemporary facility design communicates commitment to the families of the community.
- Facility design incorporates safety and ease of access for all families, visitors, and staff.
- A separate entrance is available for maternity service.
- Parking is adequate, affordable, convenient, and secure.
- Directional signage is clear and welcoming and reflects respect for families.
- There are receptionists and information desk personnel to help patients and visitors find their way.
- There are windows in the:
  a. common areas
  b. examining rooms
- Seating is comfortable:
  a. The chairs are comfortable.
  b. There is sufficient personal space.
- Nourishing snacks are available in the waiting area.
- There is sufficient space to accommodate support persons and children in the:
  a. waiting room
  b. examining rooms
  c. consultation rooms
- Public toilets with infant-changing accommodations are available.
- Posters that provide information on topics such as nutrition, avoidance of teratogenic substances, environmental hazards, safety, and the family's emotional well-being are rotated regularly.
- Educational materials on abuse are clearly displayed in exam rooms and bathrooms, and include telephone numbers of local shelters and help lines.
- A lending library, as well as free pamphlets written at educational levels appropriate for the clientele and in the language spoken by the families served, is available.
- Special adjustments are made for the handicapped.
- Information about community prenatal care services, intrapartum services, and educational programs is prominently displayed.
- The area has plants.

- Audiotapes, closed circuit TV, and computers with Internet access are:

  a. available in English

  b. available in the language(s) of the population served

  c. appropriate for the population served

- There is education space for childbirth and parenting classes:

  a. The space is designed for easy access by families and for equipment, which includes a birthing bed.

  b. There are large, carpeted classrooms for childbirth preparation classes.

  c. Public toilets are near the classrooms.

- There are conference rooms, work areas, and lounges available for staff members.

- There is office space for educators.

- There is adequate storage space for teaching aids and AV supplies.

- There is a Lactation Resource center to provide support for breastfeeding through information, pump rentals, and retail sales.

COMPONENTS OF FAMILY-CENTERED ANTEPARTUM CARE

The following components of family-centered antepartum care are designed to emphasize family participation during pregnancy:

1. There is a family-centered maternity care philosophy of care with clearly defined goals and objectives.

   a. Philosophy is developed and understood by all care providers.

   b. Philosophy is available in writing for each client family and is discussed with family members.

2. There is a multidisciplinary team approach.

   a. The team includes the woman and her family, health care providers, and the community.

   b. According to the setting, the team may include obstetricians, pediatricians, family physicians, certified nurse-midwives, nurse-practitioners, nutritionists, social workers, childbirth educators, translators and cultural mediators, and community or outreach workers.

   c. Cooperative interrelationships are developed between hospitals, birth centers, healthcare providers, and the community in an organized system of care.

3. Initial contact with the antepartum care facility is both welcoming and reassuring.

   a. The person answering the telephone and scheduling appointments has a warm telephone manner and communicates interest and concern.

   b. From the first, it is emphasized that staff members are available to answer questions at any time, not just during appointments.

   c. A hotline is available for family use, or the names of primary care providers and their telephone numbers are provided.

   d. The importance of self-care measures is communicated immediately, and follow-up information is sent by mail.

4. Timely first visit.

   a. The initial appointment is scheduled within one week of the initial contact.

   b. The woman first meets her primary care provider at each visit, while still dressed.

   c. A care coordinator is assigned to the family for the pregnancy and coordinates the plan of care.

5. Family attachment is emphasized.

   a. The woman is encouraged to bring family members with her to her appointments by:

      i. the person scheduling the appointment

      ii. the nursing staff

      iii. the primary care provider

   b. Family members and care providers are all introduced to each other upon meeting.

   c. Prior to implementing or administering examinations, procedures, treatments, or medications:

      i. explanations are routinely given

      ii. patient consent is obtained

   d. The woman and her family members are encouraged to participate in the visit.

   e. A woman's birth preferences and plan, including method of infant feeding, is developed and recorded during her pregnancy in collaboration with those whom she wishes to involve.

   f. Every woman is scheduled for the orientation to the maternity unit at a time convenient to her and her family.

   g. Each woman is given a list of the names and telephone numbers:

      i. of the hospital Ombudsman

      ii. of where she can call any hour of the day or night with questions, for information, in the event of an emergency, or when she thinks she is in labor

   h. The appointment system is flexible and can accommodate working women and family members.

   i. The woman's chart is accessible to her for reading and copying with a professional healthcare provider available for explanations and to answer questions.

   j. There is a childcare provider for mothers requesting it during prenatal visits.

   k. Fathering discussion groups are available.

   l. Parent support groups are formed.

6. Ongoing education is available.

   a. Printed instructional materials, informational posters, audio tapes and/or audiovisual materials are available as part of prenatal care:

      i.   in English

      ii. in languages other than English if there are non-English speaking populations

      iii. they are appropriate to the population served

   b. A reading list of pregnancy, childbirth preparation, and parenting books is given to each woman with information about where these books may be obtained.

   c. Each woman is given a list of community resources for childbirth education, support groups, parenting, breastfeeding, and child care with the name of the contact person and telephone number for each.

   d. A record of information/education given during appointments is included as part of the medical record and is used during hospitalization.

7. Informed decision making.

   a. Each woman/family is informed of available birth options:

      i.   an explanation of each option is given.

      ii. the woman's birth preferences and plan, including method of infant feeding, becomes part of her medical record, which is available to the in-hospital maternity unit upon admission.

   b. In addition to the assessment and evaluation of the physical well-being of the mother and of the baby, each visit includes the following:

      i.   the opportunity to express concerns

      ii. the opportunity to ask questions

      iii. anticipatory guidance

   c. Family functioning is periodically reassessed for the development of family problems, pregnancy concerns, and emotional/psychological changes.

   d. Risk and benefits are explained and family understanding is assisted via discussion.

   e. Translation services and cultural mediators are available to explain risks and benefits.

   f. Adequate time is allowed between explanations and the performance of a procedure to ensure family understanding.

   g. The Pregnant Patient's Bill of Rights and the Pregnant Patient's Responsibilities are made available and discussed with each family.

8. Childbirth education.

   a. Empowers the family by preparing them educationally, emotionally, and psychosocially for optimum childbirth experience.

Environment

a. Class size enables the following optimal learning situation:

   i.   There is individualized attention and monitoring of exercises.

   ii. There is time to respond fully to everyone's questions within the established timeframe.

b. The teacher-to-couple ratio is adequate to allow for dialogue, questions and answers, and group process.

Policy

a. There are childbirth education individual sessions or group classes for hospitalized women with antepartal complications.

b. Childbirth education program goals are written to reflect the hospital's philosophy of family-centered maternity care.

Staff Competencies

Childbirth educators are qualified as determined by the successful completion of a course or certification program.

Practice

a. There are written objectives and an outline for each class.

b. The objectives and outline for each class reflect the following:

   i.   the written goals of the hospital's childbirth education program

   ii. the principles of adult learning

   iii. engagement of the learner in his or her learning process

   iv. a variety of teaching techniques/strategies

   v.   the use of a variety of teaching tools

c. Referrals for community services and support groups are made as needed.

d. Evaluations of each class series are obtained from the participants. They are reviewed and serve as a basis for change. In addition, they are required for recertification.

e. Class series are held at varying times for the convenience of people with different work hours.

f. Printed instructional materials are available and routinely distributed as appropriate to all women:

   i.   in English

   ii. in the language(s) of the population served

   iii. as appropriate for the population served

g. Translation services are available if there are non-English speaking populations.

h. Interpreters are available for hearing-impaired women and women with other handicaps.

BIBLIOGRAPHY

American Academy of Pediatrics (AAP). 1997. Breastfeeding and the use of human milk: Policy statement. *Pediatrics* 100, no. 6: 1035–1039.

The American College of Obstetricians and Gynecologists. 1995. *Planning for Pregnancy, Birth and Beyond*, 2nd ed. Washington, DC: The American College of Obstetricians and Gynecologists.

Ashe, D. 2000. From positive to parenthood. *Nursing Management* 31, no. 10: 30–32.

Beckman, C., et al. 2000. Perceived barriers to prenatal care services. *Maternal Child Nursing* 25, no. 1: 43–46.

Bianchi, A. 2000. The emotional health of the single mother. *International Journal of Childbirth Education* 11, no. 2: 22–24.

Booth, T. 2001. *Pampers Childbirth Education Program: Teacher's Companion*. Proctor and Gamble, Pampers Parenting Institute.

Callister, L. 2001. Culturally competent care of women and newborns: Knowledge, attitude and skills. *Journal of Obstetrics, Gynecologic, and Neonatal Nursing* 30, no. 2: 209–215.

Canterino, J., et al. 1999. Domestic abuse in pregnancy: A comparison of a self-completed domestic abuse questionnaire with a directed interview. *American Journal of Obstetrics and Gynecology* 181: 1049–1051.

Center for the Advancement of Health. 2001. Pregnancy behavior and care: Enhancing infants' lifelong health. *Facts of Life* 6, no. 2: 1–6.

Corwin, A. 1998. Integrating preparation for early parenting into childbirth education: Part I—A curriculum. *The Journal of Perinatal Education* 7, no. 4: 26–33.

Fiscella, K. 1995. Does prenatal care improve birth outcomes? A critical review. *Obstetrics and Gynecology* 85, no. 3: 468–479.

Fortier, J. C., et al. 1991. Adjustment to a newborn: Sibling preparation makes a difference. *Journal of Obstetric, Gynecologic, and Neonatal Nursing* 20, no. 1: 73–79.

Haire, D. 1975. *The Pregnant Patient's Bill of Rights; The Pregnant Patient's Responsibilities*. Minneapolis, MN: International Childbirth Education Association.

Health Canada. 2000. *Family-Centered Maternity and Newborn Care: National Guidelines*. Ottawa: Minister of Public Works and Government Services.

Hill, P. 2000. Update on breastfeeding: Healthy people 2010 objectives. *Maternal Child Nursing* 25, no. 5: 248–251.

Hulsey, T. 2001. Association between early prenatal care and mother's intention of and desire for the pregnancy. *Journal of Obstetric, Gynecologic, and Neonatal Nursing* 30, no. 3: 275–282.

International Childbirth Education Association Position Paper. 1999. *The Role of the Childbirth Educator and the Scope of Childbirth Education*. Minneapolis, MN: International Childbirth Education Association, Inc.

Jeppson, E., and Thomas, J. 1994. *Essential Allies: Families As Advisors*. Bethesda, MD: Institute for Family-Centered Care.

Jordan, P. 1990. Laboring for relevance: Expectant and new fatherhood. *Nursing Research* 39, no. 1: 11–16.

Keppler, A., and Roudebush, J. 1999. Postpartum follow-up care in a hospital-based clinic: An update on an expanded program. *Journal Perinatal Neonatal Nursing* 13, no. 1: 1–14.

Klaus, M. D., Kennell, J. H. 1982. *Parent Infant Bonding*, 2nd ed. St. Louis: C. V. Mosby.

Kroelinger, C., and Oths, K. 2000. Partner support and pregnancy wantedness. *Birth* 27, no. 2: 112–119.

Lamaze International Position Paper. 2002. Lamaze for the 21st Century. *The Journal of Perinatal Education* 11, no. 1: x–xii.

Logsdon, M. 2001. Helping hands: Exploring the cultural implications of social support during pregnancy. *AWHONN Lifelines* 4, no. 6: 29–32.

Malnory, M. 1996. Developmental care of the pregnant couple. *Journal of Obstetric, Gynecologic, and Neonatal Nursing* 25, no. 6: 525–532.

Maloni, J., et al. 1996. Transforming prenatal care: Reflections on the past and present with implications for the future. *Journal of Obstetric, Gynecologic, and Neonatal Nursing* 25, no. 1: 17–23.

Maternity Center Association. 1998. *Statement of the Rights of Childbearing Women*. New York: Author.

Mattson, S. 2000a. Providing culturally competent care: Strategies and approaches for perinatal clients. *AWHONN Lifelines* 4, no. 4: 37–39.

———. 2000b. Working toward cultural competence: Making the first steps through cultural assessment. *AWHONN Lifelines* 4, no. 4: 41–43.

McFarlane, J., Parker, B., and Cross, B. 2001. *Abuse During Pregnancy: A Protocol for Prevention and Intervention*, 2nd ed. White Plains, NY: March of Dimes.

Meikle, S., et al. 1995. Women's reasons for not seeking prenatal care: Racial and ethnic factors. *Birth* 22, no. 2: 81–86.

Midmer, D., et al. 1996. *A Reference Guide for Providers: The ALPHA Form—Antenatal Psychosocial Health Assessment Form*. 2nd ed. Toronto: University of Toronto, Department of Family and Community Medicine.

Newton, N. 1963. Emotions of pregnancy. *Clinical Obstetrics and Gynecology* 6: 639–668.

Nuckolls, K., Laplan, and Ceissel. 1972. Psychosocial assets, life crisis, and the prognosis of pregnancy. *American Journal of Epidemiology* 95, no. 5: 431–441.

Office of Government Affairs, March of Dimes. 2001. *March of Dimes Data Book for Policy Makers: Maternal, Infant, and Child Health in the United States 2001*. Washington, DC: Author.

Omar, M., and Schiffman, R. 1995. Pregnant women's perceptions of prenatal care. *Maternal Child Nursing Journal* 23: 132–142.

Phillips, C. R. 1996. *Family-Centered Maternity and Newborn Care: A Basic Text*, 4th ed. St. Louis: C. V. Mosby–Year Book.

Polomeno, V. 2000. Social support during pregnancy. *International Journal of Childbirth Education* 11, no. 2: 22–24.

Raines, D., and Morgan, Z. 2000. Culturally sensitive care during childbirth. *Applied Nursing Research* 13, no. 4: 167–172.

Ramer, L., and Frank, B. 2001. *Pregnancy: Psychosocial Perspectives*, 3rd ed. White Plains, NY: March of Dimes.

Rising, S. 1998. Centering pregnancy: An interdisciplinary model of empowerment. *Journal of Nurse-Midwifery* 43, no. 1: 46–54.

Roudebush, J. 2000. The Evergreen story—Moving toward family-centered care. *Advances in Family-Centered Care* 6, no. 1: 6–11.

Rubin, R. 1970. Cognitive style in pregnancy. *American Journal of Nursing* 70, no. 3: 502–508.

————. 1975. Maternal task in pregnancy. *Maternal Child Nursing Journal* 4, no. 3: 143–153.

————. 1984. *Maternal Identity and the Maternal Experience*. New York: Springer Publishing.

Scherger, J., et al. 1992. Teaching family-centered perinatal care in family medicine, Part 1. *Family Medicine* 24, no. 4: 288–298.

Simpson, K., and Creehan, P. 2001. *Perinatal Nursing*, 2nd ed. Philadelphia: Lippincott Williams and Wilkins.

Todd, L. 1998. Reciprocal interaction as the foundation for parent-infant attachment. *International Journal of Childbirth Education* 13, no. 4: 5–8.

U.S. Department of Health and Human Services. 2000. *Healthy People 2010: National Health Promotion and Disease Prevention Objectives*. Washington, DC: Government Printing Office.

U.S. Department of Health and Human Services Public Health Service. 2000. *Healthy People 2010* (Conference edition). Washington, DC: Author.

Webster, J., et al. 2000. Measuring social support in pregnancy: Can it be simple and meaningful? *Birth* 27, no. 2: 97–101.

Westmoreland, M., and Zwelling, E. 2000. Developing a family-centered, hospital-based prenatal education program. *The Journal of Perinatal Education* 9, no. 4: 37–48.

White, M. 2000. Men's concerns during pregnancy, Part 1: Reevaluating the role of the expectant father. *International Journal of Childbirth Education* 13, no. 4: 14–17.

Family-Centered Intrapartum Care

INTRODUCTION

Family-centered care during labor and birth offers many options to the childbearing family. Although specific maternity program features will vary, a family-centered birth is as important when the pregnancy is at risk as it is when the pregnancy is normal.

The birth experience is complex and multidimensional. It includes numerous physical and psychosocial factors, with negative feelings sometimes coexisting with positive feelings (Waldenstrom et al., 1996). For most women and their families, labor and birth are natural, intimate processes wrapped in excitement and anticipation but mixed with some anxiety and fear. It is a happy time but a tense time: Will the mother have safe passage? Will the baby be OK?

One woman may fear the pain of labor and lack confidence that she will be able to cope with any pain at all. This woman may request anesthesia before labor even begins. Another woman may have a very strong desire for natural childbirth and anticipates a sense of personal achievement when she "masters" the pain of labor. Confident of her coping abilities, she may refuse any analgesia or anesthesia for labor and birth.

Given their hopes and fears, all expectant mothers and fathers need emotional support during labor (Klaus et al., 1993). Some women want their large extended families and selected friends with them for social support during labor. Other women may prefer having only their partner and/or a trained support person attend them during labor and birth.

A woman's previous experiences, emotional readiness, cultural and ethnic heritage, class, race, and age will impact her preferences for her birth experience (Vande Vusse, 1999). Not to be overlooked will be the influence of what is happening to her loved ones during this time. For example, if a woman's mother or father has recently experienced a life-threatening event, she may especially want that person with her to experience the birth of the next generation that can represent promise and hope for the future.

In other words, no two women and their families are alike, and no two births are alike. Each woman, each family, and each birth is unique.

GOAL OF INTRAPARTUM CARE

The goal of intrapartum care is to provide a safe and satisfying birth experience that supports the normalcy of childbirth and empowers the family.

DEFINITION OF FAMILY-CENTERED INTRAPARTUM CARE

Family-centered intrapartum care is a program of care that strives to keep birth normal and takes into account the roles that are unique to families as a social group: providing for nurturing and intimacy needs; helping each other in stressful situations; mutual commitment; shared history and values; and providing support to each other in major life passages (such as birth and death).

In family-centered intrapartum care, the healthcare team understands and respects the family's values, culture, and lifestyle. Family strengths and ability to work together are considered when providing care to the laboring woman. Members of the healthcare team do not make choices for the family or simply ask family members what they want. Instead, the team helps the family become clear about what they want so that the family can make informed decisions.

There will be times when it will be in the best interest of the laboring woman and her partner to have privacy. Family and friends can be helped to understand this when sensitive care providers speak as advocates for the laboring woman while at the same time recognize family needs and concerns (Tomlinson et al., 1996).

SOCIAL SUPPORT IN LABOR

Hospital visitation policies for labor and birth that arbitrarily limit the presence of family and friends overlook the importance of the social context in which childbirth occurs. When a woman enters a hospital to give birth, she is removed from her everyday life and support network. She becomes a stranger in a strange land, and this experience in itself can provoke anxiety and create a form of culture shock. This in turn causes the woman to feel dependent and vulnerable.

Social support from a woman's partner and family can help her deal with both the anxiety and the physical pain created by labor and birth (Fox and Lavendar, 1999). Knowing that family and friends are nearby, and that they care about her and her baby, communicates a message to the woman that she is not alone as she takes on the birth of the baby and her new role as a mother.

VISITATION POLICIES

It is a privilege for family members and healthcare providers to be present at the celebration of birth. Rigid rules and regulations that limit support for women during labor and birth have no place in FCMC. Instead, personalized and individualized care is at the very core of family-centered intrapartum care. The Birthplace at Gaston Memorial Hospital celebrates families, as their welcoming photos on the wall at the maternity control station illustrate in Figure 3-1.

In family-centered intrapartum care there are flexible visitation policies that encourage nonseparation of the woman and her support person during labor and birth, and that also provide her with access to family members and friends of her choice. The key words here are "her choice." During her pregnancy the woman decides who she wants with her during labor and birth. Her preferences are discussed with her care providers and recorded in her birth plan. When the intrapartum staff reviews the birth plan they can then honor the laboring woman's wishes.

While helping the woman make important decisions about visitation privileges, healthcare providers can begin a dialogue with her about the intimate experiences of labor and birth. Anticipatory guidance about the sensations of labor, the potential for exposure of "private" body parts, the options for pain control, and ways that intrapartum nurses provide labor support are important for the woman to be aware of as she decides who she wants to support her during labor and birth.

Exhibit 3-1 is a sample policy and procedure for the presence of fathers or designated significant others at a birth in a family-centered maternity care program. (See Appendix J for a full-page version of the exhibit.)

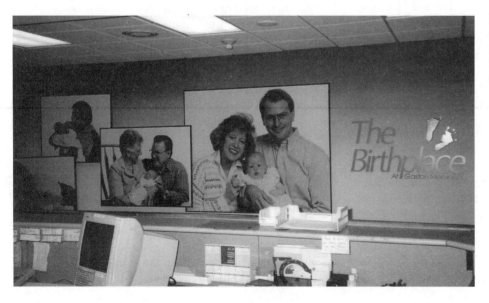

FIGURE 3–1 Celebrating families at The Birthplace, Gaston Memorial Hospital, Gastonia, North Carolina. *Photo courtesy of Gaston Memorial Hospital.*

EXHIBIT 3–1   Fathers or Designated Significant Others at Birth

---

Procedure

Provide support, lessen the mother's anxiety, and promote a family atmosphere. Facilitate the involvement of the father or support person(s) in a safe and supervised environment for birth.

Policy

Staff will welcome the father or support person(s) into the maternity unit during labor, birth, and the recovery period.

Patient Education

Explain procedures and define designated sterile areas to avoid contamination. Instruct the father and support person(s) on proper hand washing and the prevention and spreading of communicable infections.

Implementation

I.   Instruct the father (or support persons) to wash his hands thoroughly.

II. A scrub suit, shoe covers, mask, and hair cover must be worn for Cesarean births.

III. Encourage the father to observe and participate during the infant's initial assessment and care.

IV. Encourage and answer all questions.

VP Nursing

Department Chair

LABOR SUPPORT

The goal of labor support is to help a woman achieve her wishes for her birth experience through offering companionship, paying attention to her emotional needs, and actively helping her through the process (Hodnett, 1996). Five general categories of support that women have identified as helpful during labor include emotional support (encouragement, reassurance); comfort measures (massage, touch, cold or hot compresses, and so on); information, instructions and advice; advocacy (acting on the woman's behalf); and supporting the husband/partner (Hodnett, 1996).

A supportive environment is also important. The emphasis here is placed on privacy, quiet, and a minimal number of intrusions (Phillips, 1996).

Even when having epidural analgesia, women value emotional support as a top priority for their care during labor and birth. The bottom line is that a woman wants to feel cared about as an individual in one of the greatest tasks of her life: giving birth to and mothering a baby (Corbett and Callister, 2000).

Benefits

Quality labor support has measurable benefits in the outcomes of labor and birth. The continuous presence of a support person can reduce the need for pain medication, intravenous oxytocin, and episiotomy (Gagnon, Waghorn, and Covell, 1997; Klaus, Kennell, and Klaus, 1993; Vande Vusse, 1999; Simkin and O'Hara, 2002). Women given one-to-one labor support experience shorter labors, fewer epidurals, less use of forceps and vacuum extraction, fewer cesarean deliveries, and greater overall satisfaction with labor (Enkin et al., 2000). In a meta-analysis of 14 clinical trials, continuous support from a nurse, CNM, or lay person decreased use of medication for pain relief, operative vaginal birth, cesarean birth, and 5-minute Apgar scores of less than 7 (Hodnett, 2000).

Work Sampling

In spite of all the evidence of the benefits and value of labor support, however, work sampling studies found that supportive care, defined as reassuring touch, was provided only 9.9 percent of the time by nurses in 616 observations of nurses' interactions with laboring women (McNiven et al., 1992). This was true even when the maternity unit was staffed with the goal of one-to-one nurse–patient ratios during active labor. Most of the time nurses spent with patients fell into the category of providing "instruction/information" (Gagnon and Waghorn, 1996; McNiven, Hodnett, and O'Brien-Pallas, 1992).

In another work sampling study, twelve nurses were observed over six nonconsecutive day shifts on a birthing unit. A total of 404 observations were made. Results indicated that nurses spent only 12.4 percent of their total time providing supportive care to laboring women (Gale et al. 2001).

Numerous excuses to rationalize this sad state of affairs include a shortage of nurses, too many patients, not enough staff, traditional medical practices, ethical dilemmas and conflicts, limited financial resources, cumbersome documentation requirements, a medico-legal environment that rewards technical proficiency, and a generation of high-tech labor and delivery nurses who do not know how to perform labor support (Kardong-Edgren, 2001; Sleutel, 2000; Miltner, 2000). These are unacceptable excuses. The evidence is in and we cannot ignore it: Quality labor support demonstrates good birth outcomes, which have the potential to improve both the patient and nursing staff satisfaction and decrease overall costs (Kardong-Edgren, 2001; Ecenroad and Zwelling, 2000).

AWHONN Position Statement

A clinical position statement on professional nursing support of laboring women emphasizes the importance of continuously available labor support by a professional registered nurse as being a critical component to achieve improved birth outcomes (AWHONN, 2000). In this same position statement AWHONN states that it "believes it is incumbent on healthcare facilities to provide an environment that encourages the unique patient–nurse relationship during childbirth." In FCMC, quality labor support for childbearing women and their families is the first priority, and every effort is made to provide this support.

Creative Strategies for Labor Support

Nurses and physicians educated in an era of "high-tech," low-touch care can be taught the importance of supportive care and can be educated to provide labor support techniques and nonpharmacologic pain management strategies. By focusing on the potential for improved outcomes for the mother and newborn, there is the opportunity to shift nursing care that comprises indirect care activities to direct labor support activities (Miltner, 2000). This is exactly what happened at Good Samaritan Hospital in Lebanon, Pennsylvania, when a traditional maternity care unit transitioned their model of care to family-centered maternity care (Ecenroad and Zwelling, 2000).

With a supportive hospital administration and nursing director of maternal–child health nursing, this hospital nursing staff became educated in FCMC. Part of a comprehensive staff education program consisted of a 3-day workshop, "Creative Strategies for Managing Labor and Birth." In this workshop staff learned to enhance their nursing care with nonpharmacologic pain management strategies such as relaxation, massage, aromatherapy, visual imagery, maternal positioning, hydrotherapy, music, and breathing techniques (Zwelling and Anderson, 1997). Figure 3-2 illustrates a nurse and father providing support for a laboring mother at Good Samaritan Hospital. Techniques learned in the Creative Strategies class are being used.

Notebooks containing journal articles documenting evidence supporting all the creative strategies were provided for the nursing and medical staffs, with additional copies placed in the doctor's lounge. Physicians were not as willing to learn about the new labor support strategies. However, because physicians and nurses are members of the same patient care team, the CNS at Good Samaritan Hospital met with the physicians to explain the nonpharmacologic pain management strategies that the nurses were implementing. She did an excellent job of sharing the research supporting the use and benefits of these modalities and clarified that the comfort measures were nursing strategies for labor support and did not require a physician's order. Also, a seminar on labor support was provided for the physicians. The instructors were physicians who practiced FCMC at another hospital. After a lot of hard work, the medical and nursing staffs at Good Samaritan Hospital now provide physical and emotional support for laboring women and their families. This change has resulted in happy families, and greater job satisfaction and a new sense of pride for nursing staff.

Doulas

A "doula" (from Greek, meaning "in service of") provides nonmedical emotional, physical, and informational support to the childbearing woman and her family (Simkin and Way,

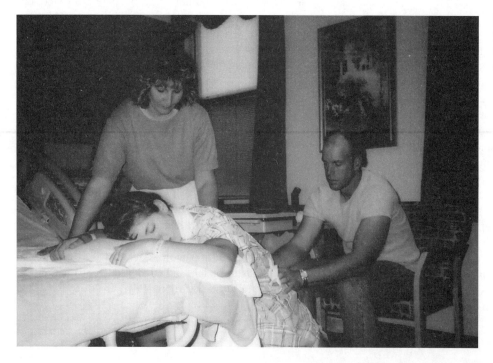

FIGURE 3–2 A nurse and father providing labor support. *Photo courtesy of Good Samaritan Hospital, Lebanon, Pennsylvania.*

1998). Private and hospital-based doula programs are being accepted in many communities throughout North America (Young, 1998). In these programs, a trained labor support specialist fills the gap that results when there aren't enough nurses to provide one-to-one labor support.

The doula also provides support, guidance, and relief for fathers during the birth process (Perez, 1998). Even when men want to take an active role in their partner's labor and birth, most do not feel qualified to act as a labor authority. Thus, the doula can take the pressure off of a father and allow him to be much more relaxed than he would otherwise be if he felt totally responsible for providing labor support. When the partner and doula work together to provide labor support, it becomes highly probable that the woman's emotional and physical needs will be fully met (ICEA, 1999).

As the scientific literature on doulas continues to expand, findings consistently demonstrate the benefits of doula support for women in labor. These benefits include improvements to the mothers' and infants' health and greatly reduced rates of medical procedures (Young, 1998; Keenan, 2000).

Boston Medical Center in Boston, Massachusetts, is a level III facility that provides care to a very diverse urban population. Many of the childbearing women served are new immigrants with little means, but with all of the wishes and hopes for a positive birth experience and a good start for the family. The hospital offers a Birth Sisters[SM] program in which every woman has access to a birth sister. The birth sister is a trained birth attendant who visits with the mother prenatally, accompanies and supports her during labor and birth, and makes one follow-up home visit to help with laundry, run errands, or care for siblings so the new mother can rest and be with her baby. The Urban Midwife Associates (UMA) developed the Birth Sisters program in 1994 as part of its overall model program. (See Appendix F for a description of the program.) Figure 3-3 shows a laboring woman with her Birth Sister providing support.

Monitrice

The "monitrice" (from French, meaning "to watch over attentively") is another labor-support professional. Generally a nurse or midwife, this individual combines labor support skills with clinical assessment skills (Perez and Snedeker, 1994). The monitrice can provide actual care to the laboring woman. She can also assist and monitor women at home during early labor and help them determine when to leave for the hospital.

PROVIDER GROUP

Physicians, midwives, nurses, doulas, monitrices, and partners and families may all be involved in caring for the woman during labor and birth. Although physicians deliver more than 92 percent of the approximately 4 million births

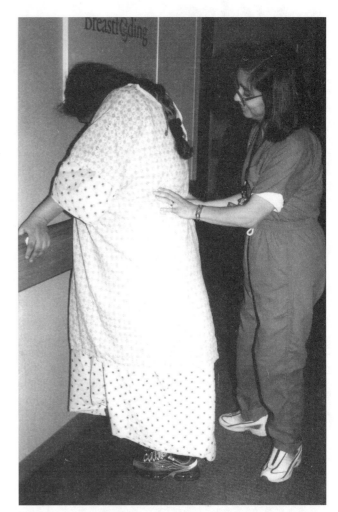

FIGURE 3–3 A Birth Sister supporting a laboring woman.
Photo by Emily Pascoe, courtesy of Urban Midwife Associates, Boston, MA.

each year in the United States, the number of births attended by certified nurse–midwives is growing, rising from 3.7 percent in 1989 to 6.7 percent in 1997 (National Vital Statistics Report, 1999).

Nurse-Midwifery

Certified nurse–midwives (CNMs) are an essential part of delivering family-centered care. Nurse-midwifery care is accepted as a reasonable option for women with low-risk pregnancies (Oakley et al., 1996).

Studies of nurse-midwifery care outcomes reported over the past 70 years document many benefits in both low- and high-risk populations. Examples of these benefits include low rates of cesarean birth and preterm birth, fewer low or very low birth weight babies, less use of oxytocin, fewer episiotomies, fewer severe lacerations, and lower instrumental delivery rates. Further, nurse–midwives incur fewer legal incidents and boast excellent maternal and neonatal outcomes (Goer, 1999; Rooks, 1997). The advantages of quality midwifery care are further enhanced by its cost benefits (Butler et al., 1993; Clark, Taffel, and Martin, 1997; Ernst, 1996; Rosenblatt et al., 1997; Oakley et al., 1996).

Women also report increased satisfaction with care provided by nurse–midwives. They describe a relationship based on respect, trust, and alliance (Kennedy, 1995). Women who use midwives often experience more personalized care that is more sensitive to their needs and desires. Indeed, midwifery care embodies the values of FCMC.

Nurse-Midwifery and Physician Partnerships

In some FCMC programs, obstetricians practice collaboratively with nurse–midwives. This arrangement can result in lower intervention rates, superior perinatal and maternal care, and improved maternal satisfaction. In addition, these practices demonstrate increased efficiency in obstetric care provision and improved financial profiles for the provider practice (Brown and Grimes, 1995; King and Shah, 1998; Walker and Stone, 1996). Collaborative practice allows each professional to do what he or she does best. Midwives can lower the obstetricians' normal obstetric caseloads, leaving them free to treat complicated or high-risk maternal cases and to perform surgery. Having female midwives available in practices where physician providers are male also provides women with access to a female provider if they wish. This is an especially attractive option to some women. If the practice of midwifery continues to grow, midwives will have an increasing impact on how pregnancy and labor are managed in the United States (Curtin, 1999).

TRENDS IN CHILDBIRTH

The first principle of FCMC recognizes birth to be wellness, not illness, and places the emphasis on striving to keep birth a normal process. This principle is founded on the belief that women's bodies were made to birth babies, and that most women can give birth with loving support and minimal intervention, if any. In fact, women have been doing so since the beginning of time.

Interventions

However, in the last decade of the 20th century, data reported on birth certificates revealed some troubling trends in the circumstances surrounding births in the United States. Changes in medical practice have altered the way in which pregnancies and labors are managed. The numbers for mothers receiving electronic fetal monitoring, ultrasound, induction, and labor stimulation have all increased, with the most dramatic increase being the doubling of the use of induction (Curtin and Park, 1999). Because induced labors are often longer than spontaneous labors, the intrapartum inpatient length of stay is increased when labor is induced compared with that of a woman who has a spontaneous birth. The medication used for induction, intravenous solutions, increased maternal–fetal monitoring, one-to-one staffing, and increased length of stay all lead to increased costs to the hospital.

Epidurals

Another trend is the use of epidural analgesia/anesthesia for pain control during labor. Epidural analgesia is rapidly becoming the most common method of labor pain relief in the United States (Caton et al., 2002). Among patients with private insurance who deliver at large hospitals, the rate of epidural analgesia for labor approaches 80 percent (Newton, 2000). The strongest advocates for labor epidurals are often the childbearing woman herself, her friends and family, nursing personnel, and anesthesiologists.

Controversy surrounds the increase in interventions and epidural usage for labor and birth. Intervention increases costs and creates the potential for iatrogenic maternal-fetal injuries (Knox, Simpson, and Garite, 1999). Epidural analgesia or anesthesia has been associated with slowed and longer labors, malposition and malrotation, increased rates of instrumental delivery, and a greater incidence of operative delivery (Traynor et al., 2000; Thorpe and Breedlove, 1996; Walker and O'Brien, 1999; Newton, 2000). Also, a higher incidence of fever in labor has been reported with epidural usage (Caton et al., 2002), resulting in treatment with antibiotics and evaluations to rule out sepsis in newborns. If the laboring mother receives antibiotics for fever, the mother–baby couplet is often separated for neonatal observation and/or antibiotics. This separation of mother and baby disrupts mother–infant bonding and breastfeeding.

Evidence from the Cochrane database suggests that epidural anesthesia for labor is a tradeoff between beneficial and harmful—and that labor support and freedom of movement in labor are beneficial (Enkin et al., 2000). (See Appendix B.)

Education

It is essential that women and families considering inductions or epidural anesthesia for labor receive information on the risks and benefits of these interventions for normal labor and birth, so that they can make educated decisions. When confronted with some type of technology or intervention, each family should receive answers to the following questions:

- What is the procedure?
- What are its benefits?
- What are its risks?
- How successful/accurate is it?
- What is the next step after the procedure?
- What are the alternatives?
- Does a decision have to be made immediately?

Only through full disclosure of information can we expect families to be able to make the decision that is right for them. At the same time, it is extremely important to teach women that there are numerous options for pain relief in labor. Nursing staff must be able to articulate the value of one-to-one care during labor as clearly as the anesthesiologist can articulate the value of epidurals for pain relief (Phillips and Fenwick, 2000).

PHYSIOLOGIC LABOR AND BIRTH

FCMC programs strive to keep birth normal. A normalcy-oriented maternity and newborn care program, developed on evidence-based, physiologic management, is key to making childbirth safer and more comfortable. The program controls unnecessary interventions and their costs, and aids in developing the family's self-confidence. It is that simple.

Positioning

In addition to quality one-on-one labor support, keeping birth normal uses ambulation and maternal positioning to make labor and birth quicker, easier, and more comfortable (Albers, Schiff, and Gorwoda, 1996; Phillips and Fenwick, 2000; Simkin and O'Hara, 2002). An upright position shortens labor (Liu, 1989), and the second stage of labor is decreased when women are in a squatting position (Golay, Vedam, and Sorger, 1993). Walking and position changes in labor help labor progress, and when given permission, women often choose their own positions of comfort as well as ambulation. The most comfortable movements and positions seem to also enhance labor progress (Simkin and Ancheta, 2000). Vertical postures such as standing or walking, sitting, squatting, kneeling, and leaning all use gravity to encourage descent of the fetus (Enkin et al., 2000). Side-lying can be very restful

for the mother. The hands-and-knees position is excellent for back labor.

The Birthing Ball

The birthing ball is a professional physical therapy ball that facilitates physiologic positions for labor. When a woman sits on the birthing ball, it allows her the freedom to rock her pelvis, change her position, and shift her weight for comfort. Figure 3-4 shows the birthing ball in use during labor. Exhibit 3-2 is a policy and procedure for use of the birthing ball at Good Samaritan Hospital in Lebanon, Pennsylvania. (See Appendix J for the full-page version of this exhibit.)

Restricting women to a supine position in bed, to allow for continuous fetal monitoring, will stop their ability to choose positions of comfort. Thus, in the absence of risk factors, continuous electronic fetal monitoring is not utilized. Instead the standard practice for low-risk women is to evaluate and record the fetal heart rate at least every 30 minutes during the first stage of labor, every 15 minutes during the second stage of labor, and every 5 minutes once the woman starts pushing (Simpson and Creehan, 2001; Albers, 2001).

Intermittent auscultation is safe and effective in low-risk pregnancies and may play a role in helping birth remain normal. Using the intermittent auscultation approach to fetal heart rate monitoring moves the nurse away from a central monitoring station and back to the woman's bedside. When this happens the nurse can again provide hands-on comfort techniques and actually nurse the laboring woman instead of nursing the equipment.

If a laboring woman must be monitored continuously, an EFM telemetry unit may be used. Utilizing telemetry leaves the woman free to walk in or outside her room or sit in the bath or shower (Simkin and Ancheta, 2000).

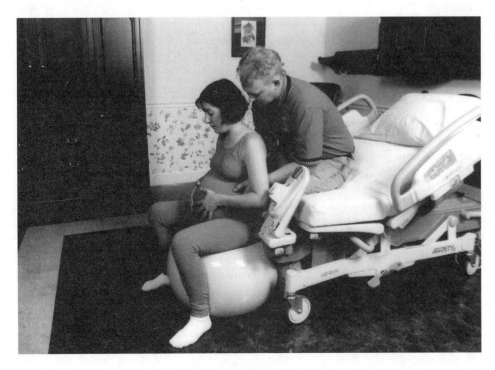

FIGURE 3–4 Use of the birthing ball during labor. *Photo courtesy of Hill-Rom.*

EXHIBIT 3–2   Policy and Procedure for Use of the Birthing Ball

---

THE GOOD SAMARITAN HOSPITAL

Section: Maternal Care

Title: Use of the Birthing Ball

POLICY

It is the policy of the Maternity Unit to provide for the safe use of the birthing ball for low-risk women in labor.

PURPOSE

To outline the safe use of the birthing ball in the Maternity Unit.

EQUIPMENT

Birthing Ball

PROCEDURE

1. The staff member is responsible to explain the safe use of the birthing ball as a labor support mechanism. These include:

    a. Support person with patient at all times during use.

    b. Actual demonstration in use of the ball with a support mechanism in place for stabilization of patient (i.e., siderail, chair).

    c. Rocking motion to be utilized—not bouncing.

    d. Patient should have bare feet flat on floor to promote stabilization.

2. The nurse should observe patient utilizing ball and subsequently document return demonstration.

3. The labor ball is cleaned using the same solutions with which all other equipment is cleaned.

4. The labor ball should be approximately 65 cm in diameter when inflated.

5. Women over 280 pounds should not use the birthing ball.

Use of the Birthing Ball reproduced here with permission of Good Samaritan Hospital, Lebanon, Pennsylvania.

Nonpharmacologic Pain Management

Before the use of anesthesia, warm teas and herbs were used as pharmaceutical agents, comforting massage and lotions were used to promote relaxation, and women taught other women about ways to cope with the pain of labor and birth. For most women, multiple pain management strategies are needed during the course of labor. There are nonpharmacologic methods and comfort measures that can be used to decrease or alter painful sensations associated with labor and birth. These methods can be classified as cutaneous techniques to relieve painful stimuli, auditory or visual techniques to block the transmission of painful stimuli, and cognitive processes to control the degree to which a sensation is interpreted as painful (Simpson and Creehan, 2001).

Cutaneous techniques include acupressure, therapeutic touch, aromatherapy, acupuncture, massage, bathing, showering and jet hydrotherapy, application of heat and cold, back rubs, counterpressure, effleurage, transcutaneous electrical nerve stimulation (TENS), and intradermal sterile water injections for back pain. Auditory or visual techniques include hypnosis, music, focal point concentration, paced breathing, distraction, and attention focusing. Cognitive processes include prenatal education, relaxation, affirmation, labor support, and imagery.

At the Flower Hospital Birth Center in Toledo, Ohio, a complementary care program supports women in labor. The therapies offered include:

- Music—tranquil, peaceful music that can be used to achieve deep relaxation.

- Imagery—visualization exercises to help the woman remain calm and feel more in control.

- Aromatherapy—diffused aromas that may enhance relaxation efforts.

- Massage—soothing touch to help relieve tension.

- Comfort aids—positioning options might include a birthing ball or beanbag chair; hydrotherapy (water in a tub or shower); and application of heat/cold to help the woman be more comfortable throughout labor.

It is explained to women that complementary care offers the opportunity to enhance the birthing experience with therapies such as massage, hydrotherapy, aromatherapy, and other care options to provide support during labor.

These therapies can be used alone as the choice of pain control, or be used in conjunction with pain control measures such as epidural anesthesia or other pain medications.

The belief statement at the Flower Hospital Birth Center follows:

We believe:

- that a woman's confidence and ability to give birth are enhanced—or diminished—by each and every person who provides care.
- you have the right to make choices about your body and the baby.
- you and your partner should know about Complementary Care options before labor so that you may request and use them to support the labor process.0

At the Woodwinds Health Campus in Woodbury, Minnesota, the Maternity Care Center staff uses complementary techniques, including aromatic oils, hand and foot massage, herbal teas, and hydrotherapy. These complementary therapies are integrated with traditional therapies to support women throughout the childbearing experience.

Sample Policy and Procedure

Hydrotherapy for Labor and Postpartum Pain Relief
When hydrotherapy is utilized for labor and postpartum pain relief, a policy for use and cleaning of the tub is necessary. Exhibit 3-3 is a sample of such a policy. (See Appendix J for the full-page version of the exhibit.)

Nutrition and Hydration During Labor

For more than 50 years it has been hospital practice to give women only ice chips during labor. The rationale for this practice was to prevent aspiration in the event that a cesarean delivery became necessary.

In 1999 the American Society of Anesthesiologists (ASA) members revised their recommendations for oral intake during labor to include clear liquids (ASA, 1999). Examples of clear liquids include water, fruit juices without pulp, carbonated beverages, clear tea, and black coffee. Flavored gelatin, fruit ice, Popsicles, and broth may also be offered (Simpson and Creehan, 2001). Because all women and all labors are unique, decisions about nutrition during labor must be made on an individual basis, in consultation with the woman.

EXHIBIT 3–3   Hydrotherapy for Labor and Postpartum Pain Relief

---

HYDROTHERAPY FOR LABOR AND POSTPARTUM PAIN RELIEF

Procedure

Use hydrotherapy as an effective source of pain relief in labor and the postpartum period.

Policy

Upon order of the provider, the maternity unit staff will initiate and maintain hydrotherapy while continuing observation and assessment of the laboring or postpartum woman.

Equipment

1. Hydrotherapy tub.
2. Doppler and aquasonic gel.
3. Thermometer.
4. Nonslip bath mat, towels, and washcloths.
5. Bath skimmer.
6. Nonabrasive cleaner.

Patient Education

Explain the procedure to the woman, orient her to the room, the tub, and the emergency call system.

Hydrotherapy includes the following benefits:

1. Effective in providing pain relief in labor.
2. Effective in relieving postpartum cramping, episiotomy pain, muscle aches associated with labor and pushing, and breast tenderness.
3. Beneficial in facilitating breast stimulation for milk production and relieving engorgement by assisting relaxation and let-down reflex.

EXHIBIT 3–3   Hydrotherapy for Labor and Postpartum Pain Relief *(continued).*

Implementation

I.   Hydrotherapy may be initiated when:

A. Maternal vital signs are within normal limits.

B. Fetal well-being has been established.

C. Status of membranes has been documented. Membranes may be ruptured or intact. May use hydrotherapy if fluid is clear or is lightly meconium stained.

D. During cervical priming with any type of prostaglandin product. (Should be used no sooner than two hours following application.)

E. The patient has an IV.

II.   Contraindications for using hydrotherapy include but are not limited to the following:

A. Patients in which tocolysis is desired.

B. Patients with heavy bleeding (more than usual bloody show or heavy lochia flow).

C. Patients with a history of precipitous or rapid labor.

D. Patients who are dilated more than 6 cm.

E. Patients with epidural catheter in place.

F. Patients with internal scalp electrode or needing close observation of fetal well-being.

G. Patients whose labors are being augmented or stimulated with oxytocin and therefore need constant fetal monitoring.

III.   Preparing the patient.

A. Obtain baseline data, including vital signs and a minimum of 20 minutes reactive fetal monitor strip. Take vital signs as follows:

1. Check and record maternal temperature every hour while the woman is laboring in the tub.

2. Check blood pressure hourly or any time the mother expresses light-headedness. If her blood pressure is low, immediately remove the mother from the tub. If her blood pressure remains stable, the mother may return to the tub.

3. Assess fetal heart rate according to ACOG guidelines for the low-risk patient (every 30 minutes in active phase of labor, every 15 minutes during second stage). If fetal tachycardia is present, cool the water or assist the mother out of the tub to cool down. If tachycardia persists, the mother must not return to tub, but needs continuous fetal monitoring.

B. Obtain an order for hydrotherapy from the primary healthcare provider.

IV.   Using hydrotherapy during labor.

A. Maintain the water temperature to not exceed 100 degrees Fahrenheit.

B. Primip mothers may remain in the tub up to four hours and multip mothers up to three hours, then reassess them out of the tub. The mother may use the jet tub during labor as long as both mother and fetus tolerate the procedure. Encourage the mother to ambulate if the labor begins to slow down.

C. Provide hydration for the mother with cold drinks (preferably apple juice or Gatorade-type replacement fluids).

D. Never leave the mother alone during hydrotherapy. Designated support persons may stay with the patient during the procedure if the nurse or provider is not present. Instruct attending support persons on using the emergency call system.

E. For greatest benefit, completely undress and submerge the mother with her breasts underwater and the jets directed so that the agitation facilitates nipple stimulation, thereby facilitating the release of oxytocin. If the patient is modest, place a towel over her during hydrotherapy.

F. Check and record the water temperature hourly. Add warm water as needed to maintain water temperature. Skim the water as needed to remove particulate matter.

V.   Using hydrotherapy during birth.

A. Have the mother assume a comfortable position for pushing. This may be sitting, squatting, or being held by her partner.

B. Provide perineum support as needed.

C. Lift the infant's head out of the water as soon as the infant is born. The infant's body may remain underwater.

D. Perform bulb suctioning and cord clamping in the usual fashion.

E. Suction the infant immediately after exiting the water. Standby suction should be available in case of unexpected meconium.

F. The infant should be submerged except for face or removed from the tub, dried and wrapped for optimal thermoregulation.

EXHIBIT 3–3   Hydrotherapy for Labor and Postpartum Pain Relief *(continued)*.

    G. Complete infant admission procedure.

    H. Have the mother exit the tub prior to delivering the placenta. Assist her to the bed or have her sit on the side of the tub.

    Note: Mother must sign designated permit.

VI. Using hydrotherapy postpartum.

    A. Maintain the water temperature between 102–104 degrees Fahrenheit.

    B. The mother must have completed the initial recovery period (one to four hours). Vital signs should be stable with no known postpartal complications existing.

    C. The mother may use the jet tub as long as she tolerates the procedure. Ask her to discontinue usage at any time deemed necessary.

    D. Do not leave the woman alone during hydrotherapy. Designated support persons may observe the woman during the procedure if a nurse or provider is not present. Instruct on using the emergency call system.

    E. Check and record water temperature every hour. Add warm water as needed to maintain the temperature. Skim the water as needed to remove particulate matter.

VII. Tub cleaning and sanitation.

    A. Clean the tub after each use even when being used by the same woman.

    B. Refill the emptied tub until the jets are covered.

    C. Add a hospital-approved cleaning agent and turn the jets on. Skim any visible matter and leave the skimmer in the tub for disinfection.

    D. Circulate the water through the system for ten minutes. Drain the tub. Refill the tub with plain water and run the jets for five to ten minutes.

    E. Drain the tub and clean the surface with a nonabrasive cleaner.

    F. Rinse thoroughly.

VP Nursing

Department Chair

A Case Study

At Lawrence General Hospital in Lawrence, Massachusetts, a physiologic model of childbirth is practiced. In May of 1995, the maternity nurse-manager and her colleagues at Lawrence General participated in a 15-month workshop on reducing hospital cesarean rates. The Boston-based sponsoring organization was the Institute for Healthcare Improvement (IHCI), which conducts breakthrough series to redesign specific clinical operational functions within hospitals. Physicians participated in developing, implementing, and monitoring guidelines as needed. Office staff were invited to luncheons and in-services to gain support for the program and to encourage women to be involved in it. Since that time the cesarean rate has dropped from 26 to 22 percent (fiscal year 2001), with the primary cesarean rate stable at 11 percent for 3 years (1998–2001).

As part of their program to reduce the cesarean rate, the Lawrence General Hospital maternity staff adopted a fundamentally different approach to birthing. They encourage women to shower, drink clear liquids, use upright positions, and walk during labor. Only low-dose "walking" epidurals are administered and as a result the epidural rate in fiscal year 2001 was just 34 percent.

Lawrence General Hospital's Birthing Suite Policy is reproduced in Exhibit 3-4. Note that women are encouraged to labor at home until they are in active labor.

Pregnant women are taught in childbirth classes that they will probably be most comfortable at home when in early labor. However, they are also instructed to come to the hospital to be checked if they wish. Lawrence General Hospital's policy on admission to a birthing room is reproduced in Exhibit 3-5.

It is exciting to witness what can happen when hospital staffs (physicians, midwives, and nurses) empower women and their families to keep labor and birth normal.

EXHIBIT 3–4 Lawrence General Hospital—Birthing Suite Policy

LAWRENCE GENERAL HOSPITAL—BIRTHING SUITE POLICY

Title: A Philosophy of Care for Women During Pregnancy and Birth

1. *General Principles*

Pregnancy and birth are very special events in the lives of women and their families. At Lawrence General Hospital, those who provide health care for women recognize that this experience is unique for each woman. We see our role as supportive of the woman and her family, understanding that ultimately the experience of pregnancy and birth belongs to them. We are guides during this natural process, but we respect the independence of each woman to determine, within reason, what is experienced on this journey toward the birth of a child. We feel privileged to participate in this experience.

We see pregnancy as a state of health, and birth as the natural consequence of the desire to bear children. While most pregnancies fall within the boundaries of normal outcome, pregnancy is not always an easy process. Some pregnancies will be altered by co-existing illness or by new problems related to the pregnancy. We will use the combined expertise of our providers to optimize the outcome of pregnancy and the experience of women and their families even when complications arise. We will encourage women to gain an understanding of the natural processes of pregnancy and birth, and to recognize variations from the normal process. We acknowledge that women who seek our care may not always see personal value in our recommendations and have the right to refuse them.

2. *Providers and Level of Care*

Pregnancy care is provided by nurse midwives and practitioners, generalist obstetricians, specialists in pregnancy complications, and family medicine physicians. We recognize and value the expertise of each of our providers and will recommend their involvement as needed to ensure optimal pregnancy outcome. Nurses, childbirth educators, and other professionals play a vital role in caring for women during pregnancy and birth. Their expertise and collaboration with physician and midwife providers greatly enhances the care we give to women. We believe that the participation of individuals in training is safe and beneficial to women, both now and for the future. We believe that providers of both genders are able to provide sensitive and satisfying care to women.

3. *Timing and Mode of Birth*

We believe that the spontaneous onset of labor defines the optimal timing of delivery for term pregnancies. We believe that induction of labor should be performed only when the health of the mother or baby will be enhanced by this intervention. We believe that vaginal birth is best for the great majority of women, including those who have previously experienced Cesarean birth. We believe that forceps delivery, vacuum-assisted delivery, breech vaginal delivery, and Cesarean birth can be utilized safely and are appropriate to use to assist a woman with birth in specific situations.

4. *The Labor Experience*

We believe that women should labor at home until they are in active labor, unless the health of mother or baby is at risk. Whenever possible, women should ambulate in labor to gain the beneficial effects of gravity and to allow them to find positions which provide them comfort. We recognize that there is much variability in the process and progression of normal labors, and will recommend interventions in labor only for significant variations from the normal process. We believe that it is our responsibility to provide comfort and pain relief to women in labor, in accordance with a woman's individual needs. We believe that intrusive monitoring should be limited to women who have specific risk and need for these technologies. We believe that the role of providers and of the woman's family is to discover how best to guide and assist the woman through labor and delivery.

Reproduced with permission of Lawrence General Hospital, Lawrence, Massachusetts.

EXHIBIT 3–5   Lawrence General Hospital Policy on Admission to a Birthing Room

LAWRENCE GENERAL HOSPITAL
DEPARTMENT OF NURSING—BIRTHING SUITE POLICY

Title
Practice Guidelines: **Admission to a Birthing Room**

Purpose
To ensure the appropriate admission of a patient to the Birthing Room by providing guidelines for assessment and disposition if the patient does not meet the criteria for true labor.

Procedure
1. The low-risk patient with the following objective findings is assumed to be in true labor and will be admitted directly to an LDR:
   - ruptured membranes and/or bleeding
   - painful contractions every 5 minutes lasting at least 30 seconds and/or a cervix > 4cms or 100% effaced.
2. The low-risk patient with the following findings may be evaluated in the observation or NST room if L&D is unavailable.
   - membranes intact
   - irregular uterine contractions > 8 minutes apart
   - no active vaginal bleeding
   - no signs of fetal distress
   - no medical or obstetrical complications
3. If the patient's status changes and she meets the criteria in #1, she will be transferred to an LDR.
4. If the diagnosis of true labor cannot be made, the patient will be allowed to ambulate for one hour and will then be reassessed. Reassessment should include a vaginal examination, palpation of contractions, and fetal monitoring with reactive NST. If criteria of #2 is still met, patient will be discharged home with NS186/NS186A Discharge Instructions.
5. If true labor has been ruled out, and it is necessary to keep the patient for observation, she may be transferred to R2 and nursing assessment will then include:
   - vital signs every four hours
   - fetal monitoring per MD order
   - FHR auscultation every shift

Reproduced with permission of Lawrence General Hospital, Lawrence, Massachusetts.

SUPPORTING FAMILY ATTACHMENT

The initial mother–infant bond marks the beginning of all the infant's subsequent attachments (Health Canada, 2000). In FCMC, the mother and her newborn baby are viewed as an inseparable unit. Immediately after birth the infant is gently dried with a warm towel and placed skin-to-skin on the mother's chest with a warm, dry cover over both of them. A stockinette cap on the baby's head retards heat loss, as does a warming light placed over mother and baby. The dry, warm covering is changed periodically.

The baby can be cared for in the mother's or father's arms. Identification tags can be placed, Apgar scores determined, and necessary injections administered while one parent holds the baby. Ophthalmic eye ointments or drops can be delayed for at least one hour (or longer, depending on the law) to allow unimpeded eye contact between parents and baby. In Figures 3-5 and 3-6, the new mother and father are becoming acquainted with their baby as the baby breastfeeds in the first 30 minutes of life.

Breastfeeding is encouraged during the immediate recovery period as early feedings are optimal for breastfeeding success. Also, when the baby sucks at the mother's breast, the secretion of oxytocin from the pituitary gland is increased, producing contractions of the uterus. As a result, the uterus begins to undergo reduction in size, uterine vessels constrict, and the placenta becomes detached from the uterine wall (Montagu, 1978). This is yet another reason why it is very important that mother and baby not be separated.

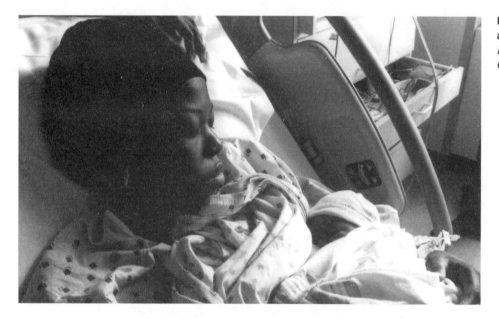

FIGURE 3–5 Becoming acquainted. *Photo by Emily Pascoe, courtesy of Boston Medical Center.*

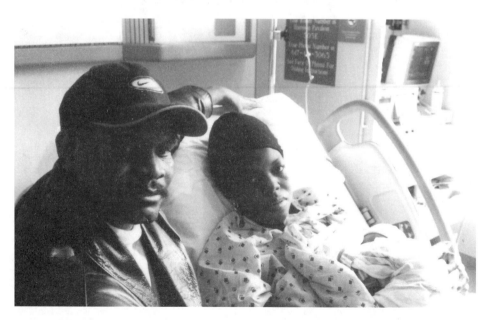

FIGURE 3–6 A family beginning. *Photo by Emily Pascoe, courtesy of Boston Medical Center.*

Newborn assessments can be done when the baby is with the mother. The care provider can describe normal physical characteristics. The father can help siblings count the baby's fingers and toes. With the newborn's eyes shaded from bright lights, the family can marvel at how the baby looks at them and responds to their attention. Encouraging interaction with the newborn sets the stage for successful attachment and integration into the family unit (Simpson and Creehan, 2001).

If the newborn must be placed in an infant warmer, the warmer should be next to the parents. This requires that medical gasses, suction, oxygen, and power plugs be available for the baby at the mother's bedside.

Sample Policy and Procedure

Bonding between Parent and Infant Exhibit 3-6 shows a sample policy that is supportive of parent and infant bonding. (See Appendix J for a full-page version of the exhibit.)

PLACE OF BIRTH

Hospital

From 1989 to 1997, almost all births in the United States (approximately 99 percent) occurred in hospitals (Curtin, 1999).

A hospital environment for birth should be safe for mothers, babies, and families. It should provide efficient layouts for staff, support family participation, and facilitate medical care. The physical environment for birth should also enhance the experience of birth through family control over their environment and provision of a nonclinical atmosphere.

Traditional Maternity Unit Design

The traditional maternity unit was divided geographically and functionally into three or four care units: Labor and Delivery

---

EXHIBIT 3–6   Bonding between Parent and Infant

BONDING BETWEEN PARENT AND INFANT

Procedure

Promote healthy attachment between parent(s) and infant through careful interventions.

Policy

All unit staff will promote parent and infant bonding, a component of family-centered maternity care, at all times.

Equipment

Radiant warmer or warming light for the newborn.

Patient Education

Encourage questions and provide parenting education during the newborn assessment.

Implementation

I.   Encourage skin to skin contact with the mother immediately after the newborn's birth.

II.   Encourage support persons to interact with the newborn by touching, holding, and talking.

III. Delay administering prophylactic eye medication until the initial bonding process has begun.

IV.   Encourage breastfeeding during the immediate recovery period as early feedings are optimal for breastfeeding success.

V.   Use the newborn admission assessment, dressing, and infant bathing as teaching opportunities. Explain all findings to the new parents.

VI.   Support the mother's caretaking efforts.

VII. Provide mother–baby care for cesarean mothers at the bedside or returning with the newborn from the holding nursery for frequent visits.

VIII. Assess bonding and document findings. Report potential maladaption to the charge nurse and infant care provider.

VP Nursing

Department Chair

(as one or two units), Postpartum Nursery, and Special Care Nursery. Each of these areas was further subdivided. For example, most traditional Labor and Delivery areas have separate Admission, Labor, Delivery, and Recovery Rooms.

Contemporary Maternity Unit Design

In recent years, many hospitals have replaced, or are replacing, traditional multiple-transfer labor, delivery, postpartum, and nursery designs with more contemporary facility designs. The contemporary model offers mothers, their partners, and their families a home-like, noninstitutional environment in which to give birth without compromising medical care, with nursing care provided by a well-integrated team of perinatal specialists and assistive staff.

The more successful contemporary obstetrical facilities offer advantages to families, nursing staff, and medical staff alike, allowing hospitals to meet customer and provider satisfaction benchmarks.

Labor–Delivery–Recovery Rooms (LDRs)

Labor–delivery–recovery rooms (LDRs), designed to accommodate the birthing process from labor through delivery and recovery of mother and baby, are equipped to handle most complications, with the exception of cesarean sections. At time of delivery, LDRs are fully equipped for uncomplicated vaginal deliveries for mother and/or baby, and are also prepared for fully operative preterm and high-risk vaginal deliveries. For these deliveries, the use of forceps, the repair of lacerations, and so on, can all be safely performed in an LDR.

Installed or portable lighting can be identical to the lighting of a conventional delivery room or operating suite. There is space and capacity for any level of infant resuscitation, from simple to complex. The rooms are equipped with LDR beds that adjust to a full range of labor and delivery positions, including semi-Fowler, lithotomy, lateral or Sims delivery, along with Trendelenburg positioning for various maternal treatments. Complications and surgical procedures can be managed without transfer.

Although regional anesthesia (spinals and epidurals) can be administered, general anesthesia is usually not given in LDRs. Equipment for the care of mothers and babies need not be stored or prepared in the patient room, but rather in a central area from which it can be moved into the patient's room as needed. Instead of moving the patient to equipped rooms, equipment and skilled personnel go to the patient.

Certain complicated deliveries (multiple deliveries, for example), cesarean births, and postpartum operative procedures are handled in operating rooms. In most facilities patients are transferred directly to postpartum rooms for recovery and care following delivery room/operative procedures, eliminating the need for specialty recovery rooms or post-anesthesia care units.

Nurses skilled in labor, birth, and recovery care for both mother and infant provide nursing care in the LDRs. Early initial care of the infant is provided in the LDR and then the mother and infant are typically transferred together out of the LDR for care elsewhere.

Following care in an LDR, mothers and infants are transferred together to either postpartum and nursery areas, or to an integrated mother–baby unit. This separation occurs at a critical juncture in the newly developing mother–baby relationship, when the mother's physical recovery is only partially complete and baby's early alert phase is well underway.

Ancillary and support service employees are kept busy by the transfer of mother and baby to the postpartum unit, because floors, walls, bathrooms, and beds must be cleaned, linen must be changed, and supplies not transferred with the mother must be discarded to make ready for the next admission of a laboring patient.

Labor–Delivery–Recovery–Postpartum Rooms (LDRPs)

Labor–delivery–recovery–postpartum rooms (LDPRs) add postpartum (and, typically, newborn) care to the LDR model. Room design and capability to handle most emergencies remain the same as in LDRs. *However, this design eliminates the move to postpartum (and nursery) after delivery and recovery because one private room is used for labor, delivery, recovery, and postpartum stay.*

In addition to being able to accommodate the majority of vaginal deliveries, these flexible rooms provide infant care areas. They may also include sleeping spaces for family members who are present for the birth, or who wish to stay to assist the new mother in learning about and assisting with infant care. An example of an LDRP room is shown in Figure 3-7.

Other functional aspects of care in an LDRP are the same as those in an LDR.

Single-Room Maternity Care (SRMC)

Many hospitals' operational objectives include a contemporary model of care that incorporates "family-centered" care principles. This well-defined model, when operated in the LDRP environment, becomes "single-room maternity care." When successfully implemented, SRMC integrates family-centered care concepts with sound business principles for optimum results for the hospital's maternity program.

SRMC requires that all care be provided in LDRP suites, which facilitate all aspects of labor, delivery, and postpartum/newborn care. SRMC is *not just a facility option*—rather, it is a comprehensive *program of care* implemented within an LDRP facility. Developed properly, SRMC achieves maximum programmatic gains and operational efficiencies for the hospital.

Development of SRMC requires considerable preparation and the concerted efforts of providers, staff, and departments throughout the hospital. It also incorporates the education of patients—to prepare them to deliver in the setting and to participate in the SRMC process—as an essential program component.

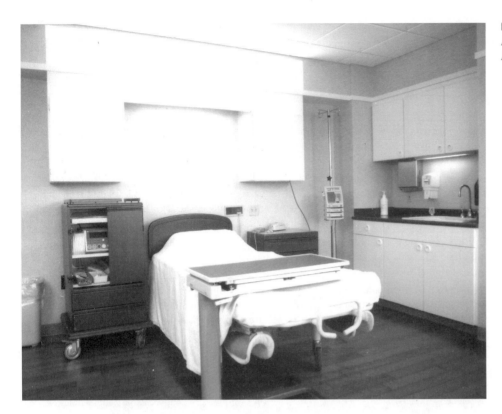

FIGURE 3–7 An LDRP room.
Photo courtesy of Mercy Health Partners, Cincinnati, Ohio.

Table 3-1 summarizes some of the critical factors that should affect selection of the "right" facility design model for a hospital. SRMC is compared with the LDR model.

Freestanding Birthing Centers

An alternative to hospital birth can be found in freestanding birthing centers for childbearing families at low risk. These centers are homelike, private places where labor and birth are treated as normal life events. The nurse–midwife or physician and an experienced labor attendant carefully and continually assess laboring women.

Controversy has surrounded the safety of giving birth in freestanding birthing centers. However, studies have found that birth centers offer a lower cost, safe, and acceptable alternative to hospital birth for selected pregnant women, particularly those who have previously had children (Scupholme, McLeod, and Robertson, 1986; International Childbirth Education Association, 2002).

Nativiti Women's Health and Birth Center in Houston, Texas, is an example of a freestanding birthing center owned and operated by a private nurse-midwifery service. Melanie Dossey, founder and director, is licensed in the State of Texas as a Certified Nurse–Midwife. Her entire professional career has been committed to the concept of midwifery—entrusting the care of childbearing women to other women who understand the experience of childbearing and its many facets— physical, medical, emotional, and spiritual:

The Birth Center exists for healthy women who are having a baby. The guiding principle at Nativiti Women's Health and Birth Center is that pregnancy is not a sickness! Birth is a wonderful and normal life event—to be experienced however and with whomever the mother wishes, within the dictates of safety for all concerned.

Nativiti is licensed by the State of Texas Department of Health, the regulating body for birthing centers. Each year a state inspector comes to review the Center for the state-defined standards of safety. The Center is also nationally accredited through the Commission for the Accreditation of Birth Centers. A voluntary process, the Certificate of Accreditation symbolizes the excellence a center has achieved in providing quality care to childbearing families. At year-end 1997 there were only 46 accredited birthing centers in the United States. Of these, five were in Texas.

The Center is equipped with a whirlpool bath, and mothers are encouraged to walk, eat, drink, and get into positions that are comfortable for *them* during labor and birth. At birth the baby is immediately placed into the hands of the mother. Each mother receives careful guidance in the first few hours after birth so that when she is discharged a few hours later, she will feel confident in her ability to breastfeed and care for her baby.

The nurse–midwife closely follows the family via phone as well as home and office visits for the first weeks of the infant's life. The family is responsible for ensuring the baby sees a pediatrician 24 to 48 hours after the birth. Besides providing a positive birth experience, the staff at Nativiti Woman's Health and Birth Center perform routine gynecological examinations, including PAP smears.

TABLE 3–1   Comparison of LDRs and LDRPs (SRMC)

Aspect	Labor–Delivery–Recovery Rooms (LDRs)	Single-Room Maternity Care (LDRPs)
Mission Effectiveness	Allows promotion of a mission that reflects the principles of family-centered maternity and newborn care.	Allows optimal promotion of a mission that reflects the principles of family-centered maternity and newborn care.
Provider Satisfaction	Often difficult for the provider who delivered the baby to locate the mother postpartum, because she and the baby have been moved. The same staff, whom the provider knows, cares for mothers and infants at every stage of hospitalization.	Locating all family members in one room makes provider rounding easier, improves physician contact with all family members, and decreases in-office (telephone) follow-up time after discharge. A hospital that attains a high level of satisfaction among patients and families also increases provider satisfaction and loyalty.
Patient and Family Satisfaction	LDRs require that every new mother be transferred to a postpartum room at some time (usually one hour) following childbirth. This transfer occurs at a critical time for physiological and psychological recovery from childbirth, and during a time when the infant achieves early alertness. This disruption of early attachment processes does not promote optimal patient care or satisfaction.	Mothers and babies are only separated on mother's request. Recognizing the importance of the first hours of a baby's life in fostering parenting and positive parent–child relationships, newborn transitional care is provided at the mother's bedside in the LDR or LDRP.
Facility Functionality and Utilization	Single-function rooms (either LDRs or postpartum rooms) must be constructed.	Construction of multipurpose patient care rooms allows for greater occupancy than single-function rooms.
Financial Performance	Multiple patient care areas are monitored by separate budgets, requiring redundant preparation and monitoring processes.	A single cost center simplifies cost accounting (including tracking of expenses by hours per patient day (HPPD) for the patient's entire LOS).
Equipment and Supplies	Locating single storage areas within each patient care unit may result in the duplication of stored equipment and supplies, resulting in higher cost and lower utilization.	Single, central storage areas serve all types of patients and their nurses. This can decrease the need for duplication of purchases and higher utilization of some equipment and supplies.
Nursing Leadership	Multiple patient care areas require multiple unit managers, each working with shift leaders assigned to that unit, to coordinate nursing care (depending on census and size of staff). Typically, clinical nurse specialists are selected for each subspecialty area.	A single patient care unit allows a single unit manager, working with a single shift leader for every shift, to coordinate the work of many nurses performing a variety of types of patient care. A single clinical nurse specialist (or staff educator) can provide all aspects of education for an entire staff of nurses.
Nurse Staffing	Typically, facility divisions create staffing divisions, resulting in retention of staff in at least two subspecialty areas (LDR and Postpartum). Core staff are allocated to each separate physical area (i.e., L&D and Mother–Baby).	A single staff of registered nurses, assisted by non-professional staff, is educationally and experientially prepared to care for women and infants throughout the entire maternity inpatient stay. Core staff are allocated to the single physical area that encompasses the SRMC suites.
Ancillary and Support Services	Transfer of mother and baby from an LDR room to a postpartum room necessitates cleaning of the LDR bed, bathroom, and room to ready them for another patient, while the patient who was cared for in that room proceeds to a clean room for continued care.	With few patients transferred out of rooms, cleaning is limited to postpartum cleanup and cleaning following discharge.
Compliance with Program and Care Standards	The World Health Organization, UNICEF, and the American Academy of Pediatrics endorse programs that minimize the separation of mothers and infants following birth. Promotion of mother–baby care and interaction may be a key element under the LDR model.	The World Health Organization, UNICEF, and the American Academy of Pediatrics endorse programs that minimize the separation of mothers and infants following birth. Promotion of mother–baby care and interaction is a key element of SRMC care.

CHAPTER SUMMARY

The experience of labor and birth is different and intensely personal for every woman. However, for most women and their families, labor and birth are natural processes.

In family-centered intrapartum care there are visitation policies that encourage nonseparation of the childbearing family during labor and birth. Quality support during labor and birth is encouraged, and every effort is made to provide that support with professional nursing and midwifery care as well as doulas and monitrices.

Physiologic support for labor and birth encourages women to shower, drink clear liquids, utilize upright positions, and walk during labor. Hydrotherapy using tubs for immersion is an effective source of pain relief in labor as are numerous other nonpharmacologic methods.

Because the mother and her newborn baby are viewed as an inseparable unit, staff supports family attachment and encourages breastfeeding in the immediate post-birth period.

Hospital maternity unit design replaces traditional multiple-transfer labor, delivery, postpartum, and nursery designs with the more contemporary labor–delivery–recovery–postpartum rooms (LDRPs). The optimal hospital maternity care program incorporates family-centered care principles in the LDRP environment and provides single-room maternity care.

FACILITY DESIGN FOR FAMILY-CENTERED INTRAPARTUM CARE

Facility design for intrapartum care provides an environment that facilitates family-centered intrapartum care.

Access
- Parking is close to the facility, adequate, and provides safe and easy access.

Admission
- Signs directing women, families, and visitors to the maternity unit are clearly placed, easy to read, and in the languages of the population served.
- There is a sign at the entrance to the maternity unit that specifically welcomes family members and support persons.
- Signs within the maternity unit are worded to reflect the facility's philosophy of FCMC.

Environment
- Walls are clean and the décor is pleasant.
- There is a sibling play area.
- Space is provided for family and support persons to have relaxation and nourishment breaks.
- There are restrooms for family and support persons.
- There are telephones and data ports available for families.
- Furnishings are comfortable.

- There is properly designed storage for supplies and equipment to minimize clutter.
- Facility design recognizes the varying cultures—cultural amenities designed into facility.
- Environmental stressors like noise, glare, and poor air quality are eliminated.

LDR or LDRP
- Design is LDR or LDRP with private shower/bath and toilet for each room.
  - There is a telephone in each room.
  - There is individual control of light and temperature within each room.
- There are an adequate number of LDRs and/or LDRPs to accommodate birth volume and length of stay.
- LDR/LDRP space is adequate to allow for access of emergency equipment and for safe emergency care.
- An infant warming light and equipment is present in the LDR/LDRP.
- There is sufficient space to accommodate:
  - family/support person(s)
  - personal possessions
  - a sofa that converts into a bed for overnight stays
  - a rocking chair
  - comfortable furnishings
  - a tape and CD player
  - videos and a VCR
  - an infant crib and supplies
  - equipment and professional personnel as needed
- There is a refrigerator, microwave, and coffee maker in each LDR/LDRP room.
- Décor is homelike and attractive and de-emphasizes the hospital environment.
- LDR and LDRP rooms have soundproofing.
- There are privacy curtains at entrances to rooms.
- There are hydrotherapy tubs available in the maternity unit for pain relief during labor.
- The birth unit's environment is safe and secure.
- There is secure storage for valuables and other possessions.
- There are handrails in the corridors.
- There is restricted access to the unit.
- There is a respite nursery.

PACU
- The PACU is located in direct proximity to the LDR/LDRP rooms, or to Triage Services, to optimize utilization of nursing staff working with women recovering from general anesthesia.

- Patient care areas are planned with efficient utilization of staff as primary outcome.

Facility Functionality
- The facility design and environment:
  - is efficient.
  - enhances privacy for women and families.
  - emphasizes noise reduction.
- A nurse locator system that does not involve overhead paging is in place.
- There is a dedicated office for the lead lactation consultant.
- Staff spaces are convenient for both staff and women in labor.
- The environment supports technical needs such as
  - fetal monitoring.
  - medical gasses.
  - monitoring of the mother.
  - epidural analgesia/anesthesia.
  - closed-circuit TV.
  - data ports.
  - electronic charting at the bedside.

COMPONENTS OF FAMILY-CENTERED INTRAPARTUM CARE

The maternity care professional team includes physicians, nurse–midwives, nurses, doulas, and monitrices. The women's personal support team comprises her partner, family, and the friends of her choice. The following components of the family-centered intrapartum care program are designed to keep birth normal and empower the family.

Admission
- Whether a day or night admit, the process is family focused.
- Provisions are in place to prevent separation of the laboring woman from her support person during parking, hospital registration, admission to the unit, triage care, and so on.
- Provisions are in place for streamlining the admissions process so family members are not separated.
- Provisions have been made for family members and/or support people who are accompanying the laboring woman to the hospital.

Family process is supported.
- There are no arbitrary restrictions on the number of family members/support people who are present for labor and birth.

Social support in labor is encouraged.
- The woman chooses those she wishes to be present to support her during:
  - labor
  - birth
  - recovery
- Siblings, who are accompanied by a responsible adult other than the woman's primary support person, are welcome to be present during:
  - labor
  - birth
  - recovery
- Support persons in the LDR or LDRP room and the maternity unit are shown.
  - where the bathroom is.
  - where they can obtain nourishment.
  - how they can help the mother.

The maternity care professional team practices evidence-based physiologic labor support and management. The team
- provides one-to-one labor and birth support.
- avoids unnecessary interventions.
- encourages self-help, questions, and self-knowledge.
- accepts attitudes and behaviors.
- makes adaptations for cultural variations.
- promotes physiologic positioning and ambulation.
- offers the option of the birthing ball for physiologic positioning.
- provides clear liquid nourishment and hydration in labor.
- provides hydrotherapy (shower, tub, Jacuzzi) for pain relief in labor.
- offers options of music for relaxation and supports paced breathing techniques.

In addition,
- Lighting can be dimmed at birth according to the parent's wishes.
- Ophthalmic eye ointment or drops administration is delayed for at least one hour after birth.
- Skin-to-skin contact of mother and infant is encouraged; a warm blanket over both mother and infant maintains newborn body temperature.
- There is no separation of the baby from the mother unless medically indicated or desired by the parents.
- Mother–baby or couplet care is provided.
- Routine procedures on the baby are done in full view of the mother or while the baby is in her arms, and are used

to instruct mother/family. The procedures include:

- weighing and measuring
- identification banding
- physical examination
- gestational age assessment
- installation of eye prophylaxis
- injections

- Provision is made for the attachment process to begin:
  - Skin-to-skin contact of mother and baby is encouraged upon delivery.
- Family members and support persons are not separated from the mother and baby during the recovery period following a vaginal birth.
- Breastfeeding mothers are encouraged to initiate breastfeeding as soon as possible after birth unless contraindicated by the physical condition of either mother or baby.

BIBLIOGRAPHY

Albers, L., Schiff, M., and Gorwoda, J. 1996. The length of active labor in normal pregnancies. *Obstetrics and Gynecology* 87, no. 3: 355–359.

Albers, L. L. 2001. Monitoring the fetus in labor: Evidence to support the methods. *Midwifery and Women's Health* 46, no. 6: 366–373.

American Society of Anesthesiologists. 1999. *Practice Guidelines for Obstetrical Anesthesia*. Park Ridge, IL: Author.

Association of Women's Health, Obstetric and Neonatal Nurses (AWHONN). 2000. *Professional Nursing Support of Laboring Women. Clinical Position Statement*. Washington, DC, Author.

Brown, S. A., and Grimes, D. E. 1995. A meta-analysis of nurse midwives and nurse practitioners in primary care. *Nursing Research* 44, no. 6: 332–339.

Butler, J., Abrams, B., Parker, J., Roberts, J., and Laros, R., Jr. 1993. Supportive nurse-midwife care is associated with a reduced incidence of cesarean section. *American Journal of Obstetrics and Gynecology* 168, 1407–1413.

Caton, D., et al. 2002. The nature and management of labor pain: Executive summary. *American Journal of Obstetrics and Gynecology* 186, S1: 1–15.

Clark, S., Taffel, S., and Martin, J. 1997. Trends and characteristics of births attended by midwives. *Statistical Bulletin of the Metropolitan Insurance Company* 78, no. 1: 9–18.

Corbett, C., and Callister, L. 2000. Nursing support during labor. *Clinical Nursing Research* 9, no. 1: 70–83.

Curtin, S. 1999. Recent changes in birth attendant, place of birth, and the use of obstetric interventions, United States, 1989–1997. *Journal of Nurse-Midwifery* 40, no. 4: 349–354.

Curtin, C., and Park, M. 1999. *Trends in the Attendant, Place, and Timing of Births, and in the Use of Obstetric Interventions: United States, 1989–1997*. National Vital Statistics Report, National Center for Health Statistics 47, no. 27: 1–12.

Ecenroad, D., and Zwelling, E. 2000. A journey to family-centered maternity care. *Maternal-Child Nursing* 25, no. 4: 178–185.

Enkin, M., et al. 2000. *A Guide to Effective Care in Pregnancy and Childbirth*. 3rd ed. New York: Oxford University Press.

Ernst, K. M. 1996. Midwifery, birth centers, and healthcare reform. *Journal of Obstetric, Gynecologic, and Neonatal Nursing* 25: 433–439.

Fox, B., and Lavendar, M. 1999. Revisiting the critique of medicalized childbirth: A contribution to the sociology of birth. *Gender and Society* 13, no. 3: 326–346.

Gagnon, A., and Waghorn, K. 1996. Supportive care by maternity nurses: A work sampling study in an intrapartum unit. *Birth* 23, no. 1: 1–6.

Gagnon, A., Waghorn, K., and Covell, C. 1997. A randomized trial of one-to-one nurse support of women in labor. *Birth* 24, no. 2: 71–77.

Gale, J., Fotheringill-Bourbonnais, F., and Chamberlain, M. 2001. Measuring nursing support during childbirth. *American Journal of Maternal Child Nursing* 26, no. 5: 264–271.

Goer, H. 1999. *The Thinking Woman's Guide to a Better Birth*. New York: Perigee.

Golay, J., Vedam, S., and Sorger, L. 1993. The squatting position for the second stage of labor: Effects on labor on maternal and fetal well being. *Birth* 20, no. 2: 73–78.

Health Canada. 2000. *Family-Centered Maternity and Newborn Care: National Guidelines*. Ottawa: Minister of Public Works and Government Services.

Hodnett, E. 1996. Nursing support of the laboring woman. *Journal of Obstetric, Gynecologic, and Neonatal Nursing* 25, no. 3: 257–264.

———. 2000. Caregiver support of women during childbirth. *The Cochrane Database of Systematic Reviews*, 2, Oxford Cochrane Library.

———. 2002. Pain and women's satisfaction with the experience of childbirth: A systematic review. *American Journal of Obstetrics and Gynecology* 186, S1: 60–72.

ICEA. 1999. Position paper: The role and scope of the doula. *International Journal of Childbirth Education* 14, no. 1: 38–45, Minneapolis: Author.

ICEA. 2002. Position statement and review: The birth place. *International Journal of Childbirth Education* 17, no. 1: 36–43, Minneapolis: Author.

Kardong-Edgren, S. 2001. Using evidence-based practice to improve intrapartum care. *Journal of Obstetric, Gynecologic, and Neonatal Nursing* 30, no. 4: 371–375.

Keenan, P. 2000. Benefits of massage therapy and use of a doula during labor and childbirth. *Alternative Therapies* 6, no. 1: 66–74.

Kennedy, H. P. 1995. The essence of nurse-midwifery care: The woman's story. *Journal of Nurse-Midwifery* 40, no. 5: 410–417.

King, T., and Shah, M. A. 1998. Integrated midwife physician practice. *Journal of Nurse-Midwifery* 43, no. 1: 55–60.

Klaus, M., Kennell, J., and Klaus, P. 1993. *Mothering the Mother: How a Doula Can Help You Have a Shorter, Easier, and Healthier Birth*. New York: Addison-Wesley.

Knox, G., Simpson, K., and Garite, T. 1999. High reliability perinatal units: An approach to the prevention of patient injury and medical malpractice claims. *Journal of Healthcare Risk Management* 19, no. 2: 24–32.

Liu, Y. 1989. The effects of the upright position during childbirth. *Image: Journal of Nursing Scholarship* 21: 14–18.

McNiven, P., Hodnett, E., and O'Brien-Pallas, L. 1992. Supporting women in labor: A work sampling of the activities of labor and delivery nurses. *Birth* 19, no. 3: 3–8.

Miltner, R. 2000. Identifying labor support actions of intrapartum nurses. *Journal of Obstetric, Gynecologic, and Neonatal Nursing* 29, no. 5: 491–499.

Montagu, A. 1978. *Touching, the Human Significance of the Skin*. 2nd ed. New York: Harper and Row.

Newton, E. 2000. Epidural analgesia, intrapartum fever, and neonatal outcomes. *Birth* 27, no. 3: 206–208.

Oakley, D., et al. 1996. Comparisons of outcomes of maternity care by obstetricians and certified nurse-midwives. *Obstetrics & Gynecology* 88, no. 5: 823–829.

Perez, P. 1998. *Doula Programs: How to Start and Run a Private or Hospital-Based Program with Success*. Katy, TX: Cutting Edge Press.

Perez, P., and Snedeker, C. 1994. *Special Women: The Role of the Professional Labor Assistant*. Katy, TX: Cutting Edge Press.

Phillips, C. 1996. *Family-Centered Maternity and Newborn Care: A Basic Text*. 4th ed. St. Louis: Mosby.

Phillips, C., and Fenwick, L. 2000. *Single-Room Maternity Care: Planning, Developing, and Operating the 21st Century Maternity System*. Philadelphia: Lippincott, Williams and Wilkins.

Rooks, J. P. 1997. *Midwifery and Childbirth in America*. Philadelphia: Temple University Press.

Rosenblatt, R., et al. 1997. Interspecialty differences in the obstetric care of low-risk women. *American Journal of Public Health* 87: 344–351.

Scupholme, A., McLeod, A., and Robertson, E. 1986. A birth center affiliated with the tertiary care center: Comparison of outcome. *Obstetrics & Gynecology* 67, no. 4: 598–603.

Simkin, P., and Ancheta, R. 2000. *The Labor Progress Handbook*. Malden, MA: Blackwell Science Ltd.

Simkin, P., and O'Hara, M. A. 2002. Nonpharmacologic relief of pain during labor: Systematic reviews of five methods. *American Journal of Obstetrics and Gynecology* 186, S1: 31–59.

Simkin, P., and Way, K. 1998. *DONA Position Paper: The Doula's Contribution to Modern Maternity Care*. Seattle: Doulas of North America.

Simpson, K., and Creehan, P. 2001. *Perinatal Nursing*. 2nd ed. Philadelphia: Lippincott, Williams and Wilkins.

Sleutel, M. 2000. Intrapartum nursing care: A case study of supportive interventions and ethical conflicts. *Birth* 27, no. 1: 38–45.

Thorpe, J., and Breedlove, G. 1996. Epidural analgesia in labor: An evaluation of risks and benefits. *Birth* 23, no. 2: 63–83.

Tomlinson, P., Bryan, A., and Esau, A. 1996. Family intrapartum care: Revisiting an old concept. *Journal of Obstetric, Gynecologic, and Neonatal Nursing* 25, no. 4: 331–336.

Traynor, J., et al. 2000. Is the management of epidural analgesia associated with an increased risk of cesarean delivery? *American Journal of Obstetrics and Gynecology* 182, no. 5: 1058–1061.

Vande Vusse, L. 1999. The essential forces of labor revisited: Thirteen Ps reported in women's stories. *American Journal of Maternal Child Nursing* 24, no. 4: 176–184.

Waldenstrom, V., et al. 1996. The childbirth experience: A study of 295 new mothers. *Birth* 23, no. 3: 144–153.

Walker, N., and O'Brien, B. 1999. The relationship between method of pain management during labor and birth outcomes. *Clinical Nursing Research* 8, no. 2: 119–134.

Walker, P., and Stone, P. 1996. Exploring cost and quality. *Journal of Health Care Finance* 23, no. 1: 23–47.

Young, D. 1998. Doulas: Into the mainstream of maternity care. *Birth* 25, no. 4: 213–214.

Zwelling, E., and Anderson, B. 1997. Labor stations: A creative teaching strategy to promote the use of multiple positions for labor and birth. *Journal of Perinatal Education* 6, no. 3: 1–9.

Family-Centered Care for Pregnancy, Labor, Birth, and Babies at Risk

THE CONCEPT OF HIGH RISK

Approximately 20 to 25 percent of pregnant women are diagnosed with complications or are considered high risk (Martin-Arafeh, Watson, and Baird, 1999). High-risk mothers and infants have a higher incidence of morbidity and mortality than does the general population of mothers and infants. Pregnancy is classified as high risk in the presence of physiologic and/or psychologic factors that have been identified as a threat to the health and life of the mother and/or the infant (Fleschler, Knight, and Ray, 2001).

The risk status of a woman and her fetus can change over the months of her pregnancy. In addition, a number of intrapartum and neonatal problems occur in women and babies without known antenatal risk (AAP and ACOG, 1997).

The concept of high risk is extremely important in maternity care because the ability to predict vulnerable mothers and babies before birth means that appropriate interventions can be made early in pregnancy, increasing the opportunity for a positive outcome. Risk assessment and prediction of outcomes from risk have been the subject of intense study. The numerous scoring systems developed to quantify risk have demonstrated varying levels of predictive power. In particular, risk assessment systems to screen for women at risk for preterm birth have been low sensitivity, with up to 60 percent of preterm births occurring in women who were scored at low risk of preterm birth (Heaman, Sprague, and Stewart, 2001).

Another factor to consider when reviewing the concept of risk is that its meaning varies according to the different perspectives of healthcare professionals and women themselves. Physicians are likely to focus on the patient outcomes of a particular disease process, whereas nurses consider the whole patient from a psychosocial perspective. Payers focus on the higher cost of the high-risk patient and emphasize the need to lower that cost. At the same time, the woman herself may perceive her risk differently than healthcare providers do (Gupton, Heaman, and Cheung, 2001).

Populations at Risk

Diverse factors must be considered when determining when a woman is at risk for adverse pregnancy outcomes (Gupton, Heaman, and Cheung, 2001). There are biomedical risk factors such as factors from her past obstetric history, medical history, and current pregnancy, and psychosocial factors such as stress, anxiety, social support, and self-esteem. In addition, there are demographic characteristics that must be taken into consideration because perinatal morbidity and mortality is higher among women of lower socioeconomic groups (Ventura et al., 1999; Gupton, Heaman, and Cheung, 2001). Poverty, poor education, social isolation, inadequate housing, cigarette smoking, substance abuse, domestic violence, poor nutrition, and neighborhood disintegration contribute to death and disability (National Fetal and Infant Mortality Review Program, 2001; Heaman, Sprague, and Stewart, 2001).

Infant Mortality Rate

The current definition of infant mortality rate (IMR) is the number of deaths before one year of age per 1,000 live births (Brosco, 1999). Although the U.S. IMR decreased to 7.2 in 1998, the data demonstrate that rates for African Americans, Native Americans, and some Hispanic subgroups are higher than the national average (National Fetal and Infant

Mortality Review Program, 2001). Infants born to poor families are still twice as likely to die as those born to families above the poverty level. There are parts of the United States where the IMR exceeds that of much poorer nations (Brosco, 1999). Studies also show that deaths due to preterm labor and low birth weight, respiratory distress syndrome, infections specific to the perinatal period, and maternal complications of pregnancy contribute disproportionately to the disparity in infant mortality (National Fetal and Infant Mortality Review Program, 2001).

MODELS OF CARE

Models of care have been developed in an effort to reduce the number of high-risk pregnancies and to improve pregnancy outcome.

Population Health Strategy

Population health strategies that integrate disease prevention, and community-wide health promotion, have demonstrated improved outcomes (National Fetal and Infant Mortality Review Program, 2001). A report on a decade of fetal and infant mortality review programs in the United Staes documented a wide range of community actions that improved service systems and community resources for women, infants, and families. (To learn more about the fetal and infant mortality review process, contact the National Fetal and Infant Mortality Review Program at email address nfimr@acog.org or phone (202) 863-2587.)

In Canadian health care, the focus is moving from remediation of problems to prevention of risk and promotion of improved health and well-being (Heaman, Sprague, and Stewart, 2001). Canada's publication of national guidelines for maternity care focuses on a family-centered approach to care and shifts thinking and practice to a wellness and prevention perspective (Health Canada, 2000).

Organizational Models

Providers, health plans, government agencies, employers and employee coalitions, and other organizations are especially focusing on reducing preterm births and cesarean birth rates. A review of the best practices is identified by top-scoring plans from NCPA's Quality Compass database. Also, feedback about programs admired by others in the field revealed that these practices have targeted one or more of the following strategies:

- Facilitating early entry into prenatal care

- Actively screening for risk factors

- Using case managers to monitor higher-risk women more closely

- Educating women to be more actively involved in their own care and clinical decisions

- Challenging physicians to find strategies to reduce cesarean birth rates (Athena Healthcare Communications, Inc., 1998)

Each of these strategies is an essential component of a family-centered maternity care program.

THE HIGH-RISK FAMILY

When a hospitalized woman, such as the woman in Figure 4-1, is labeled as high-risk, the attitudes of the healthcare providers often reflect that classification. Family-centered maternity care practices are frequently limited to the "normal" childbearing woman and her family. One can visit hospitals where there are two separate hospital units and two distinct philosophic approaches to care for these two designated childbearing populations. For high-risk women, care for labor, birth, and postpartum is provided in "Obstetrics." For low-risk women, care is provided in a unit identified as "Family-Centered Care."

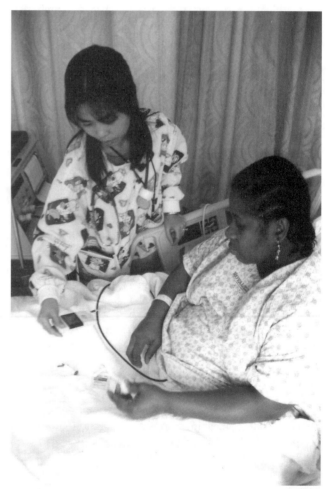

FIGURE 4–1 A high-risk patient: An antenatal diabetic mother on bed rest. *Photo by Emily Pascoe courtesy of Boston Medical Center, Boston, Massachusetts.*

This approach to care may actually cause increased stress and anxiety for the high-risk woman and her family. High-risk families need family-centered care as much or more than those families with normal pregnancies. This is an extremely stressful time for the family and the special psychosocial challenges of a high-risk pregnancy make family-centered care essential.

Developmental Tasks of Pregnancy

Pregnancy involves physiological and psychological stress for all families. All expectant parents must accomplish certain developmental tasks in order to adjust to the physical and emotional changes of pregnancy. The following describes these developmental tasks:

1. In the first trimester (incorporation), a woman must accept the pregnancy and incorporate it as a part of her.
2. In the second trimester (differentiation), she must recognize the fetus as an individual, thus differentiating it from herself.
3. In the third trimester (separation), in preparation for birth, a woman must be able to let the fetus go...separating it from herself.

Expectant fathers often have similar developmental tasks, having first to accept and then to separate from the fetus in order to parent.

High-risk pregnant women and their families have special tasks to accomplish in addition to the developmental tasks necessary for all expectant families. These are tasks related to illness and tasks related to the combination of pregnancy and illness. Persons who are ill must adapt to the sick role, accept an uncertain outcome, and adapt to chronic illness. Tasks of women who are both ill and pregnant include:

1. Loss of the ideal or perfect pregnancy
2. Adaptation to antenatal hospitalization and family separation
3. Frequent visits to a clinic, physician's office, or maternal-fetal medicine service
4. Undergoing special tests and procedures
5. Integration of "I'm sick" with "I'm pregnant" (Martin-Arafeh, Watson, and Baird, 1999).

Psychological Effects of High-Risk Pregnancy

Stresses that occur normally in pregnancy are amplified in the high-risk pregnancy. The psychological effects of high-risk pregnancy may be denial, blame and guilt, feelings of failure, and ambivalence. In addition, high-risk families may focus on the uncertain outcome of pregnancy and thus experience great anxiety and fear (Martin-Arafeh, Watson, and Baird, 1999).

Treatment Stressors

Women and their families report many emotions and feelings as a result of complications from their pregnancies. Treatment for the high-risk condition can be stressful (Martin-Arafeh, Watson, and Baird, 1999). A pregnant woman experiencing complications may delay the adaptation to pregnancy and have difficulty making a successful role transition to motherhood (Cunningham, 2001).

Antepartum Bed Rest Although there is conflicting evidence on the effectiveness of antepartum bed rest in preventing preterm birth, it is widely prescribed as one of the plans of care for preterm labor. When a woman is placed on bed rest, family members assume increased responsibilities (Cunningham, 2001), and there can be adverse effects on an older child or children that are already at home (Maloni and Ponder, 1997). Along with various physiological sequelae, researchers have found that the emotional effects of bed rest can include anxiety, sensory deprivation, stress, and depression. The expectant mother often feels isolated, lonely, and helpless (Maloni, Brezinski-Tomasi, and Johnson, 2001).

Support groups, various telephone and Web site support groups, and programs can provide emotional support. Referral to social service and other community agencies that assist parents is very important. Also, supportive care of the partner whose mate is at high-risk is needed. Noted expert Judith A. Maloni has created extensive resources for women and their families coping with the stresses and struggles of a complicated pregnancy and with the recommendation of bed rest.

Antepartum Hospitalization Women may be hospitalized early in the pregnancy for problems such as placenta previa, diabetes, premature rupture of membranes, or management of multiple gestations. These women may remain hospitalized for the duration of their pregnancies. Separation from family members, fear of where the pregnancy will lead, and loss of control over their day-to-day lives are all significant stressors for these women and their families (Katz, 2001).

Childbirth classes for an inpatient population can assist in relieving loneliness, boredom, and powerlessness (Campbell and Hart, 1994; Katz, 2001). The stress of hospitalization and feelings of dependency can be reduced by giving the woman and her family opportunities to control their environment by decorating their hospital room with personal possessions. There are antepartum hospitalization programs in which mothers are encouraged to wear their street clothes instead of hospital gowns. Routine medications such as vitamins and stool softeners are left at the bedside for self-administration. Family members are included in planning care, and the woman schedules her own day instead of being "routinized" into hospital schedules. Arts and crafts, magazines, television, audiotapes, computer with Internet access, and books can be available for diversional activities. Families can be encouraged to bring in meals and share them with the pregnant woman. Having access to a refrigerator and a microwave also allows the woman to eat at times she wishes rather than on a hospital schedule (Katz, 2001).

Visits to the neonatal intensive care units and anticipatory counseling are also important parts of these programs. If the illness extends beyond the hospital stay, it is especially important that both the woman and her family be instructed in health care, and be referred to the appropriate community resource(s) for support during the pregnancy and follow-up after discharge. A library of information and resource material on the antepartum unit can be established for the family's use.

Listening to what hospitalized antepartum women really feel about waiting can give direction to nursing care. Actively listening to women and supporting their efforts to carry their babies to full term is essential nursing practice (Thornburg, 2002).

Children in high-risk families may develop a variety of problems. They may have difficulty sleeping or coping with separation from their mother if she is hospitalized for an extended period of time. Parents, feeling anxious about their children at home, may become overprotective and overindulgent. If the mother returns from the hospital without the baby, the children at home may feel they have harmed their sibling by their thoughts. If the parents are having difficulty coping with the high-risk baby, their over-attentiveness to their sick baby may limit the time and energy available for the other children.

Pregnancy after Perinatal Loss

Women who have experienced a perinatal loss have learned that a successful pregnancy is not guaranteed. When these women are pregnant again, feeling anxious, nervous, and scared is to be expected. Although often cautiously optimistic about their pregnancies, these women may experience anxiety about the potential for another loss, feelings of guilt, grief, and resistance to attachment (Côté-Arsenault, Bidlack, and Humm, 2001).

Because pregnancy after perinatal loss is not an easy experience, women need supportive pregnant care. Healthcare providers must acknowledge women's past losses, and be responsive to their individual needs and concerns during subsequent pregnancies.

Of course, fathers and other family members also need support. The need of a grieving father to express his feelings may conflict with the traditional male role, in which he is expected to be strong and support his partner (Samuelsson, Rådestad, and Segesten, 2001). Thus, the father may become the "forgotten mourner." It is important to acknowledge men's grief and give a respectful response.

Postpartum Depression

Up to 90 percent of all new mothers will experience an episode of "baby blues," which occurs in the days and weeks immediately following childbirth. This condition is characterized by sudden mood swings, which range from euphoria to intense sadness, and includes feelings of despair, anxiety, and irritability. The woman experiencing baby blues will cry for no apparent reason, feel out of sorts and restless, and experience mild anxiety; she may sometimes have trouble with eating or sleeping. The baby blues last no more than the first six weeks postpartum and may disappear as quickly and suddenly as they appeared, without medical treatment (Sanford, 2002).

Ten to 20 percent of women who give birth experience postpartum depression, most often six to eight weeks after delivery. This depression often interferes with a woman's ability to function. One of the major challenges in dealing with postpartum depression has been early recognition. Undiagnosed postpartum depression can result in tragedy, sometimes in the form of maternal suicide or infanticide that makes headlines (Beck et al., 2000). There is a significant risk to babies of mothers with postpartum depression because the mothers are simply not there for their babies.

Early intervention is essential. In screening, it is important to recognize that women who have experienced a high-risk pregnancy, previous infertility, previous postpartum depression, and stressful labor and birth are at risk for postpartum depression. A nonsupportive partner or stress related to family, marriage, occupation, housing, or other events during pregnancy can also contribute to the risk of postpartum depression. Also, women with a past history of depression not related to pregnancy are at risk. Screening for postpartum depression begins prenatally with identification of potential risks. It is important that the woman at risk and/or diagnosed with postpartum depression receive appropriate counseling, treatment, and support.

CESAREAN BIRTH

Although there is a great deal of variation among hospitals, cesarean births in the United States account for between 21 and 22 percent of all births at the time of this writing. At the same time, the rate of vaginal birth after previous cesarean delivery (VBAC) has leveled off at between 34 and 35 percent (Curtin, Kozak, and Gregory, 2000). Cesarean birth is a major surgical procedure that entails increased maternal and fetal risks (Enkin, Keirse, and Chalmers, 1992).

Psychological Integration of the Cesarean Birth

A decade or more ago, women experiencing an unplanned cesarean birth reported troubled feelings about their cesarean births, such as disappointment, frustration, guilt, depression, failure at not having delivered "normally," feelings of being cheated, feelings of intrusion from the surgical procedure, and alteration in body image. Fathers excluded from participation in cesarean births reported feelings of isolation, inadequacy, failure, and being cheated. They often felt left out and reported difficulty relating to their baby.

In contrast, the findings of more recent research suggest that the negative emotions after cesarean birth may no longer be as profound. Instead, women have reported happiness about the birth of a healthy baby, but with continuing disappointment about having to have a cesarean birth (Reichert, Baron, and Fawcett, 1993). This change in women's response to cesarean birth has been attributed to the "normalizing" effect of the high rate of cesarean birth and the efforts of childbirth educators to include cesarean birth in prenatal classes. Whatever the reason, women still experience disappointment and require continued attention and sensitive care that takes into account their special needs.

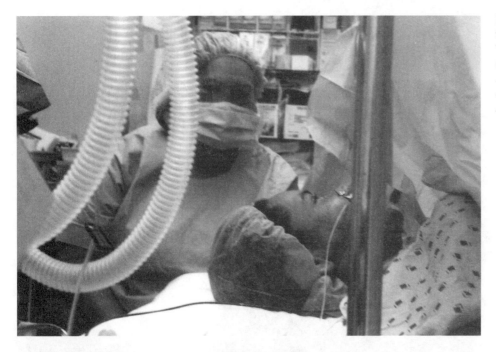

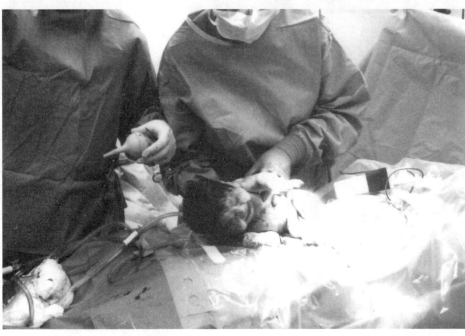

FIGURE 4–2 Photos from a family-centered cesarean birth. The birth mother and her sister share in welcoming the baby. *Photos by Emily Pascoe, courtesy of Boston Medical Center, Boston, Massachusetts.*

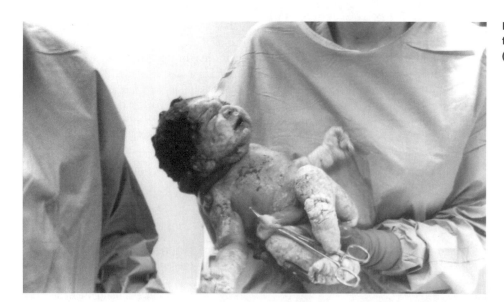

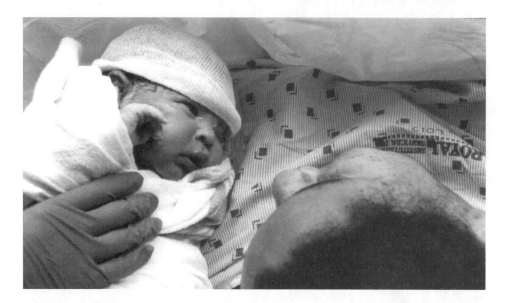

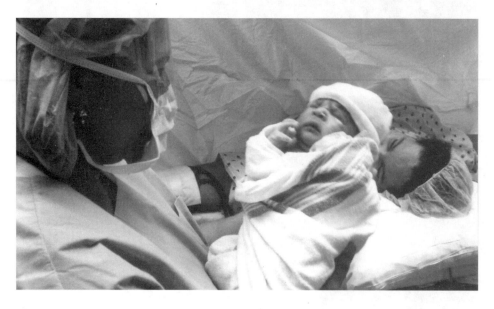

FIGURE 4–2 Photos from a family-centered cesarean birth (*continued*).

Family-Centered Cesarean Birth

Care of parents experiencing a cesarean birth should be family-centered rather than surgery-centered. (See Figure 4-2.) In an effort to focus on the birth and not the operative procedure, the term *cesarean delivery* or *cesarean birth* should become common usage rather than the more familiar, surgically oriented term *cesarean section*. The rationale is that, although the mother is experiencing an abdominal rather than a vaginal birth, she is still giving birth.

It is essential to provide prenatal and postpartum education regarding cesarean birth and to minimize separation of mother, father, and child at the time of the delivery. The cesarean delivery is a birth experience and must be incorporated as such when family-centered care is provided. The goal is a positive birth experience, regardless of the type of delivery.

Presence of Father or Support Person In hospitals where family-centered maternity care has been extended to the cesarean birth family, there is no evidence of harm to mother, father, or baby. Research on fathers' presence during cesarean births has shown no adverse outcome. There is growing evidence that their presence improves the post-cesarean behavioral responses of the families.

The experience of cesarean birth, either elective or emergency, provokes anxiety for most women and families. A number of options, however, can be made available to facilitate a family-centered cesarean birth. These are summarized in Exhibit 4-1.

Policies and procedures for care of a mother following a cesarean birth are included in Exhibits 4-2 and 4-3. Note that family attachment with their infant is encouraged. (See Appendix J for the full-page versions of these exhibits.)

EXHIBIT 4–1   Options fo Facilitate Family-Centered Cesarean Births

- Admit the woman to hospital for an elective cesarean on the morning of the birth, so that family members can spend the previous night together.
- Enable father/partner/support person to remain with the mother during the physical preparation.
- Provide a viewing window into the cesarean operating room for family members; include stools for children.
- Provide regional anesthesia where possible and explain the differences between regional and general anesthesia.
- Enable father/partner/support person to be in the cesarean birth room in nonemergency situations. (There is controversy regarding the support person's presence during emergency situations. Further evidence is needed to assess this area.)
- Provide a mirror and/or ongoing commentary from a staff member for mother and family.
- Enable photographs or videos to be taken, if even one parent is unable to witness the birth.
- Free the mother's hands from restraint, thereby allowing contact with her partner and the baby.
- Provide the opportunity for both parents to interact with the baby in the cesarean birth room and/or the postanesthetic recovery room.
- Provide an opportunity for the mother to breastfeed in the cesarean birth room or the postanesthetic recovery room.
- If father/partner chooses not to be in the cesarean birth room, replace him/her at the mother's side with a support person. Give the father/partner the baby to hold as soon as possible. Have the staff describe the birth experience to the father/partner.
- Assess the baby's condition individually to avoid time alone in an incubator in the nursery, whenever possible.
- If the baby must go to a nursery for special care, have the father/partner accompany the baby to the nursery and remain with the infant until both are reunited with the mother.
- Keep the mother informed of the status of the baby in the nursery (if the baby must go to a nursery for special care).
- Reunite the family in the postanesthetic recovery room.
- If it is difficult to reunite the family in the postanesthetic room, judge each mother's condition individually with an eye to reuniting the family as soon as possible.
- Ask the father/partner to be in the postanesthetic recovery room to tell the mother, if she has had a general anesthetic, about the birth.
- Provide time alone for the family in those first critical hours after cesarean birth.
- Institute mother/baby nursing as soon as possible and do not routinely separate mothers and babies.
- Include the family in the teaching of caretaking skills.
- Include siblings according to their and the family's wishes.

EXHIBIT 4–2 **Postcesarean Birth Recovery Care**

Procedure

Provide safe, effective care of new mothers immediately following cesarean birth.

Policy

An RN shall recover the cesarean mother for a minimum of one hour or until vital signs are stable and the course of recovery is normalized.

Equipment

1. Blood pressure monitoring equipment.
2. Thermometer.
3. Stethoscope.
4. Pulse oximeter.
5. Heart rate monitor.
6. Respiration monitor.
7. IV pole, fluids, and supplies.
8. Suction and catheters.
9. Oxygen and nasal cannula or mask.
10. Warm blankets.
11. Washcloths and towels.
12. Sanitary pads and belt.
A. Waterproof under-buttocks pads.
B. Crash cart.

Education

Explain the procedure to the woman and her family and answer their questions prior to the cesarean. Reassure and inform the new mother and her family during the recovery period. Limit visitors only if the mother requests.

Implementation

I. Observations and documentation.

    A. On the woman's arrival from the OB/OR suite, observe and chart the following:

        1. Vital signs.

        2. Level of consciousness.

        3. Subjective experience of pain.

        4. IV fluids:

            a. Type and number of bottles.

            b. Added medications.

            c. IV site and condition.

            d. Amount absorbed.

        5. Operative site:

            a. Cesarean and/or episiotomy site.

            b. Dressing—dry and intact.

            c. Drainage—(lochia) amount, type, and color.

        6. Drainage tubes:

            a. Type.

            b. Location.

            c. Amount of drainage.

            d. Type and color of drainage.

EXHIBIT 4–2 **Postcesarean Birth Recovery Care** *(continued).*

    7. Type of anesthesia administered.

    8. Medications and fluids used in the OR.

    9. Physician's orders checked and completed.

   10. Fundus:

       a. Location.

       b. Condition—firm, boggy, firm with massage.

B. Check and record every 15 minutes x 1 hour or until stable. Notify the physician of any abnormal findings. (After one hour or when the woman is stabilized, see Postsurgical Recovery Assessment, or follow the physician's orders.)

    1. Vital signs.

    2. Fundus:

       a. Location relative to umbilicus.

       b. Condition—firm, boggy, firm with massage, etc.

    3. Lochia—amount, appearance of episiotomy, if applicable, for swelling, hematoma.

    4. Condition of dressing.

    5. Mobility and sensation.

C. Check for bladder distention. Assess the catheter for patency if urine is less than 30cc per hour. Document the procedure, amount, and color. Pink- or blood-tinged urine may indicate bladder trauma. Notify the physician if urine output is less than 30cc per hour.

D. Give peri and catheter care as needed.

E. Check and record the new mother's temperature. Notify the physician if her temperature is above 100.4°F. Document notification and any orders received.

II. Special care required to maintain an airway after receiving a general anesthetic.

A. Using an oral airway.

    1. Stay at the bedside of a woman with an oral airway.

    2. Observe respirations for quality.

    3. Observe color—oxygen may be started if ordered.

    4. Suction PRN. Deep suction may cause bleeding.

    5. Airway removal:

       a. Wait until the woman either gags slightly or makes an effort to remove the oral airway herself.

       b. Never remove an oral airway forcefully; doing so may break her teeth.

       c. Never attempt to remove an oral airway if it is loose and she does not respond. Use nasal airways for women with caps or without an oral airway whose respirations are inadequate.

B. Administering oxygen.

    1. Regulate the oxygen flow rate and concentration to maintain the SaO_2 greater than 90 percent or as ordered by anesthesia. If unable to maintain SaO_2 greater than 90 percent, notify the anesthesiologist.

    2. Oxygen may be discontinued as ordered by anesthesia personnel.

    3. Have suction equipment set up and available. The woman may become nauseated and vomit. Suction as needed.

C. All women who receive general anesthesia will have their SaO_2 monitored with a pulse oximeter. Monitoring with a pulse oximeter may be discontinued as ordered by anesthesia personnel.

_____

VP Nursing

_____

Department Chair

EXHIBIT 4–3   Postcesarean Recovery Assessment

Procedure

Prevent postoperative complications. Provide adequate post-partum care. Promote family attachment.

Policy

An RN will assess the new mother and maintain proper care and management after a cesarean birth.

Equipment

1. Cardiac monitor.
2. Pulse oximeter.
3. Blood pressure monitor.
4. Thermometer.
5. OB recovery assessment sheet.
6. Postpartum supply pack.
7. IV pole or infusion pump.
8. Basin.
9. Nurse call button.

Implementation

I. Admission assessment.
   A. Check the woman's vital signs.
   B. Assess each body system, with particular attention to:
      1. Respiration—quality, frequency, and regularity.
      2. Circulation—the amount of bleeding from incision and lochia.
      3. Cardiac function—pulse, blood pressure, and rhythm strip.
      4. Urinary and genital—quantity of output and color.
      5. Fundal assessment—tone. Administer oxytocin, if prescribed.
      6. GI system—intake, abdominal distention, and bowel sounds.
II. Provide comfort measures for the new mother.
   A. Provide analgesics as ordered by physician
   B. Position for comfort.
   C. Explain splinting of the incision.
III. Begin postpartum and postoperative instructions. Document.
IV. Promote early interaction between the mother, father, and their infant. Document.
V.   Reunite the family in the recovery as soon as possible.
VI. If the baby must go to the nursery for special care, keep the mother informed of the status of the baby.
VII. Include siblings according to the family's wishes.

VP Nursing

Department Chair

FAMILY-CENTERED NEONATAL INTENSIVE CARE

In caring for the family of a high-risk baby, the goal should be to send a well baby home as a family member, not as a stranger. Parents of a high-risk baby may lose their child through death or relinquishment (adopting out the baby), or they may be presented with a premature or defective child, thus losing the perfect child of their dreams. In the immediate newborn period, the holding, touching, and eye-to-eye contact important in establishing parent–infant attachment often have to be delayed so that immediate life support measures can be initiated. Prolonged separation from the infant not only may threaten the attachment process, but also may increase the potential for future problems, such as failure to thrive and neglect (Bialoskurski, Cox, and Hayes, 1999).

Separating a mother and her baby during the first week of the child's life involves much emotional strain for the mother (Nystrom and Axelsson, 2002). Whenever a baby is in an intensive care unit, the other family members also need special nursing care. The high-tech environment of the neonatal intensive care unit (NICU) and the infant's dependence on complex technology for life support can make parents feel helpless and dependent on the healthcare professionals (Dobbins, Bohlig, and Sutphen, 1994; Hughes et al., 1994; Epps and Nowak, 1998). Prolonged hospitalization in the NICU is particularly stressful for the family, leading to distress in most aspects of their lives (McGrath, 2001).

Parents, siblings, and grandparents should be encouraged to visit their baby in the nursery and to participate in the care. Because the parents are responsible for providing life-long physical and emotional care, they and their infant must be treated as a unit from the very beginning. The basic belief at the core of family-centered neonatal intensive care is that the infant's family members are the best people to care for and nurture their child (Fenwick, Barclay, and Schmied, 1999). See Figure 4-3.

When parents cannot be present in the NICU, low cost videoconferencing technology can connect families at home to the NICU. Parents can then see their babies on their home computer screen.

The Principles of Family-Centered Neonatal Care

In response to problems identified by parents, medical professionals, ethicists, academics, and journalists, a conference was held June 27 through 29, 1992, in Burlington, Vermont. The result is a document that addressed the participants' concerns about the way babies and their parents were being treated in neonatal intensive care units (NICUs).

The parents of critically ill newborns and professionals involved with high-risk infants and their families advocated a family-centered approach to treatment in NICUs. The following "Principles for Family-Centered Neonatal Care" were drafted to encourage families to participate as fully as

3. In medical situations involving very high mortality and morbidity, great suffering, and/or significant medical controversy, fully informed parents should have the right to make decisions regarding aggressive treatment for their infants.

4. Expectant parents should be offered information about adverse pregnancy outcomes and be given the opportunity to state in advance their treatment preferences if their baby is born extremely prematurely and/or critically ill.

5. Parents and professionals must work together to alleviate the pain of infants in intensive care.

6. Parents and professionals must work together to ensure an appropriate environment for babies in the NICU.

7. Parents and professionals should work together to ensure the safety and efficacy of neonatal treatments.

8. Parents and professionals should develop nursery policies and programs that promote parenting skills and encourage maximum involvement of families with their hospitalized infant.

9. Parents and professionals must work together to promote meaningful long-term follow-up for all high-risk NICU survivors.

10. Parents and professionals must acknowledge that critically ill newborns can be harmed by overtreatment as well as by undertreatment, and we must insist that our laws and treatment policies be based on compassion. We must work together to promote awareness of the needs of NICU survivors with disabilities to ensure adequate support for them and their families. We must work together to decrease disability through universal prenatal care.

When these principles of family-centered neonatal intensive care are translated into actions, families are empowered. They become true partners with healthcare professionals in the care of their special babies. Family-centered neonatal care is a relationship-centered system of care for fragile infants and their families.

DEVELOPMENTAL CARE

Developmentally sensitive care for preterm infants was introduced in the early 1980s (Als et al., 1986). However, it has only been since the early 1990s that this approach has been adopted in progressive neonatal units across North America (Petryshen et al., 1997). A remaining challenge is to find ways to introduce developmental care principles into most neonatal intensive care nurseries (Gretebeck et al., 1998).

Als (1992) defined "developmentally appropriate" as provisional care that is individualized and behavioral—developmental in nature. Basing care in the NICU on the infant's developmental strengths while supporting their efforts

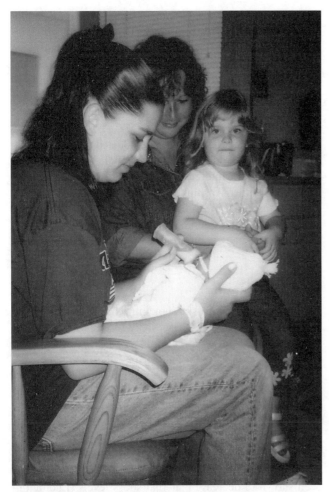

FIGURE 4–3 Feeding a preterm baby in the hospital special care nursery. *Photo courtesy of Good Samaritan Hospital, Lebanon, Pennsylvania.*

possible in caring for and making decisions for their hospitalized newborns, help caregivers respect the diversity of family values and beliefs, and help parents and professionals form mutually beneficial and supportive partnerships in the NICU and beyond.

Principles[1]

1. Family-centered neonatal care should be based on open and honest communication between parents and professionals on medical and ethical issues.

2. To work with professionals in making informed treatment choices, parents must have available to them the same facts and interpretation of those facts as the professionals, including medical information presented in meaningful formats, information about uncertainties surrounding treatments, information from parents whose children have been in similar medical situations, and access to the chart and rounds discussions.

---

[1] From Harrison, H. 1993. The principles for family-centered neonatal care. *Pediatrics* 92, no. 5: 643–650.

toward developmental gains embodies the developmental care approach (Dobbins, Bohlig, and Sutphen, 1994). Two major goals of developmental care are to individualize care by (1) decreasing infant disruptions and handling by caregivers, and (2) modulating or attenuating infant responses to the care they received. Use of developmentally supportive techniques allows healthcare providers in NICUs to become proactive in providing care that is cost-effective and improves medical and neurobehavioral outcomes (Ashbaugh, Leick-Rude, and Kilbride, 1999).

Benefits

Infants receiving individualized developmentally supportive care have been found to experience improved outcomes, including less need for assisted ventilation and supplemental oxygen, earlier oral feeding, faster and greater weight gain, fewer intraventricular hemorrhages, shorter hospitalization, lower hospital charges, and better neurobehavioral outcomes, as well as improved parent–infant interactions, when compared with infants receiving standard NICU care (Ashbaugh, Leick-Rude, and Kilbride, 1999; Westrup et al., 2000; Petryshen et al., 1997). In one study, costs of nursing care for infants receiving developmental versus conventional care were reduced because the move from the NICU to the transitional unit occurred earlier and their nursing intensity needs were lower (Petryshen et al., 1997).

Clustering Care

Because rest is an important feature for normal growth and development, ensuring periods of undisturbed rest is important for high-risk infants. In the provision of developmental care, clinical interventions are coordinated or "clustered" to certain limited periods to prevent interruptions during infant sleep. Care is planned to decrease infant disruptions and handling by caregivers, and modulating or attenuating infant responses to the care they receive (Peters, 1999). Positioning and bundling the infant to prevent disorientation and to promote self-regulation are also important. Making a nest in the incubator can make it easier for the infant to assume a flexed position, thus facilitating self-soothing/consoling behaviors.

Physical Environment

The traditional NICU is characterized by bright, loud environments and sensory overload. Research has shown that this type of an environment can actually have a detrimental effect on an infant's development. A reduced stress NICU environment is more supportive of normal growth and development, and may lead to improved outcomes (Committee to Establish Recommended Standards for Newborn ICU Design, 1999). In developmentally sensitive care, the environment is structured so that light and noise levels are reduced and individually controlled at each bed space. Cycling between normal and low light levels in the

NICU has been suggested as one way to support development of mature day/night rhythms (Peters, 1999).

Also, modern NICU design promotes family participation by increasing accommodations for families. There are rooms for families to stay for extended periods of time so that they can be close to their babies and participate in care practices. Space for education and relaxation of staff is also a priority.

Many hospitals have already remodeled or are currently designing single-room neonatal care units. One such unit can be found at Children's Hospital and Regional Medical Center in Seattle, Washington, where single-room neonatal care was instituted in 2000. In that facility, the most significant impact of single-room care was the improved ability to control each baby's environment (Brown and Taquino, 2001).

Kangaroo Care

Kangaroo care (skin-to-skin holding) is an intervention that meets developmental care criteria by fostering neurobehavioral development (Ludington-Hoe and Swinth, 1996). During kangaroo care, the mother or father holds the baby (wearing only a diaper) skin-to-skin, covering him or her with the parent's own clothing or a towel.

Studies have demonstrated that skin-to-skin contact had no adverse effects but did have positive effects on physiological parameters in preterm infants (Föhe, Kropf, and Avenarius, 2000; Mellien, 2001; Ludington-Hoe and Swinthe, 1996; Engler et al., 2002). Also, kangaroo care has been shown to decrease maternal stress levels (Ludington-Hoe and Swinthe, 1996), increase maternal milk volume, and improve milk letdown (Anderson, 1991).

A policy for implementation of kangaroo care can be found in Exhibit 4-4. (See Appendix J for the full-page version of this exhibit.)

Family Care

Family-centered care is integral to developmental care, with parents encouraged to be equal members of the care-giving team. Parents are helped to understand their infant's signals and recognize their infant's unique needs. Staff encourages the family's early and continuous participation in caregiving in order to foster positive parental interactions.

WellStar Health System Cobb Hospital in Austell, Georgia, designed a developmentally sensitive program, nursery, and family rooms shortly after developmentally sensitive care was introduced to North America. The Special Care Nursery is an important component of a comprehensive family-centered maternity care program at this hospital. The Statement of Philosophy for their Special Care Nursery clearly articulates the staff's belief in developmentally sensitive care. That philosophy statement is found in Exhibit 4-5.

The mission of the Neonatal Intensive Care Unit at Gaston Memorial Hospital reflects the family-centered philosophy of the hospital's full maternity service, known as

EXHIBIT 4–4   Kangaroo Care

Policy

To facilitate parent/infant closeness by promoting increased physical contact, to ease psychological burdens imposed by a premature birth, and to aid parents to feel more confident in responding to their infant's needs.

The procedure of skin-to-skin Kangaroo care (KC) will be used in the SCN.

Implementation

1. Receive or verify provider's orders to initiate KC.

2. Place rocking chair with pillows for support in draft-free private area.

3. Instruct parent to wear a medium weight blouse that can zip or button over the infant's back or have mother undress to waist and wear a cover gown. The infant's back is then covered with a warmed receiving blanket folded in fourths.

4. Place a hat on the infant's head, remove all other clothing except the diaper.

5. After explaining all procedures to the mother, have her sit in the rocking chair, position pillows for comfort, and place the baby upright onto her chest, between her breasts, from under the bottom of the blouse (so the leads, cords, and wires do not obstruct the view of the baby). Adjust oxygen if used. (The baby may need less oxygen flow under the mom's blouse as it acts like an oxygen "hood").

6. Obtain baseline vital signs (axillary, T, RR, HR, O_2 saturation) on the infant and take them again 20–30 minutes after KC initiated. Some infants warm up to an individual threshold at which they begin to squirm. If this happens, take the infant's temperature. Repeat vital signs checks when infant returned to incubator.

7. Give mother as much support as she needs. Emphasize that she is not hurting the baby. Stay close to the isolette during Kangaroo care for the first few days, until she tells you that she can be left with other nurses monitoring the baby.

8. Teach the mother how to hold, handle, breastfeed, and care for her baby, as well as to recognize and respond to behavioral cues. For example, teach the mother that if the infant shows such signs as finger splaying, extended limbs, tongue extension, or averted gaze, then she should withdraw some stimulation, such as rocking, singing, or talking, and offer such activities one at a time. As Kangaroo care progresses over weeks, encourage the mother to take control over care-taking activities.

9. If temperature is ± 37°, unfold the blanket covering the infant's back so only 2 folds are against the infant. Reassess the temperature in another 10 minutes.

10. If the infant is bottle feeding, offer the bottle when the infant begins to move his/her head from side-to-side.

11. Encourage the mother to take breaks as needed, usually at least every 2 hours. The mother can participate in Kangaroo care for as long or as briefly as she wishes, but the level of satisfaction and knowledge about the baby seem to be improved as more time is spent with baby.

12. If infant shows signs of unrest (not attributable to hunger, burping, and/or elimination) that persists for more than 5 minutes or if infant is in physiologic compromise (sustained desaturating, color changes, respiratory distress, HR instability, irritability), remove from KC.

13. Document initiation of, use of, and modifications to this policy.

14. Document start and stop times, vital signs, topics discussed, parental concerns, infant's behavioral and physiological responses to Kangaroo care.

Additional Information

Supportive Data

1. Breastfeeding mothers who give Kangaroo Care (KC) are inclined to produce more milk.

2. Infants given KC have adequate oxygenation.

3. Infants are warmer when being held in KC than when in open air cribs, so heat loss is not a real concern.

4. There is no rationale to support policies limiting and dictating incremental increases in the amount of time spent in KC. In many European sites, 4–5 hours per KC session is recommended to allow maximum benefit from KC.

5. Infants are shown to have fewer episodes of periodic breathing and apnea.

6. Infants receiving KC have had earlier hospital discharges.

7. Dressing/undressing and movement from crib to mother and back can be physiologically stressful to preterm infants. *At least one hour of KC at a time is recommended.*

EXHIBIT 4–5   WellStar Cobb Hospital Neonatal Intensive Care—Statement of Philosophy

The staff of the Special Care Nursery believe our tiny patients are our future therefore we commit ourselves to a family-centered approach of care through...

Special Care

Supportive Service—	We will assist families in providing as much support and knowledge of community resources as available.
Patience—	Existing on a day to day basis when you parent an ill child is very difficult. We promise all parents patience and understanding of your ever-changing world.
Environment—	We promise to provide a safe environment with tender hands, soft sounds, and easy lighting to promote positive developmental outcomes.
Communication—	As parents, you are our partners in caring for your little one(s). We promise open and honest communication to encourage an atmosphere of trust and growth for you as parents and us as professionals.
Individualized Care—	Each baby develops in his/her own unique way. We commit ourselves to provide individualized care recognizing the baby's own developmental signals.
Accountability—	As staff, we will take initiative in clinical, economical, and ethical decision making to provide appropriate services to our patients.
Liaison—	We will use a multidisciplinary team approach including the family to facilitate return of the infant to the family unit as quickly as possible.
Compassion—	We promise to show sensitivity to the needs of our patients, parents, and their extended families.
Acknowledge—	We will acknowledge parents' diversities and points of view. We will show respect by recognizing each one's uniqueness. We believe parents should be involved in decision making regarding their infant's care and actively participate in that care.
Respect—	Each of us can expect to be treated with respect and dignity. We promise to maintain strict confidentiality and promote as much privacy as possible.
Excellence—	We are committed to excellence. Each of us works to the best of our ability to deliver high quality health care...delivered with a human touch. Each member of our team is expected to strive toward our common goal of professionally serving and caring for others.

Source: Special Care Nursery Statement of Philosophy courtesy of WellStar Health System, Cobb Hospital, Austell, Georgia.

The Birthplace. The Mission Statement for the Neonatal Intensive Care Unit is shown in Exhibit 4-6.

At Gaston Memorial Hospital parents participate in daily NICU rounds and together with the healthcare team discuss the optimal plan of care for their baby.

Staff Education

A comprehensive quality improvement process, guided by a unit-based newborn developmental specialist, can facilitate the transition of a NICU program from provider-centered to family-centered (Ballweg, 2001). As the NICU becomes family-centered, its staff and direct caregivers must be educated about the rationale for, and practice of, developmentally sensitive care for neonates.

All neonatal care providers must be included in the education program. These include neonatologists, staff and transport nurses, neonatal nurse practitioners, clinicians, respiratory therapists, ancillary unlicensed staff, the neonatal dietician, social worker, occupational therapist, phlebotomists, radiology technicians, housekeepers, and even the project architect. The education program enables all staff members to optimize the use of the NICU environment, and to see the vision and future direction of the unit and all its caregiving practices. This education is pivotal to the success of the program.

EXHIBIT 4–6   The Birthplace Neonatal Intensive Care—Mission Statement

We recognize the special care infant to be a unique individual with distinct needs. We are committed to providing competent and tender care to support the physiologic, developmental, psychosocial, and educational needs of infants and their families.

We respect the importance of the family and encourage their involvement and support in their infant's care.

Source: Mission statement courtesy of Gaston Memorial Hospital, Gastonia, NC

The NIDCAP® (Neonatal Individualized Developmental Care and Assessment Program) has been used to train selected staff in the NIDCAP approach to assessment and care. This assessment program includes systematic observation of infant behaviors before, during, and after caregiving. Professional staff, who have been trained to perform these assessments, describe their observations and follow them with individualized recommendations for caregiving (Ashbaugh, Leick-Rude, and Kilbride, 1999).

Children's Medical Ventures (a Novametrix Company) has the Wee Care Program of hands-on training in developmental care for the entire staff (see Appendix G, Resources for Information on Family-Centered Maternity Care). The Wee Care team will travel to a hospital and provide classroom teaching and a week of hands-on demonstration of practical skills.

BREASTFEEDING THE NICU INFANT

The health benefits of breastfeeding extend to preterm infants as well as their mothers. Breastfeeding is less physiologically stressful than bottle feeding. Preterm infants can better maintain their transcutaneous oxygen pressure and body temperature while breastfeeding than while bottle feeding (Meier et al., 1994). Episodes of hypoxia and hypothermia may be more prevalent while bottle feeding than while breastfeeding. Infants show better coordination of suck, swallow, and breathing during breastfeeding (Riordan and Auerbach, 1999). Oral feeding readiness may be determined by gestational age, clinical stability, tolerance of enteral feedings, ability to swallow own secretions, and no noted pauses in breathing during nonnutritive sucking bursts on a pacifier or finger.

Sample Guidelines

With proper planning, counseling, and follow-up, many mothers of infants in NICUs can successfully breastfeed their infants. Healthcare providers must provide timely, evidence-based management strategies for achieving successful outcomes. Guidelines, policies, and procedures for breastfeeding the NICU infant follow in Exhibits 4-7 through 4-12. (See Appendix J for the full-page versions of these exhibits.)

EXHIBIT 4–7   Guidelines for Initiating and Establishing Breastfeeding for the NICU Infant

---

Breastfeeding Unit Guide

1. The NICU parent should be encouraged to provide skin-to-skin holding as soon as medically stable. Good positioning; adequate support of the head, trunk, and neck; and proper body alignment allow the infant to explore the breast.

2. If needed, mom may pump before bringing baby to breast to decrease forceful let-down.

3. Utilizing test weights, when possible, assist in more accurately determining the need for supplements.

4. Feedings will be determined by physician order. Ad-lib feeds are encouraged to promote neurobehavioral organization and normalize the infant feeding pattern. Ad-lib refers to whenever the baby exhibits hunger cues such as rooting or sucking on hands. These feedings may be as often as every 1 to 3 hours during the day. Breast milk has a digestion time of approximately 90 minutes. This feeding process is made in an attempt to imitate the possible feeding pattern at home after discharge.

5. In preparation for discharge, "nesting" should incorporate a continuous 24 hour period to better simulate the home situation. Ideally, suggested feeding routines should take into account realistic expectations of the mother's 24-hour caregiving ability. When ordered, this may include clustering care and allowing 4–5 hours of uninterrupted sleep at night.

6. Mothers should be referred to lactation services for breastfeeding follow-up after discharge.

A suggested routine to assist in establishing breastfeeding may include:

1. First breastfeeding week, offer breast ad-lib for exploration and initial attempts to latch, maintaining nutritional requirements with gavage feeding.

2. Second breastfeeding week, offer breast ad-lib and utilize test weights for verification of amount ingested. Test weighing includes a cloth diaper only weight on hospital grade electronic scale. Two weights are taken, one pre- and one post-breastfeeding to determine intake 1GM-1cc. Supplement as necessary to meet nutritional requirements.

3. Beginning the third breastfeeding week, assessment will be made regarding supplemental feedings anticipating discharge. Focus feeding volume on total 24-hour intake rather than each individual feed.

4. Colostrum/breastmilk is always the first choice of supplement. It is helpful to question a mother regarding family history of milk allergies or sensitivities before feeding anything other than breastmilk. Unnecessary exposure to artificial baby milk may trigger food sensitivities.

5. Alternate feeding methods may be used after proper instruction.

6. If supplementation is offered by bottle, use a firmer, standard size and/or orthodontic nipple when possible to slow the flow of liquid. This allows the caregiver to support the infant in pacing the feedings and coordination of suck, swallow, and breathe. Red preemie nipples are not recommended because they flow too fast and can also interfere with the baby's ability to coordinate suck, swallow, and breathe.

7. Assist the infant to pace feedings, if needed. To pace, the infant is to be held in a supported sitting position, and the bottle is held horizontally with enough milk in the tip of nipple to avoid swallowing air. Feeding stimulation should begin at the baby's lips, encouraging baby to open mouth and pull nipple in rather than forcing nipple in with no feeding cues.

Source: Guidelines for Initiating and Establishing Breastfeeding for the NICU Infant, courtesy of Barbara Ford, RN, IBCLC.

EXHIBIT 4–8   Nursing Policy: Assisting the NICU Breastfeeding Mother

Policy

Assistance and instruction will be offered to staff and parents in providing the best possible nutrition and the best method of feeding the preterm infant.

Procedure

1. The mother will be supported in her personal goals regarding breastfeeding her infant.

2. Parents will be encouraged to provide Kangaroo Care when ordered. The physical contact with the baby is also important to the mother as it helps to increase her milk supply and improve the milk let-down.

3. Non-nutritive sucking will be encouraged to provide comfort, promote neurobehavioral organization, and increase oral-facial muscle tone and strength. Non-nutritive sucking helps increase ability to provide good intra-oral pressure for effective breastfeeding.

4. If supplementation is offered by bottle, use a firmer, standard size or NUK nipples when possible, to slow the flow of liquid. Red, premie nipples are not recommended.

5. Only appropriate size and type pacifiers should be used. Bottle nipples should not be used as pacifiers.

6. Mothers should be referred to lactation services for breastfeeding following discharge.

7. See NICU Breastfeeding Unit guide for specific suggestions regarding establishing breastfeeding for the NICU infant.

8. Milk should be thawed slowly to room temperature before feeding to infant. Microwave thawing is not allowed nor high temperatures of water as valuable nutrients are destroyed in the process.

9. It is recommended that milk refrigerators or freezers accessible to the public should have locks to protect against sabotage.

10. To avoid using the wrong milk, the container should be checked as when giving meds to verify correct patient identification.

11. The integrity of the container will be confirmed before feeding stored breastmilk to infants.

12. When possible, use colostrum or breastmilk for the first feedings.

Source: Assisting the NICU Breastfeeding Mother policy, courtesy of Barbara Ford, RN, IBCLC.

EXHIBIT 4–9   Guidelines for Breastfeeding the Preterm Infant in NICU

- When Kangaroo Care is initiated, the baby may begin suckling on a breast that was emptied by pumping up to one hour prior to the feeding.

- When the infant is able to take in some "low flow" milk, the mother will pump out milk from one breast (about 7 to 8 minutes), then nurse. The milk remaining in the breast is called "hind" milk and is much higher in calories and fat content than the "fore" milk. This may be repeated on the second breast if the baby will nurse for 20 minutes.

- When the infant is able to coordinate sucking and breathing, the mother no longer needs to express milk prior to the feeding and should nurse at least 20 to 30 minutes total on one breast or both.

- A *small* nipple shield may be necessary to help the infant maintain a latch-on. The nipple shield will help to increase the effectiveness of the infant's suck by remaining in the correct position in the infant's mouth.

- The infant is best held in a "football" or clutch hold, which in turn offers support to the entire body, neck, and head. A pillow would provide additional support to the mother's back and under the arm holding the baby. A footstool could also be used if available.

- It is essential to weigh the baby on a gram scale before and after the feeding to determine how much milk the baby is getting.

- When the infant is able to take to all feedings at the breast, the infant may nurse on demand or ad lib, providing the infant is consuming the prescribed amount according to weight and nutritional requirements. The neonatologist or CNP can estimate this amount for each 8- or 24-hour period.

- Mothers are to be reminded to pump after each breastfeeding while the infant is in the hospital. The lactation consultant will formulate a discharge plan for the mother at the time of the infant's discharge.

- In the mother's absence, tube feedings should be given by an auto syringe that has been upended rather than by "gravity" feeds. This allows the lipids or higher calorie portion of the breast milk to be pushed out first as it naturally rises to the top.

Note: Three studies done in 1988, 1993, and 1995 demonstrated that preterm infants who served as their own controls for breastfeeding and bottle feeding had more stable measures of $TCPO_2$ and body temperature during breastfeeding than during bottle feedings. These data suggest that the more stable patterns of oxygenation for breastfeeding than for bottle feeding are a result of less interruption of breathing during breastfeeding.

Source: Riordan, J., and Auerback, K. 1999. Breastfeeding and Human Lactation 2nd ed. Sudbury, MA: Jones and Bartlett, 449–481. Guidelines for Breastfeeding the Preterm Infant in NICU courtesy Barbara Ford, RN, IBCLC.

EXHIBIT 4–10 Guidelines for Feeding Expressed Breast Milk to Infants in the NICU

Be aware that various methods of infant feeding have implications regarding breastfeeding. Some methods make breastfeeding more difficult for the mother/infant dyad. Proper handling of breastmilk enhances the unique benefits of breastmilk for the preterm infant. Frozen expressed breastmilk retains many important antibodies, and is nutritionally superior to commercial formula for feeding of preterm infants.

Suggested process for obtaining optimal benefits of mother's milk:

1. Check container to verify name and integrity of container.
2. When using frozen expressed milk use oldest milk first.
3. To thaw
   a. Rapid thawing may be done either by holding the bottle of milk under cool or lukewarm running tap water or by allowing milk containers to stand in warm water until thawed. The water level should not touch the bottle cap.
   b. Basins of warming or thawing milk should never be left in the sink where they may become contaminated.
   c. Bottle warmers using dry heat may be used according to manufacturer's instructions. Settings should not overheat the milk. Human milk should only be warmed to body temperature. Gentle swirling is also recommended to re-suspend fats.
   d. To avoid using the wrong milk, milk for each infant should be thawed and warmed separately.
4. When gavage feeding with a pump, tilt the tip of the syringe at an upward angle. The fat rises to the top, allowing the rest of the milk to push the fat in first. This limits how much fat is lost along the lumen of the tubing and syringe.
5. Bolus feeding has benefits even in small amounts. Less nutrients and fats are lost if infusion is not spread over several hours. Bolus feeding reduces the threat of infection by infusing the milk over a shorter period of time.
6. If gavage feeding, offering a drop or two of expressed breast milk to baby's lips or on a pacifier stimulates the mouth to secrete amylase and other digestive enzymes. This helps promote digestion.
7. Coordinate Kangaroo Care with gavage feeding times so infant will associate the smell and touch of a caregiver (preferably mother) with nutritive satiation. Hold the infant in breastfeeding positions as he nears breastfeeding readiness.
8. Feed colostrum of breastmilk as the first feedings whenever possible to colonize the gut with "good" bacteria.

Source: Guidelines for Feeding Expressed Breastmilk to Infants in the NICU courtesy Barbara Ford, RN, IBCLC.

EXHIBIT 4–11 Collecting and Storing Breast Milk for the NICU Infant

Information for mother to properly collect and store her milk:

1. Wash hands thoroughly with soap and water when preparing to express milk and before handling milk collection equipment.
2. Wash the breast once a day during the bath or shower. No other breast cleaning is required.
3. Take care not to sneeze or cough on equipment.
4. Place collection devices on the breasts. Express milk for approximately and no more than 15 minutes at a session, 8–10 times a day. Go no longer than 6 hours at night without pumping.
5. Milk may be stored in several different containers. Glass, polycarbonate (clear, hard plastic), or polypropylene (cloudy, hard plastic) containers are recommended. Bags such as Medela CSF bags are acceptable.
6. In the first few days or if milk supply is low, mom may combine milk from more than one pumping, as long as it is collected in the same day. Chill milk before combining because pouring warm milk over cold milk can re-warm the first milk. Ask your baby's nurse to tell you how much milk to put in a container.
7. Label containers with the infant's name, time, and date of expression.
8. Expressed milk should be refrigerated immediately, within 1 hour of expressing.
9. Refrigerate or freeze milk until it is transported to the hospital for infant feedings. Milk that will not be used completely by 48 hours after expression should be frozen.
10. Pump kits (parts that come in contact with milk) should be taken apart and cleaned after each use with hot, soapy water, rinsed well, and air dried. At home, washing in a dishwasher is also acceptable. Pump parts may be placed in a rolling boil for 10 minutes one time a day if desired.
11. Transport expressed milk to the NICU in an insulated bag. If chilled milk will be used within 48 hours, mom may pack milk on ice. If transporting frozen milk, use freezer gel packs (not ice) to insure the frozen state. Since milk freezes at a lower temperature than water, the ice may thaw the milk somewhat.
12. When the mother arrives with refrigerated or frozen milk for her infant, the staff will ensure that the milk is correctly labeled.
13. Place the milk in the refrigerator or freezer.

Source: Collecting and Storing Breast Milk for the NICU Infant, courtesy of Barbara Ford, RN, IBCLC.

EXHIBIT 4–12   Process of Providing Breast Milk for the NICU Infant

Policy

Assistance and instruction will be offered to the mother of the NICU infant to provide expressed breastmilk, assuring that the infant will receive the optimum immunological and nutritional benefits of mother's milk.

Procedure

1. Mothers will be assisted by staff to begin pumping as soon as possible after delivery or when the baby is admitted to the NICU. Preferably this will occur within 6 hours if mother is medically stable.

2. It is crucial to stimulate the breasts early and often to establish an adequate milk supply and a bond when separated from the infant.

3. Mothers will be instructed in the proper collection of breastmilk for the NICU infant.

4. Mothers will be instructed in the proper storage and transportation of breastmilk for their NICU infant. Mothers will be provided with written instructions to take home regarding pumping, collection, and storage procedures.

5. Hospital pumps in the NICU area used by multiple mothers should be cleaned daily using a hospital-approved germicide. See infection control guidelines.

6. Staff will only accept milk that is properly labeled.

7. Freezers and refrigerators that store human milk should be plugged into the hospital emergency power supply (red plugs). If a red plug is not available the temperature will be checked when the power is restored.

8. Milk is to be stored at 40 degrees F. and the refrigerator shall have a thermometer contained inside and easily visible.

9. Milk should be thawed slowly to room temperature before feeding to infant. Microwave thawing is not allowed nor high temperatures of water as valuable nutrients are destroyed in the process.

10. It is recommended that milk refrigerators or freezers accessible to the public should have locks to protect against sabotage.

11. To avoid using the wrong milk, the container should be checked as when giving meds to verify correct patient identification.

12. The integrity of the container will be confirmed before feeding stored breastmilk to infants.

13. When possible, use colostrums or breastmilk for the first feedings.

Source: Process of Providing Expressed Breast Milk for the NICU Infant, courtesy of Barbara Ford, RN, IBCLC.

GRIEF

It is vital for healthcare professionals to understand the grieving process and their own reactions to profound loss. The feelings of powerlessness evoked in the presence of death and overwhelming grief take an emotional toll. People need humanizing responses in order to recuperate and restore their emotional balance.

Premature Birth

The birth of a premature infant is an acute emotional crisis. To establish a healthy relationship with their premature baby, parents must prepare for the possible death of the baby (anticipatory grief), acknowledge their failure to deliver a full-term infant, and learn the special needs of the premature baby.

The parents of a premature infant must face the fact that their child is less than perfect at the same time that they must accept the reality of the baby's early arrival. The earlier a pregnancy is interrupted, the greater the likelihood of a strong emotional reaction.

Congenital Anomalies

The parents of a baby born with a defect not only lose their anticipated perfect infant, but also are faced with a bereavement that endures indefinitely. In caring for families of the defective child, staff members must explain tests, allow time for ventilation of feelings and questions, discuss feelings, help parents prepare explanations for friends and relatives, and refer parents to public health and other community resources and to parent support groups. These parents require understanding, compassion, and education from healthcare professionals.

Death

Regardless of cultural background, the death of an infant can create an overwhelming crisis for parents. Grandparents, siblings, other family members, and friends may also mourn the loss. Dealing with fetal and infant death is not easy either for families or for their healthcare providers. When a fetus dies in the antepartum period, the mother often makes excuses for her baby's failure to move. When fetal death has been confirmed, she experiences anger and fear. The baby's father may have a difficult time understanding the reality of the fetal death because he had not felt the fetus move as the mother has. There is a time lag for paternal acceptance of both the pregnancy and the death because women have been found to attach earlier and more intensely to the fetus than men. This disparity of emotions can lead to problems between the parents (DiMarco, Menke, and McNamara, 2001).

When fetal death occurs during the intrapartum period, the purpose of the prenatal period is missing. These parents grieve over the loss of someone whom they have never had an opportunity to know. They grieve for the loss of an entire lifetime with their child.

Response to Death

Response to infant death is similar for parents and health-care professionals: (1) denial, (2) anger, (3) bargaining, (4) depression, and (5) acceptance, with an undercurrent of hope throughout. Factors that affect an individual's ability to deal with death include prior experience or education regarding death, the extent to which expectant parents believe that medical care is a safeguard against all complications, the availability of a support system, and the interpersonal communication skills of the people involved. Other factors that influence grief include cultural and ethnic heritage, religious beliefs, and the person's socialization and emotional development.

Physical symptoms of grief may range from loss of appetite and fatigue to aching arms. Many mothers talk of their arms "hurting" from not being able to hold their baby. Emotional symptoms of grief span a broad spectrum from guilt and depression to an all-encompassing sense of futility.

The Good Samaritan Hospital in Lebanon, Pennsylvania, has perinatal bereavement services. Their perinatal loss policy and procedure is reproduced in Exhibit 4-13. (See Appendix J for the full-page version of this exhibit.)

EXHIBIT 4–13   The Good Samaritan Hospital

Policy

It is the policy of The Maternity Unity to provide care to the family experiencing perinatal loss.

Procedure

It is the responsibility of all Nursing personnel to assist the family in the grief process. Nursing and Social Services must work closely in order to meet the requests of the family. If Social Services is not available, all concerns of the family are the responsibility of the nursing staff. Pronouncement of the death is the responsibility of the physician.

1. Initiate a Perinatal Loss Checklist as soon as it is evident that a fetal or neonatal death is imminent.

2. Begin a Perinatal Loss Admission folder providing complete chart including forms, death, and memorial certificates needed. Also found in folder, "When Hello Means Good Bye" should be given shortly after arrival on unit. Pink rose should be placed on patient door at this time. Place sympathy card in chart pocket. Nurses caring for the family may personally sign the nursing unit sympathy card. Address and place card in outgoing mail upon patient discharge.

3. Notify Social Service and/or Nursing Supervisor regarding the situation.

4. One-on-one nursing care prior to and in the initial hours following delivery should be followed whenever possible. The same nurse should be assigned to the patient whenever possible if her stay extends past 24 hours.

5. Select a Memento Memorial Box from bereavement supplies and place items to be used in photos in the box; i.e., baby ring, stuffed animal, baby block, and outfit.

6. Parents should be encouraged to see and hold their baby. The opportunity to have their baby remain in the crib at their bedside or held continually while family members visit is helpful in the grieving process. If they desire the baby to be removed from the room the body can be taken to the morgue or placed wrapped, on ice, and held in the soiled utility room until the family wants the body to hold again. In that case the body can be heated under an infant warmer for a few minutes to remove the ice/chilled feel of the body. Body must be picked up by the funeral home within 24 hours after delivery. Special attention should be given to not rush the family in their short time with their baby.

7. Offer parents the opportunity to bathe the baby or assist staff with the bathing and dressing of their baby. This can be done right on the mother's bed or bedside table to make it physically easier for her. Vaseline on a small piece of cotton or gauze can be placed in mouth and in nostrils if fluid is leaking from body.

8. Encourage parents to name their babies. Staff should refer to the baby by name whenever possible, i.e., "Would you like to help me bathe Michael?" Memorial Certificate should be completed and given to the patient before discharge from hospital.

9. Babies are to be dressed in an outfit provided by the family or by the hospital. Photos are to be taken by staff using a roll of film from the bereavement supply cabinet. In addition, a First Photo Bereavement Consent is obtained and First Photos are taken according to the directions.

   a. A consent is obtained—explain the package is free of charge and will arrive in approximately 3 weeks. White copy placed in package—yellow copy is placed on bulletin board in Assistant Clinical Manager's office—take care to include phone number on the yellow copy for follow-up.

   b. A new role of First Photo Film is used—up to 8 photos taken—enclose film and consent in preprinted package and place orange bereavement sticker on outer package.

Source: Perinatal Loss Policy and Procedure, courtesy of Good Samaritan Hospital, Lebanon, Pennsylvania. Reproduced with permission.

EXHIBIT 4–13 **The Good Samaritan Hospital** *continued*

    c. Mail same day.

    d. In the event a parent does not want the photos they are to be kept on file on the nursing unit for parents at a future date. While the First Photos require a consent—staff can take a roll of film for the family to later have access to. Family will be told the photos will be here for them if they desire them in the future.

10. Using film from the bereavement supplies closet, take photos of family members holding the baby and of the baby alone: dressed and at least two naked photos.

    a. Give special detail to using mementos that the family can later have to touch in remembrance of their baby i.e., stuffed animal, baby ring provided, baby block, door rose, offer to use wedding rings, religious medals or cross from mother. Return all items used in photos, including clothing and blanket to the mother's memorial/memento box.

    b. Take family photos that capture emotion.

    c. Refer to bereavement photo album for examples of how to take meaningful photos and what to avoid. There are instructions in the book.

11. Footprints:

    a. Plaster of paris and shells for an indented footprint: supplies in bereavement cabinet. Follow directions on plaster of paris container.

    b. When plaster print complete, place ink footprints on the identification certificate, the memorial certificate and inside the "memorial ring card" if it fits. (If having difficulty with the ink application on smooth feet, use the ink pad provided with the bereavement supplies—always do inking after the plaster print.

    c. Hand print can be alternative when necessary.

12. Lock of hair may be obtained if the parent desires some taken. Offer option to cut the hair themselves.

13. Infant ID bracelet: One on the body, one on the body wrap, and mother's on the foot print ID with baby footprints placed on permanent chart. Mother's signature obtained on Hollister ID. Mother may request infant ID from the funeral home.

14. Baptism of infant may be done by nurse, family, or minister/priest. See policy on Infant Baptism. Shell may be used to hold the water—holy water is in the bereavement supply cabinet. If a shell is used for water, place the shell in their memento box as a keepsake.

15. SHARE pamphlet should be given by staff in event Social Services is not available. This is in admission folder. Ask if SHARE may send them newsletters. If they say yes—check that their name may be placed on the mailing list on the perinatal loss check list.

    Ask if they would like a SHARE parent to contact them. Explain what SHARE is: a local group of parents who have experienced loss and support one another. Check appropriate space on perinatal loss check list and contact SHARE parent whose number is listed in the rolodex under SHARE parents.

16. Funeral arrangements must be made for every infant over 16 weeks gestation. The parents should select the funeral home. Suggest they ask older relatives for assistance with this task if having difficulty with a decision. Information about "Baby Land" located in Annville where the burial plot is at no cost to parents is also available in bereavement notebook.

    a. Some families desire to build their own casket. By Pennsylvania Law the body must first be treated with a chemical. Families can provide their own casket but the body will need to be treated and the death certificate filed by a funeral home. See Bereavement notebook on this topic.

17. Physician is responsible to discuss the option of autopsy and genetic studies with the family. Do not place infant and placenta in formalin if autopsy requested. Autopsy permits are on file in the nurse's station. If under 16 weeks a consent does not need to be signed; send placenta with the fetus and a pathology slip and notify the pathology lab. If greater than 16 weeks, send the fetus, the placenta, and lab slip and consent to the lab together. Also complete laboratory slips for chromosome analysis. Specimens for the chromosome analysis are to be obtained by the physician and placed in Hanks solution (found in OB med room refrigerator). Contact lab if no solution on unit prior to delivery. It is the responsibility of the lab pathologist to notify the funeral director when the autopsy is completed. The death certificate must accompany any fetus (16 weeks or greater) when sent for autopsy.

18. Patient is given option to transfer off the maternity unit. Pink rose placed on door again at time of transfer. May hold baby again on med-surg if she transfers. Refer to #5.

19. Provide family with as much privacy as possible. Unlimited visiting for family members as the parents desire. Encourage spouse to spend the night with patient. Family may have baby with them as long as they desire during the 24 hours period prior to leaving for funeral home.

20. A green fetal death certificate is completed on all stillborns of 16 weeks gestation or greater. Copy placed on mother's chart. A regular Death Certificate is completed if the infant is born alive in addition to a birth certificate. See policy on Fetal Death Certificates. A copy is placed on the infant chart and the original accompanies the body to the morgue and funeral home.

21. The Delaware Transplant Program must be notified of every stillborn and infant death. This can be done by the unit coordinator or the supervisor. Notify coroner's office in accordance with Pennsylvania Law.

EXHIBIT 4–13   The Good Samaritan Hospital *continued*

22. All mementos are given to parent to take home. If parents do not desire to take the mementos, they are kept in storage on the maternity unit and offered again at a later date. Mementos are kept indefinitely.

23. Infant measurements—weight, length, head, and chest circumference—should be obtained and recorded on the delivery record. If an infant death occurs after 24 hours of age these measurements should be redone at that time and recorded on infant chart.

24. Preparing for the morgue: Undress baby and return the clothing to the parents. Baby should have ID bracelet on arm or leg. Wrap baby in a hospital baby blanket and then a blue Denison wrap. Affix label with baby name to the outside wrap. Use addressograph with mother's name if none available for baby. Mark label with mother's name, date, and sex of baby if known. Tape second ID bracelet to outer wrap securely.

25. Notify Security to meet you at the morgue. Log the baby name in the morgue log book. Security will assist you with this task. Place body in the cold closet along with the death certificate. Call funeral home to notify them the body is now in the morgue ready for release. Do not call funeral home for release if the parents are planning to hold the baby again before discharge.

26. Review discharge instructions found in perinatal loss admission folder with parent prior to discharge. DO NOT give the standard "New Beginnings" DC booklet.

27. Document all pertinent information regarding the infant's death in Nurses' Notes.

　a. Date and time that heart rate and respirations ceased.

　b. Date and time that physician was notified of same if not present.

　c. Date and time that physician pronounced infant death.

　d. Disposition of body:

　　1. Date and time to morgue or lab.

　　2. Date, time, and name of funeral home if pick-up time known.

　e. Infant care given prior to disposition.

　f. Parent contact, interventions, and outcome.

28. Return any personal items belonging to parents and document the same, i.e., cross necklace used for photos.

29. All portions of the Perinatal Loss Checklist should be as complete as possible. Perinatal Loss Checklist should remain on the mother's chart so communication of all interventions is clear to all staff members in regard to interventions complete and those still needing completion. Information documented on the checklist does not need to be documented a second time in the nurses' notes. Include additional information not placed on checklist in nurses' notes.

　a. Copy of Perinatal Loss Checklist to be placed in the Bereavement Notebook.

　b. Copy of Perinatal Loss Checklist is to be sent to Social Services: "attention Ginger" on inter-hospital mail envelope.

30. Maternity Phone Call follow-up sheet should be placed in bereavement follow-up notebook for staff person assigned to grief follow-up to use to call patient after discharge from hospital. When call is completed, white copy is sent to medical record for permanent chart, pink copy to physician's office, yellow copy remains in bereavement book.

Children and Death

Although there are many variables in a child's concept of death, it is possible to identify some common childhood reactions to the dying process. Death has the least significance to infants under 6 months of age. Although toddlers cannot conceptualize death, separation creates anxiety for them. Between the ages of 2 and 7, children think in concrete concepts. For example, they may believe that lying very still equates with dying while moving around again means life. Early school-aged children find it difficult to differentiate between wishes and what really happens ("I wished that he would die . . . and he did, so I killed him.") When dealing with families of dying infants, it is important to include siblings, because they also need help to cope with their grief.

Helping Families

Healthcare providers can listen to the grieving family, anticipate their needs, and help them with decision making. As families regain a sense of control, they are better able to acknowledge and accept their loss. Parents can be encouraged to see and hold and spend time alone with their baby. They need to be given information on burial options, autopsy, and grieving (Cohen, 2001).

Providing mementos or keepsakes for families, such as bracelets worn by the baby, hand- and footprints, and photos or locks of hair can serve as tokens of remembrance and assign meaning to the experience (Alexander, 2001).

Referrals to support groups and mental health practitioners should be made as needed. Just being there to support the parents and expressing sympathy through touch and nonverbal emotions can be very helpful. A telephone call or home visit after hospital discharge is important in order to determine how things are going once everyone is home.

Support Groups

Throughout the United States there are volunteer groups of parents who have lost an infant and want to help other families in their time of crisis. These volunteers can speak from experience as they provide reassurance and information concerning the emotions involved in the grieving process. They offer individual visits to bereaved parents, monthly group meetings to share experiences and support each other, telephone or in-hospital visits, resource libraries, in-service seminars for professionals, and training programs for their volunteers.

Grief is a very individualized emotion, and not all individuals may benefit from a support group. When suggesting a support group, timing and a caring approach are essential (DiMarco, Menke, and McNamara, 2001).

CHAPTER SUMMARY

High-risk families need family-centered care as much or more than families with normal pregnancies. Stresses that occur normally in pregnancy are more intense in the high-risk situation. Feelings of failure and fear of the uncertain outcome of pregnancy can create anxiety for these childbearing families.

Antepartum hospitalization and pregnancy after perinatal loss bring their own unique stressors. In each of these circumstances, emotional support and active listening are essential to meet the needs of all family members.

Care of parents experiencing a cesarean birth should be family centered rather than surgery centered. The presence of the father or support person at a cesarean birth can improve the post-cesarean behavioral responses of families.

The goal of family-centered neonatal intensive care is to send a well baby home as a family member, not as a stranger. In family-centered neonatal intensive care units (NICUs), developmental care of the neonate is practiced with developmental care principles incorporated into day-to-day operations. Breastfeeding the NICU infant is encouraged, and evidence-based management strategies are used to achieve success.

Helping families through the grief process may be the biggest challenge in family-centered maternity care. People need humanizing responses to recuperate and restore their emotional balance.

FACILITY FEATURES FOR FAMILY-CENTERED CARE FOR PREGNANCY, LABOR, BIRTH, AND BABIES AT RISK

Facility design for care of high-risk mothers and babies provides a safe environment for medically fragile mothers and babies. The design must provide:

- security and privacy
- space for family members
- space for staff

NICU

Promote family-centered care:

- Provide a welcoming, comfortable, home-like setting and decrease visiting restrictions

- Provide family support spaces, including a waiting area, overnight transition room, and lactation room:
  - Cupboards for parent belongings.
- Provide family space and privacy at each infant's bedside, and provide upholstered stools and rockers or recliners:
  - Minimum dedicated floor space for each NICU bed should be 120 square feet.
- If possible, provide neonatal care in single rooms.
- Provide "nesting rooms" for families of preterm or sick babies to remain overnight for instruction prior to discharge.
- Provide support areas for families:
  - kitchen
  - lockers
  - bathroom facilities
  - breastfeeding rooms
  - sibling play areas

Provide a developmentally supportive environment for infants:

- Move sickest babies away from doors, sinks, and phones
- Decrease overall light levels
- Respect quiet at night
- Include day–night cycling of natural light
- Provide individually controlled light at each bed space
- Decrease noise level to 50 db or less:
  - Use visual alarms in conjunction with low-level audible alarms.
  - Put pagers on vibrate mode.
  - Insulate the walls, floors, and ceilings.
  - Install carpeting to absorb sound.
  - Use noise-reducing ceiling tiles.
  - Protect the incubator tops with thick cloths.
  - Don't play radios or CDs.

Reduce stress and improve efficiency of caregivers:

- Provide a workstation within the NICU.
- Provide a staff lounge.
- Provide an efficient, organized space for staff at each infant's bedside:
  - wireless communication systems
  - charting at the bedside
- Provide private rooms for babies if possible.

COMPONENTS OF FAMILY-CENTERED CARE FOR PREGNANCY, LABOR, BIRTH, AND BABIES AT RISK

The following components of family-centered care for pregnancy, labor, birth, and babies at risk are designed to support the family through a very stressful experience.

After Cesarean Birth

- There is no separation of the baby from the mother unless medically indicated or desired by the mother.
- Women having cesarean birth may see and touch/hold their babies immediately after birth unless contraindicated by the physical condition of either mother or baby.
- Family members and support persons are not separated from the mother and baby during the recovery period.
- Breastfeeding mothers are encouraged to initiate breastfeeding immediately after birth unless contraindicated by the physical condition of either mother or baby.
- Women having a cesarean birth are routinely given the option of conduction anesthesia in order to be awake for the delivery.

Postpartum

Individualization of Care/Options Offered for Special Care Needs
If the baby is transferred to another hospital:

- The mother/parents see and touch the baby before they are separated.
- If possible, a family member accompanies the infant.
- A picture is taken of the infant before transfer and given to the mother/parents.
- The mother/family is given the name of a contact person and telephone number at the hospital to which the infant is being transferred, from whom information, support, and education can be obtained.
- Specific procedures for communication between health-care professionals at the two hospitals are established, which will provide continuity of care for both baby and mother/family.
- The case is reviewed to ascertain if the neonatal outcome could have been anticipated and in-utero transfer achieved as the preferred practice whenever possible.

Women who give up their babies for adoption:

- Are encouraged to see and hold their baby.
- Are assisted with their plans:
  - for the baby
  - for themselves
- Are assisted in their grief process.

There is a written, planned, family-centered follow-up program for mothers in the following groups:

- Baby died in the hospital or was stillborn.
- Baby was in the Neonatal Intensive Care Unit.
- Baby was transferred to another hospital.
- Baby was born with congenital anomalies.
- In-hospital assessment revealed risk for maternal neglect or child abuse.

If the baby is in the Neonatal Intensive Care Unit:

- Techniques are used to personalize the baby.
- Parents are encouraged to visit at any time.
  - rooming-in for either father or mother if possible
- Siblings and grandparents are encouraged to visit.
- Parents are encouraged to participate in:
  - feeding their baby
  - daily care of their infant
  - decision-making regarding the care of their child
- Continuity of the professionals giving care to the baby is provided.
- Mothers are assisted in obtaining, storing, and delivering their breastmilk.
- Mothers are encouraged to verbalize their fears, guilt, doubts, grief, joys, and learning needs.
- Referral to appropriate support groups is offered to the woman/family.
- Social services are offered to the woman/family as appropriate.
- Assistance is given in locating affordable overnight accommodations when parents are from a distance.
- Prior to discharge:
  - a home assessment is done, if needed
  - parents have mastered necessary care-taking skills
  - in-hospital rooming-in is available for learning care-taking skills needed in the home setting

If the baby is stillborn or dies in the hospital:

- Opportunity is provided for:
  - privacy for the woman/family to hold their baby while he/she dies and grieve
  - seeing, holding, and touching their baby
  - taking pictures of their baby
  - having their baby's identification items and other keepsakes/mementos
  - explanations of their baby's birth and death
  - the mother and father or support person to be together day and night as desired
- The woman is given her choice of remaining on the maternity unit or being moved to another unit.

- There is a marker on the woman's door that indicates a death has occurred.
- Help is provided regarding:
  - naming their baby
  - baptism or other religious rite
  - autopsy
  - cremation or burial
  - funeral or memorial service
  - grief process
- Referral to grief support groups is offered the woman/family.
- Autopsy permits and cremation forms are worded sensitively.

BIBLIOGRAPHY

Alexander, K. 2001. The one thing you can never take away: Perinatal bereavement photographs. *The American Journal of Maternal/Child Care Nursing* 26, no. 3: 123–127.

Als, H. 1992. Individualized, family-focused developmental care for the very low-birthweight preterm infant in the NICU. In Friedman, S. L., and Sigman, M. D. (Eds.) *Advances in applied developmental psychology*, vol. 6: *The Psychological Development of Low-Birthweight Children.* Norwood, NJ: Ablex Publishing Company: 341–388.

Als, H., et al. 1986. Individualized behavioral and environmental care for the very low birth weight preterm infant at high risk for bronchopulmonary dysplasia: Neonatal intensive care unit and developmental outcome. *Pediatrics* 78: 1123–1132.

American Academy of Pediatrics and American College of Obstetricians and Gynecologists. 1997. *Guidelines for Perinatal Care.* 3rd ed. Washington, DC: Author.

Anderson, G. C. 1991. Current knowledge about skin-to-skin (kangaroo) care for preterm infants. *Journal of Perinatology* 11, no. 3: 216–226.

Arnold, L. 1999. *Recommendations for Collection, Storage, and Handling of Mother's Milk for Her Own Infant in the Hospital Setting.* 3rd ed. Denver: The Human Milk Banking Association of America, Inc.

Ashbaugh, J., Leick-Rude, M., and Kilbride, H. 1999. Developmental care teams in the neonatal intensive care unit: Survey on current status. *Journal of Perinatology* 19, no. 1: 48–52.

Athena Healthcare Communications, Inc. 1998. *Models of Care* 1: no. 2. Available online: www.modelsofcare.com.

Ballweg, D. 2001. Implementing developmentally supportive family-centered care in the newborn intensive care unit as a quality improvement initiative. *Journal of Perinatal and Neonatal Nursing* 15, no. 3: 58–73.

Beck, C. T., et al. 2000. Postpartum depression screening scale: Development and psychomatic testing. *Nursing Research* 49, no. 5: 272–282.

Bialoskurski, M., Cox, C., and Hayes, J. 1999. The nature of attachment in a neonatal intensive care unit. *Journal of Perinatal and Neonatal Nursing* 13, no. 1: 66–77.

Biancuzzo, M. 1999. *Breastfeeding the Newborn: Clinical Strategies for Nurses.* St. Louis, MO: Mosby, Inc.

Brosco, J. 1999. The early history of the infant mortality rate in America: A reflection upon the past and a prophecy of the future. *Pediatrics* 103, no. 2: 478–484.

Brown, P., and Taquino, L. T. 2001. Designing and delivering neonatal care in single rooms. *Journal of Perinatal and Neonatal Nursing* 15, no. 1: 68–83.

Campbell, L., and Hart, M. 1994. A need for childbirth preparation program for hospitalized antepartum patients. *International Journal of Childbirth Education* 9, no. 3: 20–21.

Cohen, J. 2001. From grief to action: Meeting the needs of bereaved families. *AWHONN Lifelines* 5, no. 1: 11–13.

Committee to Establish Recommended Standards for Newborn ICU Design. 1999. Recommended standards for newborn ICU design. Report of the fourth consensus conference on Newborn ICU design, January 28–30, 1996, Clearwater Beach, Florida.

Côté-Arsenault, D., Bidlack, D., and Humm, A. 2001. Women's emotions and concerns during pregnancy following perinatal loss. *American Journal of Maternal Child Health* 26, no. 3: 128–134.

Cunningham, E. 2001. Coping with bed rest: Moving toward research-based nursing interventions. *AWHONN Lifelines* 5, no. 5: 51–55.

Curtin, S., Kozak, L., and Gregory, K. 2000. U.S. cesarean and VBAC rates stalled in the mid-1990s. *Birth* 27, no. 1: 54–57.

DiMarco, M., Menke, E., and McNamara, T. 2001. Evaluating a support group for perinatal loss. *The American Journal of Maternal/Child Nursing* 26, no. 3: 135–140.

Dobbins, N., Bohlig, C., and Sutphen, J. 1994. Partners in growth: Implementing family-centered changes in the neonatal intensive care unit. *Children's Health Care* 23, no. 2: 115–126.

Engler, A.J., et al. 2002. Kangaroo care: National survey of practice, knowledge, barriers, and perceptions. *American Journal of Maternal Child Nursing* 27, no. 3: 146–152.

Enkin, M., Keirse, M., and Chalmers, I., eds. 1992. *A Guide to Effective Care in Pregnancy and Childbirth.* Oxford: Oxford University Press.

Epps, S., and Nowak, T. 1998. Parental perception of neonatal extracorporeal membrane oxygenation. *Children's Health Care* 27, no. 4: 215–230.

Fenwick, J., Barclay, L., and Schmied, V. 1999. Activities and interactions in Level II nurseries: A report on an ethnographic study. *Journal of Perinatal and Neonatal Nursing* 13, no. 1: 53–65.

Fleschler, R., Knight, S., and Ray, G. 2001. Severity and risk adjusting relating to obstetric outcomes, DRQ assignment, and reimbursement. *Journal of Obstetric, Gynecologic, and Neonatal Nursing* 30, no. 1: 98–109.

Föhe, K., Kropf, S., and Avenarius, S. 2000. Skin-to-skin contact improves gas exchange in premature infants. *Journal of Perinatology* 5: 311–315.

Gretebeck, R., Shaffer, D., and Bishop-Kurylo, D. 1998. Clinical pathways for family-oriented developmental care in the intensive care nursery. *Journal of Perinatal and Neonatal Nursing* 12, no. 1: 70–80.

Gupton, A., Heaman, M., and Cheung, L. 2001. Complicated and uncomplicated pregnancies: Women's perception of risk. *Journal of Obstetric, Gynecologic, and Neonatal Nursing* 30, no. 2: 192–201.

Harrison, H. 1993. The principles for family-centered neonatal care. *Pediatrics* 92, no. 5: 643–650.

Health Canada. 2000. *Family-Centered Maternity and Newborn Care: National Guidelines*. Ottawa: Minister of Public Works and Government Services.

Heaman, M, Sprague, A., and Stewart, P. 2001. Reducing the preterm birth rate: A population health strategy. *Journal of Obstetric, Gynecologic, and Neonatal Nursing* 30, no. 1: 20–29.

Hughes, M., McCollum, J., Sheftel, D., and Sanchez, G. 1994. How parents cope with the experience of neonatal intensive care. *Children's Health Care* 23, no. 1: 1–14.

International Lactation Consultant Association (ILCA). 1999. Evidence-based guidelines for breastfeeding management during the first fourteen days. April, 12, 20.

Katz, A. 2001. Waiting for something to happen: Hospitalization with placenta previa. *Birth* 28, no. 3: 186–191.

Ludington-Hoe, S., and Swinth, J. 1996. Developmental aspects of kangaroo care. *Journal of Obstetric, Gynecologic, and Neonatal Nursing* 25, no. 5: 691–703.

Maloni, J., Brezinski-Tomasi, J., and Johnson, L. 2001. Antepartum bed rest: Effect upon the family. *Journal of Obstetric, Gynecologic, and Neonatal Nursing* 30, no. 2: 165–173.

Maloni, J., and Ponder, B. 1997. Father's experience of their partner's antepartum bed rest. *Image: Journal of Nursing Scholarship* 29, no. 2: 183–188.

Martin-Arafeh, J., Watson, C., and Baird, S. 1999. Promoting family-centered care in high risk pregnancy. *Journal of Perinatal and Neonatal Nursing* 13, no. 1: 27–42.

McGrath, J. 2001. Building relationships with families in the NICU: Exploring the guarded alliance. *Journal of Perinatal and Neonatal Nursing* 15, no. 3: 74–83.

Meier, P. P., Engstrom, J. L., Chrichton, C. L., Kavanaugh, K. L., Mangurten, H. H. 1994. A new scale of in-home test-weighing for mothers of preterm and high risk infants. *J. Hum Lact.* 10: 163–168.

Mellien, A. 2001. Incubators versus mother's arms: Baby temperature conservation in very-low-birth-weight premature infants. *Journal of Obstetric, Gynecologic, and Neonatal Nursing* 30, no. 2: 157–164.

National Fetal and Infant Mortality Review Program. 2001. *Fetal and Infant Mortality Review (FIMR): A Tool Communities Can Use to Identify and Address Issues Related to Health Disparity in Infant Outcomes*. Washington, DC: Author.

Nystrom, K., and Axelsson, K. 2002. Mothers' experience of being separated from their newborns. *Journal of Obstetric, Gynecologic, and Neonatal Nursing* 31, no. 3: 275–282.

Peters, K. 1999. Infant handling in the NICU: Does developmental care make a difference? An evaluative review of the literature. *Journal of Perinatal and Neonatal Nursing* 13, no. 3: 83–109.

Petryshen, P., Stevens, B., Hawkins, J., and Stewart, M. 1997. Comparing nursing costs for preterm infants receiving conventional vs. developmental care. *Nursing Economics* 15, no. 3: 138–145.

Reichert, J., Baron, M., and Fawcett, J. 1993. Changes in attitudes toward cesarean birth. *Journal of Obstetric, Gynecologic, and Neonatal Nursing* 22, no. 2: 159–167.

Riordan, J., and Auerbach, K. 1999. *Breastfeeding and human lactation*. 2nd ed. Sudbury, MA: Jones and Bartlett.

Samuelsson, M., Rådestad, I., and Segesten, K. 2001. A waste of life: Father's experience of losing a child before birth. *Birth* 28, no. 2: 124–130.

Sanford, D. 2002. Postpartum depression: The most frequent complication of childbirth. *International Journal of Childbirth Education* 17, no. 1: 10–13.

Thornburg, P. 2002. "Waiting" as experienced by women hospitalized during the antepartum period. *The American Journal of Maternal Child Nursing* 27, no. 4: 245–248.

Ventura, S., et al. 1999. Highlights of trends in pregnancies and pregnancy rates by outcome: Estimates for the United States, 1976–96. National Vital Statistics Reports, 47, no. 29: 1–9. Hyattsville, Maryland: National Center for Health Statistics.

Westrup, B., et al. 2000. A randomized, controlled trial to evaluate the effects of the newborn individualized developmental care and assessment program in a Swedish setting. *Pediatrics* 105, no. 1: 66–71.

CHAPTER FIVE

Family-Centered Mother–Baby Care

INTRODUCTION

In traditional maternity care mothers and babies are separated after birth. Mothers are cared for on a postpartum unit by nurses specializing in postpartum care, while babies are cared for in a well baby or central nursery by nurses specialized in nursery care. In this fragmented pattern of postpartum care the focus is on tasks such as regularly measuring and recording vital signs, administering medication, and tending to housekeeping duties as well as the daily hygiene of mother and baby. The pattern of care is more suitable for sick people than for new mothers.

Our Big Failure

Rubin observed some 25 years ago that the postpartum period was our big failure because care focused on "tasks" and little attention was paid to the psychosocial needs of mothers and their families (Rubin, 1975). This is still true in today's traditional maternity care. In these programs, postpartum care is often eclipsed by the attention given to labor and birth.

Postpartum Satisfaction Surveys

When evaluating traditional hospital nursing care, it is not unusual to find new mothers praising the care they received in labor and delivery, but then expressing disappointment in care they received postpartum. On postpartum satisfaction surveys, common comments include: "I seldom saw a nurse after the baby was born," or "I wasn't taught enough about care of myself or my baby," or "I had to ask again and again for my baby but the nurses were too busy to bring him to me from the nursery."

Lack of Respect and Follow-Up

At the same time that postpartum patient satisfaction surveys rank poorly next to labor and delivery, postpartum nurses often feel frustrated. With postpartum hospital stays of one to two days, there is little time for all the routine tasks and rituals of traditional postpartum and newborn care. Also, within the hospital system, postpartum nursing is not given as much respect as the nursing expertise required to deal with the faster paced labor and birth. The prevailing belief is that most new mothers are well and just resting, so there is little for a nurse to do. As a result, postpartum may be the first unit from which staff are pulled when there are personnel needs elsewhere in the hospital.

Extending beyond the brief period of postpartum care in hospitals, many women report not feeling themselves again until well into the first year after childbirth (Mercer, 1986). Assuming the new role of mother while resuming the demands of her past role is hard work and requires social support (McVeigh, 2000). Again, the traditional maternity program often fails at providing any support as new mothers are expected to leave the hospital and immediately care for themselves and their children with no follow-up from hospital to home.

MOTHER–BABY CARE

Family-centered maternity care recognizes the importance of the postpartum period for family formation. Postpartum begins about an hour after expulsion of the placenta and includes the following six weeks. This is a critical transitional time for a woman, her newborn, and her family on psychological, emotional, and social levels. Healthcare professionals play an important role in helping mother and baby safely through their physiologic transition. Of equal importance is the role that healthcare professionals play in helping the new mother transition to her new maternal identity, and also helping the new father and other family members transition to their new roles (Pridham et al., 1991).

Goals of Mother–Baby Care

In the provision of family-centered mother–baby care there are goals that change the care from a hospital focus to a family focus. These goals are to:

- Promote the health and well-being of the mother, newborn, and family.

- Observe the mother and newborn in order to identify maternal and neonatal complications.

- Provide professional assistance to the family during a time of great adjustment.

- Promote breastfeeding establishment and maintenance.

- Help the mother feel cared for, respected, confident, and capable about basic self- and newborn care.

- Send families home from the hospital having begun the process of forming a strong attachment with their new baby.

In order to develop the postpartum mother–baby program of care and achieve the above goals, all care providers must understand the rationale for changing from traditional postpartum and nursery care to mother–baby care. That rationale is grounded in the developmental work that lays down the foundation for healthy family relationships.

Developmental Tasks of Postpartum

The developmental tasks of postpartum include physical restoration; emotional exploration of pregnancy, birth, and role change; attachment work; assumption of the care-taking role; and redefinition of relationships within the family (Todd, 1996).

Physical Restoration (Mother) Following pregnancy and birth, a mother's reproductive system returns slowly to a nonpregnant state. Among the key aspects of this process are: the involution of the uterus, the release of lochia, and the healing of the vagina, cervix, and perineum. The process of physical adaptation affects all major body systems and the establishment (or suppression) of lactation. Many of the warning signs and complications of the postpartum period tend to appear in the first days and week after birth (AWHONN, 1996). According to the World Health Organization (WHO), care should include the prevention, detection, and early treatment of complications and disease and the provision of advice and services on breastfeeding, contraception, immunization, and maternal nutrition (WHO, 1998).

A fundamental need of a new mother is rest and recovery from the physical demands of pregnancy and the birth experience. She needs pampering: someone to care about her and her needs. A calm environment, comfortable bed, nourishment, a warm bath, and a back rub can go a long way in helping a new mother feel cared for and special.

Emotional Exploration The emotional exploration that follows birth is part of a complex psychological process that helps turn women into mothers and men into fathers. If a mother feels her labor and birth went well and hospital conditions were adequate for her needs, she is more likely to experience satisfaction in parenting and to have mental and physical energy to learn about infant and self-care (Rubin, 1984). Women and men need an opportunity to review their birth experience with the healthcare professionals who supported them during labor and birth. Such dialogue allows for resolution of any confusion or questions about what happened during the labor and birth. If the couple is feeling disappointed because the labor and birth did not proceed according to their expectations, they can express their feelings. Or, if they are pleased with how they handled labor and birth, those feelings can be affirmed. In this way new parents are able to come to closure on their labor and birth experience. Nonjudgmental support, communication, and active listening make an important contribution to parents' perception of how well labor and delivery went (Pridham et al., 1991), and subsequently to the couple's transition to parenting.

If the new parents participated in a childbirth preparation program, they also need the opportunity to share their birth experience with the teacher and classmates. Birth report forms are good forums for telling their birth story. Postpartum mom and baby or dad and baby groups offer other opportunities to talk about and work through any concerns about the birth experience.

At Gaston Memorial Hospital there is an ongoing "Mommy and Me" class held each week. Mothers bring their babies to class and share their experiences with other mothers. By observing babies similar in age to their own, mothers also learn about normal growth and development first-hand. A class schedule for the "Mommy and Me" program can be found in Exhibit 5-1.

In addition, postpartum groups can provide needed postnatal support systems. Men and women can explore the changes that pregnancy, birth, and parenthood have brought to their lives and the meaning of those changes. Interacting with others in their transition to parenthood reinforces parents' new roles and helps everyone involved make the major adaptive changes required.

At Moses Taylor Hospital in Scranton, Pennsylvania, "Baby & Me" groups for new parents and their babies are held several times each month. An examples of a class description is shown in Exhibit 5-2.

EXHIBIT 5–1   Class Schedule for a "Mommy and Me" Program

The Birthplace Gaston Memorial Hospital

Mommy and Me

Classes held each Wednesday morning 10:00–11:30 A.M.

The Birthplace classroom

March 28	Infant Massage
April 4	Infant CPR
April 11	Developmental Play
April 18	Postpartum Exercises
April 25	Community Day/Resources
May 2	Nutrition/Life as a New Mother
May 9	Infant Massage
May 16	Infant CPR
May 23	Developmental Play
May 30	Speech

Source: Class schedule courtesy of Gaston Memorial Hospital, Gastonia, North Carolina.

EXHIBIT 5–2   Class Description for a "Baby & Me" Program

Baby & Me: Group for New Parents and Their Babies

Join other new parents and babies from noon to 1:30 P.M. in our Family Waiting Lounge. You will be able to share both expected and unexpected changes your new baby has made in your life. Share encouragement, parenting tips, and concerns with other new parents. Develop friendships for yourself and your child. This informal group is free and includes discussion of such topics as: feeling overwhelmed and exhausted, infant care and development, body image, relationship changes, colic relief, sick care, infant massage, and other topics as decided by the group. A light lunch will be provided.

Source: Class description courtesy of Moses Taylor Hospital, Scranton, Pennsylvania.

In addition, parent–infant massage classes are conducted at Moses Taylor Hospital. Each series of classes consists of three sessions, held monthly. A description of these parent–infant massage classes can be found in Exhibit 5-3.

Attachment Work   Attachment is the process of forming an enduring bond between parents and babies (Todd, 1998). Attachment behaviors that occur postpartum are a continuation of a process that began during pregnancy, continues through birth, and grows over a lifetime.

Attachment work is what parents and babies do to get to know one another and form their own unique relationship.

EXHIBIT 5–3   Class Description for a Parent–Infant Massage Class

---

Parent-Infant Massage Classes
Come Join the Fun!

The Family Birthing Suite at Moses Taylor Hospital is now offering a series of classes on Infant Massage. Massage has many benefits for both infant and parents. It provides important tactile stimulation for babies, emotionally nourishes them, and helps to stimulate all physiologic systems. It helps relieve discomfort such as teething and colic. Infant massage can help babies learn to relax and sleep better.

Infant massage especially contains all the elements of bonding and helps parents to feel more confident in their role as parents. It also provides a special time for parents to relax and unwind after a busy day.

Source: Class description courtesy of Moses Taylor Hospital, Scranton, Pennsylvania.

Because the attachment process in the first hours and days of life is reciprocal and almost completely sensory in nature, the mother and baby must be together for attachment work to occur (Phillips and Fenwick, 2000; Todd, 2001). They must touch each other, sense and smell each other, and be close so the magic can happen.

Attachment is facilitated by skin-to-skin and eye contact, delay of certain "routine" procedures in the first hours after birth, early breastfeeding, and time immediately after birth for the parents to be alone with their baby. While holding their new babies skin-to-skin, fathers have said, "When he opens his eyes and looks at me, I think he knows me already." Other activities in the process of maternal–infant attachment include listening to one another, recognizing one another's odor, moving in rhythm with one another, and parents and babies giving each other feedback in response to stimulus.

Nonseparation of mother and baby from the moment of birth offers the best opportunity for attachment work to succeed. Separating parents and infants for any reason challenges attachment work. (See Figure 5-1.)

When care is provided in the mother–baby model, the care providers assist the parents in recognizing the normal behavior of their infant. Instructing the parents and other family members about the "unique characteristics" and state-related behavior of "their baby" makes the unpredictable infant more predictable (Todd, 1998, 2001).

Exhibit 5-4 is a sample policy/procedure to help nursing staff provide care that promotes bonding between parent and infant. (See Appendix J for the full-page version of the exhibit.)

Social support plays an important role in attachment (Blank et al., 1995). The presence of the father or other family member offers moral support that is very powerful in helping the mother's attachment process.

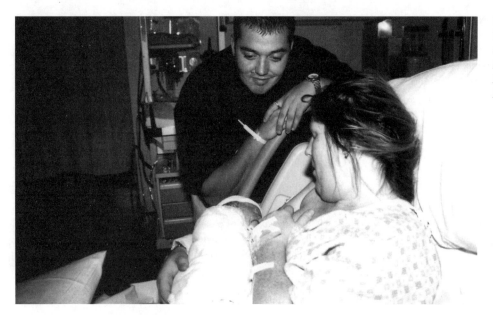

FIGURE 5–1 Within minutes of birth, the new family is becoming acquainted. *Source: Photo by Emily Pascoe, courtesy of Boston Medical Center, Boston, Massachusetts.*

EXHIBIT 5–4   Bonding between Parent and Infant

BONDING BETWEEN PARENT AND INFANT

Procedure

Promote healthy attachment between parent(s) and infant through careful interventions.

Policy

All unit staff will promote parent and infant bonding, a component of family-centered maternity care, at all times.

Equipment

Radiant warmer or warming light for the newborn.

Patient Education

Encourage questions and provide parenting education during the newborn assessment.

Implementation

I.   Encourage skin-to-skin contact with the mother immediately after the newborn's birth.

II.   Encourage support persons to interact with the newborn by touching, holding, and talking.

III.   Delay administering prophylactic eye medication until the initial bonding process has begun.

IV.   Encourage breastfeeding during the immediate recovery period as early feedings are optimal for breastfeeding success.

V.   Use the newborn admission assessment, dressing, and infant bathing as teaching opportunities. Explain all findings to the new parents.

VI.   Support the mother's caretaking efforts.

VII.   Provide mother-baby care for cesarean mothers at the bedside or return with the newborn from the holding nursery for frequent visits.

VIII. Assess bonding and document findings. Report potential maladaption to the charge nurse and infant care provider.

_____

VP Nursing

_____

Department Chair

Assuming the Caretaking Role Before a woman can assume the care-taking role, she goes through two phases of maternal tasks that are reflected in observable behaviors and attitudes: the taking-in phase and the taking-hold phase (Rubin, 1961). As first described by Rubin, the taking-in phase lasts for two to three days and the taking-hold phase begins on the third day and lasts approximately 10 days (Rubin, 1961). Nursing literature generally accepts Rubin's framework of "peripheral change"; however, the timelines for the changes have been found to be faster in the last decade. Data from Ament's study support a taking-in phase lasting only for the first 24 hours after delivery. The duration and peak of the taking-hold phase were not determined in this study (Ament, 1990). Cultural and personal habits and beliefs also affect each woman's psychological changes and therefore the following description of the three phases of the postpartum period is useful only as a relative guideline.

Three Phases of the Postpartum Period During the *taking-in phase*, which occurs in the first 24 hours after delivery (Ament, 1990), physical recovery is also occurring. The mother is passive and dependent, needing to be mothered herself. She is fatigued after the hard work of labor and needs nourishment, rest, and sleep. However, she also needs her new baby so that the attachment process can continue.

Following the taking-in phase, women go through the taking-hold and letting-go phases. It has been generally accepted that these phases last 3 to 14 days each. In the *taking-hold phase* the woman regains control over her body and assumes the mothering role. She has recovered her energy and again asserts her independence and autonomy.

In the *letting-go phase*, the woman establishes new maternal role patterns, incorporating the necessary changes in personal and family life. While centering on her baby and the baby's needs, she begins to return to her nonpregnant state.

For a woman to assume the caretaking role, she will need "mothering"—rest, nourishment, support, and lots of contact with her baby. This is a tremendous challenge for physicians and nursing staff. It requires a care model designed on the philosophy of FCMC. The traditional practice of focus on tasks will not provide what new mothers need from their caregivers.

Redefining Family Relationships The addition of a new baby to a family changes each family member's relationship with one another. Women may fear inadequacy, loss of marital intimacy, isolation, and constant responsibility of caring for the baby and others (WHO, 1998). Fathers and siblings may feel the loss of the mother's attention and affection. The father's sleep patterns may be disrupted causing fatigue and stress at work. Also, changes in the new mother's sexual availability may be disturbing to the new father. It has been found that men take on the identity of father more slowly than women take on the identity of mother. Supporting the new father as he gets to know his infant helps the baby become more "real" to him (White, 2002).

New parents have to cope with these changes in self, relationships, and routines while redefining relationships with parents and friends. Men become fathers and grandfathers. Women become mothers and grandmothers. Children become brothers and sisters, and numerous other roles change for family members and friends. As family members adjust to their new roles, they can benefit from the supporting solidarity of the family unit (Brazelton and Cramer, 1990).

This postpartum period is a magical time when individual people become families in their own unique way. Men and women of diverse cultural groups may demonstrate their own special behaviors and thus, caution must be taken in interpreting maternal and paternal behavior of different cultural groups. It is best to ask a family member or close friend of each mother about her unique cultural norms, because cultural variations may differ from textbook descriptions (Symanski, 1992).

THE MOTHER–BABY CARE MODEL

FCMC programs change the traditional practice of separating mothers and babies after birth. Instead, families are cared for as a unit. In order to facilitate the developmental tasks of postpartum, the model of care provided combines postpartum and nursery care into mother–baby care. The postpartum unit is replaced by a mother–baby unit designed to promote nonseparation of mothers and babies. The nursery is replaced by a much smaller baby holding or respite area. Some hospital staffs have named this space "the baby lounge."

Nursing Model

In order to provide mother–baby care, postpartum and nursery nurses are cross-trained to become mother–baby nurses. In mother–baby nursing, one nurse cares for both the new mother and her newborn as an interdependent couplet. Other family members are included in the care process as appropriate. Such an arrangement can avoid duplication of services and overlap of responsibility. Each nurse is assigned to care for three to four mother–baby couplets and is responsible for giving shift-to-shift reports on her mother–baby couplets.

The mother–baby nurse integrates the mother's and newborn's physical care with the education needed in both maternal self-care and care of the newborn. Attachment work is fostered through nonseparation of mother and baby. The mother–baby nurse role models and demonstrates infant care. In addition, the mother–baby nurse teaches parents about the state-related behavior of their unique baby.

Exhibit 5-5 is the Policy and Procedure for nursing care of a mother and newborn from Mercy Hospital in Fairfield, Ohio. The goal of the practice identified in this policy and procedure is nonseparation of mothers and babies in the postpartum period. An example of a maternal self-care instruction policy is shown in Exhibit 5-6. (See Appendix J for the full-page versions of these exhibits.)

EXHIBIT 5–5   Policy and Procedure for Nursing Care of a Mother and Newborn from Mercy Hospital

POLICY & PROCEDURE

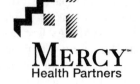

A general principle or plan that outlines expectations of a person or group in a defined situation, including a series of steps or a course of action used to complete the process and achieve an expected outcome.

MERCY™
Health Partners

START DATE: 5/96

REVIEW DATE: 10/04   **REVISED DATE:**   10/01

OWNERS: Women's and Children's Services

SCOPE OF CARE: Women's and Children's Services

TITLE: Mother Baby Care

PURPOSE: To provide standards for mother-baby nursing care from birth through discharge.

POLICY: Mother-baby couplet care is provided by the perinatal staff at the Mercy Family Birth Centers in accordance with national standards and within the framework of family-centered care.

PROCEDURE (steps/flowchart/decision algorithm)

I.   Recovery period/Transition: when possible, care is provided with minimal interruption of family bonding.

    A.   Maternal recovery—Recovery is complete when vital signs and assessments indicate the mother is stable

        1.   Reassemble bed, place in low position with side rails up and call light within reach.

        2.   Maternal vital signs and assessments are done every 15 minutes X 4, then 1 hour later.

            a.   Vital signs include: pulse, respirations, blood pressure, with a temperature X 1 during recovery. Vital signs are taken more frequently as indicated.

            b.   Fundus, lochia, and perineal status are assessed q 15 min. Also included during the recovery period are assessments of pain/comfort level, maternal infant attachment process, safety measures, IV, bladder, and effects of anesthesia.

        3.   Encourage every opportunity for parent-infant interaction and support early breastfeeding as appropriate.

        4.   Provide comfort/treatment measures as appropriate including warm blankets, ice to perineum, pain medication or medication for bleeding, bladder catheterization and the offering of food/fluids when patient is stable.

    B.   Newborn transition:

        1.   A TPR and assessment will be done at least 3 times with in the first 2 hours of life. This assessment will be done more frequently as indicated.

        2.   Complete newborn assessment. Complete gestational age assessment if there is a question of mom's dates, no prenatalcare, or dates inconsisitent with general newborn assessment.

        3.   Verify notification of newborn physician's office of birth, presence of risk factors and any abnormal findings.

        4.   Thermoregulation may be maintained by skin to skin contact, swaddling with warm blankets, or radiant warmer.

            a.   If radiant warmer is used: apply servo-control probe to the infant's abdomen, but not over liver.

Source: Courtesy of Mercy Hospital, Fairfield, Ohio. Reproduced with permission.

EXHIBIT 5–5   Policy and Procedure for Nursing Care of a Mother and Newborn from Mercy Hospital (*continued*)

Cover the tip of the probe with a temperature probe cover. Care must be taken to keep the thermometer probe in constant contact with the infant's skin.

b. Take axillary temperature when placing under the warmer and prior to removing from the warmer. Verify temperature rectally if axillary temperature is <97.6 or >99.6.

c. If the infant has a low temperature, set the servo-control to 36.5 (97.8). Axillary temperatures should be monitored frequently until temperature is normal.

d. The plexigalss sides of the bed should remain upright.

e. If the infant is repositioned, the temperature probe should be in direct line with the heat source.

f. Initial bath with soap may be given when infant's condition has stabilized and the axillary temperature is above 98.4.

　　1) Make every effort to minimize heat loss by giving the bath quickly and drying the infant thoroughly.

　　2) Assess temperature 30-60 minutes after the bath.

5. Glucose screen and Hematocrit screen per policy.

6. Newborn transitional period is complete when vital signs and assessments indicate newborn has stabilized.

II. Continued Care of Mother-Baby Couplet. ALL women receive THE BABYKIND GUIDE BOOKLET and this is used as a reference for specific teaching.

A. Maternal care following vaginal delivery (for care following Cesarean Delivery see Perioperative Care for Cesarean Patients policy)

1. After mother's condition has stabilized, nursing assessments and vital signs are done every 8 hours for duration of hospitalization. Assessments are done more frequently as indicated.

2. Educate the patient about good handwashing techiniques and the importance of handwashing after pericare, before caring for her infant, and after each infant's diaper change.

3. Perineal care

a. Instruct patient in appropriate perineal care and the use of a peribottle.

b. Methods of perineal pain reduction include cold packs, witch hazel pads, hydrocortisone cream, Epifoam and sitz baths. These methods may be used singularly or in combination to provide needed pain relief as ordered by physician/CNM.

c. Administer pain medication as needed.

4. Breast care

a. Breasts should be washed with water and a clean cloth daily during shower. No soap is necessary.

b. Breastfeeding mothers will be assessed for nipple irritation or breakdown and will be taught how to examine and care for her breasts during lactation (Refer to "Breastfeeding", and "Use and Cleaning of Breast Pumps" policies).

c. Educate non-lactating mothers on decreasing any stimulation of the breasts.

d. Discuss the engorgement process with patient.

5. Voiding

a. Assess the bladder frequently for distention along with assessment of fundus deviation

b. Offer bedpan if patient is unable to ambulate. When effects of anesthesia have worn off,

EXHIBIT 5–5   Policy and Procedure for Nursing Care of a Mother and Newborn from Mercy Hospital (*continued*)

encourage ambulation to bathroom with assistance.

    c. Educate patient on methods to promote voiding such as running water, pouring water over the vulva, or the use of sitz baths.

    d. Encourage patient's comfort level and administer pain medication (i.e. Ibuprofen) if patient has difficulty in voiding

    e. If patient remains unable to void, catheterize as ordered.

6. Rest

    a. Care including comfort measures, assessments and feedings.should be clustered when mother is awake

    b. Maternal rest should be encouraged and quiet periods protected.

7. Pain management continued as in recovery period.

B. Infant care

1. Nursing assessment and vital signs (TPR) are to be done every 4 hours X 24 hours and then every 8 hours thereafter.

2. Heat loss is minimized by dressing the infant with a hat, t-shirt and 2 blankets.

    a. If the infant's temperature is less than 97.6 with no extrinsic reason, methods to warm baby include wrapping in warm blankets, skin to skin contact or placing uncer radiant warmer. Reevaluate temperature hourly until above 98.

    b. If the infant"s temperature is above 99.6 wrap the infant loosely and reevaluate temperature hourly until 98.6. Evaluate maternal temperature.

    c. Notify physician of infants with a sustained decreased or elevated temperature.

3. Bathing: after the initial bath, an infant may be bathed with warm water every other day.

4. Weigh daily

5. Umbilical cord is to remain clean and dry. Remove cord clamp when cord is dry.

6. Infant feeding

    a. Breast feeding: place infant to breast as soon as possible after birth and then feed on demand (8-12 times in 24 hours). Refer to "Breastfeeding" Policy.

    b. Bottlefeeding: feed with preferred formula as soon as possible after birth and then feed on demand every 3-4 hours.

7. Infant identification

    a. Every infant should have two identification bands on.

    b. If for any reason the infant is taken out of the mother's room, her identification band and the infant's will be compared upon return of the infant to the room. (Refer to Safety, Identification and Security Policy)

8. If infant is to be circumcised refer to Circumcision policy.

9. Newborn Screening Test

    a. Infants discharged after 24 hours of age will have blood drawn prior to discharge.

    b. Infants discharged prior to 24 hours of age will have the initial Newborn Screen drawn before discharge and an additional Newborn Screen kit will be sent home with the parents. Instruct the parents to have the test repeated before the infant is two weeks of age.

10. Complete High Risk Hearing Questionnaire and make referrals as indicated.

EXHIBIT 5–5   **Policy and Procedure for Nursing Care of a Mother and Newborn from Mercy Hospital** (*continued*)

11. Assess infant for jaundice before discharge and draw specimen for bilirubin test if baby is jaundiced. Notify physician of results of test prior to discharge.

III. Discharge of Mother-Baby Couplet

A. Educational assessment

1. Have mother complete discharge instruction sheet and review the topics with her that she has identified.

2. Complete teaching sheet on mother and infant.

3. When possible include family members/significant others in teaching.

4. Have mother sign teaching sheet.

B. Verify before discharge:

1. Mother has "BabyKind Guide Booklet" and a copy of signed teaching sheet.

2. Mother has prescriptions.

3. Birth certificate Information sheet complete.

4. Photos are taken of baby.

5. Baby has voided and stooled.

6. Cord clamp has been removed if appropriate

7. Discharge orders are written for both mother and infant.

7. RhoGam has been given if candidate.

8. Rubella has been given as indicated.

9. Hearing Screening Questionnaire has been completed.

10. Second Newborn Screening form is provide if indicated.

11. Mother verifies understanding to have or make appointments with both her and infant's health care providers.

12. Mother's numbered band and one of Infant's matching bands removed and attached to baby's chart.

C. Each mother is discharged per wheelchair with infant in her arms.

1. The mother is wheeled tocar by hospital personnel.

2. Parents place the infant(s) in the car seat(s). (See Car Seat policy)

D. A discharge note is made on the mother's and infant's records which includes: time/date of discharge, how they were discharged, with whom they were discharged, and their condition upon discharge.

IV. Mother Discharged Prior to Infant:

A. Instruct mother to keep her infant identification band on.

B. Give the mother the nursery phone number and encourage parents to call and/or visit frequently.

C. Teaching sheet is placed on infant's chart for completion prior to infant's discharge.

V. Infant Discharge Separate From Mother:

A. Complete Social Service, Mother/baby home visit, and Public Health Referrals if indicated.

EXHIBIT 5–5   Policy and Procedure for Nursing Care of a Mother and Newborn from Mercy Hospital (*continued*)

B. Validate that educational assessment are complete (refer to teaching sheet). Have mother or other primary care giver sign the teaching sheet. Give copy of teaching sheet to care giver.

C. Verify identification of the person to whom the infant is:

1. Infant discharged to mother:

   a. Mother has identification bands: compare identifying information on both mother and infant; cut mother's numbered band, and a matching one from infant and attach to infant's chart.

   b. Mother does not have identification bands: verify identification of the mother with a picture ID; obtain driver's license number from the mother and document number in designated area; cut one band from infant and attach to the infant's chart.

2. Infant discharged to person other than mother:

   a. Have mother sign the Consent to Release Child Form (obtained from the Social Service Department)

   b. Verify identification of person infant being discharged to with a picture ID; obtain the driver's license number from the person and document in infant's chart.

   c. Hospital personnel will transport the infant from the unit to the outside front door.

VI. Mothers wishing to dismiss their infants against medical advice must sign release form. Every effort will be made to discourage this action. The Shift Lead, mother and infant health care providers, and Social Service/Discharge Planning Department. will be notified of parents considering this.

VII. **Documentation will include assessments, nursing interventions, and evaluation of care given.**

• **DESIRED OUTCOME:** Mothers and infants will receive comprehensive physical and psychological care with optimal opportunity for family bonding and attachment and will be appropriately discharged in stable condition.

• **PERSONNEL:** Physician, CNM, NNP, RN, PCA.

• **EXCEPTIONS:** Critical situations involving mother or neonate may not allow continuous mother-baby couplet care.

• **ADAPTATIONS:** This policy contains information previously held in Intrapartum Nusing Policy and replaces Infant Discharge Separate from Maternal Discharge Policy.

• **REFERENCES:**

American Academy of Pediatrics and American College of Obstetricians and Gynecologists (Eds.). (1997). *Guidelines for Perinatal Car*e, 4th Edition.

Egbert, Robin, and Peggy Foster, (2001). *The BabyKind Guide to Caring for You and Your Newborn Baby,* 2nd Edition. Cincinnati: Mercy Health Partners Greater Cincinnati.

Olds, Sally B., Marcia London, and Patricia Ladewig. (1999). *Maternal Newborn Nursing, A Family and Community Based Approach,* 6th Edition. New Jersey: Prentice-Hall Health.

Pilliterri, Adele. (1999). *Maternal and Child Health Nursing, Care of the Childbearing and Childrearing Family,* 3rd Edition. Philadelphia: Lippincott.

Simpson, Kathleen Rice, and Patricia A. Creehan. (2001). *Perinatal Nursing,* 2nd Edition AWHONN. Philadelphia: Lippincott.

• **DEFINITION OF TERMS: None**

EXHIBIT 5–6   *Breast Care for Breastfeeding Mothers*

BREAST CARE FOR BREASTFEEDING MOTHERS

Procedure

Support and educate the breastfeeding mother to help ensure that the newborn has an adequate supply of breast milk and that the risk of bacterial contamination is reduced.

Policy

Staff will provide all breastfeeding postpartum mothers with information on breast care, including information on the electric and/or manual breast pump, breast milk expression, and storage

Equipment

1. Non-toxic nipple cream (preferably containing lanolin), if ordered.
2. Electric breast pump and/or manual pump.
3. Warm compresses.
4. Ice packs.
5. Discharge teaching checklist.

Patient Education

Provide breastfeeding education and nursing support. Encourage and answer all questions. Document teaching on the discharge checklist.

Implementation

I. General breast care.

   A. Instruct the mother to wear a supportive bra immediately after delivery.

   B. Offer nipple cream with instructions on its use. Apply cream to the nipples and areolas after feeding and wipe off with a tissue before feeding (if toxic or infant refuses to nurse). Use sparingly.

   C. Instruct the mother to wash her breasts with warm water only. Avoid soaps or perfumes on the nipples to prevent cracking.

   D. Allow breasts to air-dry completely after feeding. Apply dry bra pads.

   E. Instruct the mother to apply warm compresses if her breasts become engorged. Massage her breasts prior to feeding. This will assist with milk expression and emptying.

II. Support needs.

   A. Initiate breastfeeding early.

   B. Assist the mother in correctly positioning the infant at her breast.

   C. Encourage a demand-feeding schedule.

   D. Do not offer the infant supplemental feedings unless medically indicated and/or ordered by the infant care provider.

   E. Teach the mother to use techniques to stimulate milk letdown: deep breaths, visualizing the infant, sensory stimulation such as baby items or baby smells. The nurse of the mother's partner may massage the mother's shoulders to enhance relaxation.

   F. Offer psychological support.

VP Nursing

Department Chair

It takes one nurse providing care to a mother and baby at the mother's bedside to optimize the limited time of hospitalization. Even if the baby is at the mother's bedside when a postpartum nurse cares for the mother and a nursery nurse cares for the baby, the subtle opportunities and interactions to facilitate attachment work can be missed. This shift in emphasis is often difficult because nurses are accustomed to being postpartum or nursery nurses. With experience, however, most nurses find increased satisfaction in becoming mother–baby nurses rather than being confined to a functional specialty. Mother–baby nurses claim that it is easier to provide couplet care than to provide separate postpartum and nursery care. They like the bond they establish with the families and feel they are closer to their patient than they were in the traditional system of care. The family, too, benefits from the continuity of care they receive during the postpartum period—care that may continue after discharge when the mother–baby nurse makes herself available via telephone or is able to visit the family at home.

Physician Model

Making the transition to mother–baby care can also be difficult for pediatricians. Historically, they have known the nursery as the place for infants, not the mother's room. There is often concern about the safety of the infant in the mother's room, as well as the perception that examining newborns at the mother's bedside may be too slow and "scattered."

The realities are that examining the infant and teaching the mother at the same time saves physicians' time. Mothers are encouraged to write down their questions when they occur to them and then ask their physician during the daily visit. Examining babies at the mother's bedside gives the mother the opportunity to ask questions of the physician and saves calls to the office with questions that could have been answered in the hospital. In addition, the newborn exam at the bedside stimulates some questions that the parents ordinarily might not ask. The physician can also be proactive and answer questions before they are even raised.

When mother–baby care is implemented successfully, physicians find that daily patient rounds are efficient and that they actually do not spend more time in hospital than they did prior to mother–baby care.

A well-designed care system with adequate lighting, equipment, patient and nurse locator boards, and documentation systems is essential. Of course, the most important part of the equation is well educated, skilled mother–baby nurses, capable of safely caring for mother and baby in the mother's room.

Myths about Mother–Baby Nursing

Critics of mother–baby nursing claim that the new mother will not be able to sleep with the baby in her room at night. The work of Keefe (1987) refutes that by demonstrating that mothers actually slept more soundly with their babies at their bedsides instead of in the nursery. In another study, when asked the cause of awakening from their first postpartum sleep, new mothers often identified that the nurse awakened them, not the baby (Lentz and Killien, 1991).

In the following excerpts of surveys of new mothers at Good Samaritan Hospital in Lebanon, Pennsylvania, the fallacy of this myth is exposed:

- Para 4 (age 34 years)
  "I liked having the baby with me. I will admit that I almost sent her to the nursery the first night cause I was so tired but she settled and slept well so it was fine anyway.

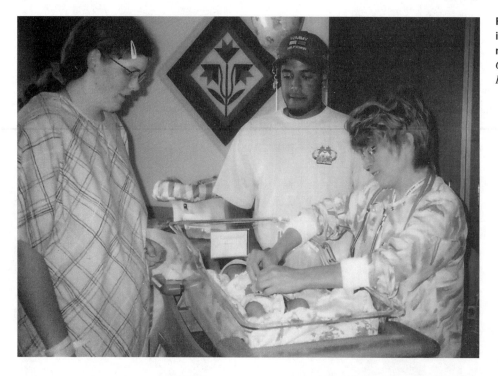

FIGURE 5–2 Parents reviewing infant care with their mother–baby nurse. *Source: Photo courtesy of Good Samaritan Hospital, Lebanon, Pennsylvania.*

I had a daughter in your hospital 12 years ago and this was a big difference. 12 years ago she was taken from me right after birth and I did not see her again for hours. When she came out it was just to feed. This was so much nicer this time."

- Para 3 (age 26 years)

"I liked having the baby with me a lot. Nights were not a problem. He ate then went right back to sleep."

- Para 1 (age 18 years)

"I loved having the baby right there. It was no problem having her in the room at night. I just enjoyed looking at her all the time—couldn't believe how wonderful she was."

- Para 2 (age 31 years)

"Having the baby with me went real well. I thought maybe this would be a problem when I realized the baby was going to stay with me, but it wasn't at all—actually I didn't want my baby to ever leave me when the times the baby was taken! I liked this stay better than my stay a few years ago—this way was actually easier because last time my baby came out just to breastfeed and you brought him. This time I fed my baby more frequently and now this time my breasts aren't as hard and I find I can deal with her better than my first one."

- Para 3 (age 29 years)

"Having the baby with me was wonderful. This was such a change from the last time. This was my mother's seventh grandchild and she so enjoyed holding the baby and spending time with the baby—she did not get to do that with the other grandchildren. Once in a while she got a close peek with the others but she did not get to hold them—she could only look at them through the glass window, so this was a real treat for my mother."

- Para 1 (age 26 years)

"I loved the baby with me. It was really nice. The one night she was fussy so I put her in bed with me and she stopped and slept right in my bed with me. I had great nurses they were the best. One night the baby kept fussing so my nurse took her out and cup fed her then brought her right back."

- Para 1 (age 15 years)

"It was good having the baby in the room all the time. Nights were good too. The first night he didn't like sleeping in the plastic box so I put him in bed with me—the nurse helped me. I kept him in the room all the time. My nurse let me watch the picture being taken and I picked the one I liked best. His blood work was done in my room."

- Para 9 (age 37 years)

I was impressed with everything! I was dreading coming in and having twins but it was wonderful. Everyone was so friendly. I loved having the babies stay right there with me. They were no problem at night and the nurses were a big help too. I thought it was nice that they stayed with me—after all you may as well get used to it right from the start."

Another myth about mother–baby care is that new mothers will want their babies in the nursery instead of their rooms because they will "want to rest." Consumer research consisting of both focus groups and telephone surveys of 5000 women over a 10-year period indicated that 85 percent of the women surveyed wanted their babies at their bedsides and preferred mother–baby nursing over the traditional separate postpartum and nursery care (Phillips and Fenwick, 2000).

And once again excerpts of surveys of new mothers at Good Samaritan Hospital help to dash this myth:

- Para 2 (age 22 years)

"This is the second baby I had at your hospital and I liked it this time a lot better. I loved having my baby in the room. Last hospital stay my son was on IV therapy for low blood sugar and I had to visit him in the nursery…he never came to my room so this was great having her right there by my side."

- Para 1 (age 19 years)

"I like having the baby with me. It went well. One night the baby cried a lot and my nurse took her out but then brought her back when she was asleep. I thought it went well."

- Para 4 (age 34 years)

"I really enjoyed having my baby in the room all the time. It was so different from three years ago when they just gave her to me for a short time. This was great and he was so good at night! I had no problems at all. My other children came in yesterday and checked him out head to toe in the hospital room and that was fun. The baby and I were not separated at all in the hospital."

- Para 1 (age 20 years)

"I was in such awe in the hospital. I could hardly believe she was actually here. Having her in my room helped reality hit me cause I couldn't pass her off to someone else I had to face learning how to take care of this baby. One night I asked the nurses to take her back to the nursery for the night. Later I woke up and felt like I had to go see her. I walked to the nursery and asked to have her back. Here I wanted her with me after all! I just felt better with her right there. It was a good experience."

Of course, babies cannot just be brought to new mothers' rooms and left there. In the prenatal period, the mother and family need preparation for mother–baby care and all the care they will receive in the hospital They will need an understanding and appreciation of the developmental tasks of postpartum and the importance of parent–infant interaction in the first days of life.

When admitted to the mother–baby unit, parents will need further explanation of the care model. Northeast Medical Center in Concord, North Carolina, distributes the welcome shown in Exhibit 5-7 to new parents on their mother/baby unit. This handout from Northeast Medical Center reinforces the importance of mother–baby care for family formation.

EXHIBIT 5–7   A Welcome to New Parents on the Mother/Baby Unit

---

NORTHEAST MEDICAL CENTER

"Supporting the Miracle of Life"

Welcome to the Mother–Baby Unit

We believe that having a baby is a family affair and that our services are best provided in a family-centered approach. Members of your family will be included in this experience as much as you desire. We are here to support, help and provide education to you and your family.

Most infants are able to remain in the Labor Delivery and Recovery Room with their families after birth. A nurse will assess both mother and infant and provide their care. Families will be included in the care of the infant from the moment of birth, as much as you want them to be involved. You and your infant will be moved together to the Mother–Baby Unit, where a mother–baby nurse will assume your care. Keeping the baby in your room helps to teach you and your family how to care for the baby and allows time for the many questions you have as a new (or experienced) parent. You learn about your baby's needs, responses and personality. Research tells us that bonding between the mother and the baby occurs through tactile means (hearing, seeing, touching, smelling). This is why it is important to both the mother and the baby to be physically close together. Having the nurse immediately available should reassure you that all your individual needs, physical, emotional and instructional, are being met by one nurse who knows you as a family unit.

In preparation for feeding or holding the infant, please wash your hands with soap and also have visitors wash their hands before holding the infant. Practice good hand-washing after toilet use, after using the sitz bath and after changing pads. Also, wash hands before and after applying medication to your breast, changing the baby's diaper or clothing or feeding your baby. This helps prevent transmission of infections to your baby.

Mothers who are breastfeeding will receive assistance and support from the staff and our lactation consultants. Your baby should nurse every 2–3 hours and on demand. If you choose to bottle feed, the nurse will give you formula of your choice in ready to feed bottles. The nipple should be attached just prior to feeding. It should remain clean and a fresh bottle should be used with each feeding. Please discard any bottles that have been open for more than an hour. Babies usually feed 6–8 times a day (about every 3–4 hours). Please record any feedings or diaper changes on the record supplied to you by the nurse.

For safety, please do not leave your baby unattended at any time. If for some reason you can not take care of your baby and you have no family or visitors with you, please let the nursing staff know and they will care for your infant. Please place your baby on its side or back in the bassinet when not being held. Research has proven that this reduces the incidence of Sudden Infant Death Syndrome (SIDS). For safety and security reasons, all babies must be in their crib if you are strolling the hallway.

We strongly encourage you not to smoke around your new baby. While you are here, an outdoor area has been provided for smoking. Please ask your nurse for directions. For the protection of you and your infant, we request that you not visit other units in the Family Center or main hospital while you are a patient here.

You will be asked for information by the registration clerk to prepare the official birth certificate. Mothers will be asked to verify and sign this birth certificate. If you have questions, the clerk will be happy to answer them for you.

A staff member from First Impressions will visit you in your room to discuss baby pictures. The pictures will be taken in your room and you will receive proofs immediately. After you choose the packet you wish to purchase, the pictures will be printed and ready for you before you go home. There is also a procedure for you to share the pictures with family and friends on a web site. Ask the photo representative for information. If you want your baby dressed in a special outfit for the picture, please bring it in and we will be sure the baby is dressed the way you wish. This also applies to special blankets, hats, etc. If you do not have a special outfit, the photo staff will provide a clean outfit for your baby to wear for the picture. We want your baby's first picture to be special!

Your baby's doctor will be coming to your room to examine your baby in the mornings and this will provide you with an opportunity to ask questions. Some of the doctors also have an office nurse who will make rounds and answer your questions.

We are pleased that you have selected us to provide your care at this special time in your life. Research and experience have clearly shown us how to promote and nurture happy, healthy families and this is our goal as providers of care to women and infants in our community. We are committed to Family Centered Maternity Care at Northeast Medical Center.

The Staff of the Maternity Center

Source: Northeast Medical Center, Concord, North Carolina. Reproduced with permission.

Benefits of Mother–Baby Care

In *A Guide to Effective Care in Pregnancy and Childbirth*, 3rd edition, a register of controlled trials in perinatal medicine covering data over more than the past 25 years, the authors found routine restriction of mother–infant care and routine nursery care for babies in hospitals to be an ineffective or harmful form of care, demonstrated by clear evidence (Enkin et al., 2000). (See Appendix B.) In contrast to the ineffective or harmful practice of restricting contact, mother–baby care provides many benefits to parents, hospitals, and staff. These benefits are summarized in Exhibits 5-8, 5-9, and 5-10.

Facility Design

In developing family-centered care, many hospitals are designing facilities and procedures whereby nurses can closely observe newborns without separating the babies from their parents. In situations where the maternity unit is designed in a separate Labor-Delivery-Recovery (LDR) Unit and a mother–baby unit, the baby stays with the mother in the

EXHIBIT 5–8 Benefits of Mother–Baby Nursing to Family and Baby

- Provides an environment for the parents to learn about their baby's responses and sleep-wake cycles.
- Facilitates earlier establishment of biologic rhythms with flexible feeding and sleeping according to individual baby's needs.
- Helps mother sleep better with baby at her side.
- Fosters successful breastfeeding and, thus, aids in postpartum involution.
- Decreases incidence of infant cross-infection.
- Provides individualized, one-to-one attention.
- Promotes the mother's role and bonding and attachment.
- Increases educational opportunities.
- Fosters continuity of care and reduction of confusion of messages between caregivers.
- Promotes the mother's learning about her infant and self-care capabilities.
- Increases maternal self-confidence in caring for her infant.
- Eliminates anxiety about whether the baby is receiving proper care. Mother knows quality of care because she sees it.
- Maintains high patient care standards.

Source: Harvey, 1982; Keefe, 1987; Mansell, 1984; Norr, Roberts, and Freese, 1989; Panwar, 1986; Vestal, 1982; Watters, 1985; Watters and Kristiansen, 1995; Wilkerson and Barrow, 1988.

EXHIBIT 5–9 Benefits of Mother–Baby Nursing to the Staff

- Increases skills and knowledge base, thus making nurses more marketable.
- Diversifies skills.
- Streamlines responsibilities for care and teaching.
- Increases nursing value to the hospital.
- Increases nurses' personal involvement and responsibility for patient care and self-learning.
- Increases accountability.
- Improves communication between family and caregivers.
- Replaces fragmented care with continuity of care.
- Eliminates duplication of services.
- Facilitates discharge planning.
- Increases efficiency and productivity.
- Improves interdisciplinary communication and teamwork.
- Increase job satisfaction through the provision of individualized care.
- Provides a more stimulating work environment.
- Elicits positive comments from families.
- Enhances image in the community due to family observation of professional skills.

Source: Harvey, 1982; Keefe, 1987; Mansell, 1984; Norr, Roberts, and Freese, 1989; Panwar, 1986; Vestal, 1982; Watters, 1985; Watters and Kristiansen, 1995; Wilkerson and Barrow, 1988.

EXHIBIT 5–10 Benefits of Mother–Baby Nursing to the Hospital

- Eliminates unnecessary rules and enhances support of justified institutional policies.
- Increases openness between community and hospital in assessing institutional quality and commitment to care.
- Improves image in the community.
- Increases favor for preventive approach to care for managed care contracts.
- Reduces nursing staff turnover through job enrichment.
- Increases staff productivity and flexibility and reduces costs.
- Adapts easily to individual family needs.
- Increases patient satisfaction.

Source: Harvey, 1982; Keefe, 1987; Mansell, 1984; Norr, Roberts, and Freese, 1989; Panwar, 1986; Vestal, 1982; Watters, 1985; Watters and Kristiansen, 1995; Wilkerson and Barrow, 1988.

LDR, and is assessed and cared for there for the first two hours. The baby is breastfed and snuggled with the mother for warmth, instead of lying in a warmer for several hours. The infant and mother are then transferred to the mother–baby unit together, where a mother–baby or couplet nurse cares for them. Infants who are grunting or retracting at delivery, or who have obvious problems that require immediate attention, are cared for in the holding area or special care nursery, if available.

Exhibit 5-11 is a copy of the newborn admission record used at Northeast Medical Center. The facility design is Labor-Delivery-Recovery Rooms (LDR) and a Mother–Baby Unit. Newborns are not separated from their mothers, thus, the nurse who supported the mother through labor and birth completes the newborn admission assessment in the LDR.

Daily shift assessments of the newborn are done at the mother's bedside as the nurse teaches. The documentation form used at Northeast Medical Center is shown in Exhibit 5-12.

In hospitals practicing single-room maternity care (SRMC), the baby remains with the mother and family after birth and does not have to leave the Labor-Delivery-Recovery-Postpartum (LDRP) room unless the baby needs special care (Phillips and Fenwick, 2000).

The LDRP room's temperature is maintained at a level that prevents excessive cooling of the infant, and the baby is dried and placed skin-to-skin on the mother's or father's chest, with a warm cover over them. A dry stockinette cap on the baby's head retards heat loss, as do warmed blankets and a warming light placed over mother (or father) and baby.

Staff can care for the baby in the mother's or father's arms. Nurses can place identification tags, determine Apgar scores, and inject medications while one parent holds the baby. If the infant is at risk, unstable, or requires a greater degree of physical attention, nurses can place an infant warmer next to the mother's bed. This allows the baby to be next to the mother, at the side of her bed, where she can observe her baby's care.

Cost Savings

Mother–baby nursing is a different way of thinking about care for families and is not merely a different way of organizing work for nurses. Mother–baby nursing offers a link between quality of care and cost containment. By practicing this form of nursing, professional time is optimized. In conventional, separate postpartum and nursery staffing, each staff member uses time and energy problem solving, only to find that the other group has begun a similar task. For example, on a questionnaire completed by postpartum staff members in one hospital, teaching basic newborn care was identified as a primary duty. The nurs-

ery staff identified teaching newborn care as their function, too. Thus, both groups were teaching this subject, with no mechanism to assure continuity. Similarly, documentation of the family's ability to care for the newborn and their reaction to the newborn was charted by both sets of nurses. Mother–baby nursing eliminates such redundancy and decreases the possibility of conflicting information being given.

Historically, census swings on obstetric units often result in staffing problems. When nursery and postpartum nurses are cross-trained, greater scheduling flexibility is possible. As a result, both decreased overtime and decreased reliance on supplemental staff are possible benefits to the facility. Cost savings are possible with mother–baby nursing because of increased nursing productivity. In addition, the potential for increased job satisfaction as nurses recognize challenges and rewards from their nursing care can account for savings in the human resources budget through reduced attrition and diminished need for orientation of new staff (Phillips, 1997).

Rooming-In

Rooming-in and mother–baby nursing are not the same care model. Rooming-in was begun in the 1940s as an alternative to separation of mothers and babies in postpartum units and nurseries. When the baby "roomed-in" with the mother (instead of being in the nursery), the parents had an opportunity to have their baby with them to the extent they wished.

Although preferred by many women and endorsed by professional organizations, rooming-in was only an option for new families. It did not become standard practice. Some families did not choose rooming-in because it required the mother to provide most of the infant's care when the baby was at her bedside. Because the postpartum nurse was not responsible for the baby, the mother would have to call on the nursery nurse to help her with infant care. At times when the nursery nurse was busy in the nursery and could not come to the mother's bedside, the mother might have to wait a long time for help or answers to her questions. This created stress for inexperienced new mothers, and thus they chose to stop rooming-in or did not request it at all.

Mother–baby care is not a program option. It is standard practice in FCMC and mother–baby, or couplet, nurses are available to care for mother and baby together day and night.

In mother–baby nursing, care plans are designed and implemented that are consistent with the new family's needs and values. In this way, mother–baby care can be provided for families with varying physical, social, and cultural needs.

EXHIBIT 5–11 Newborn Admission Record

_____ Die Cut Area! _____

Newborn Admission Record
(See also Newborn History and Physical Record and Delivery Record)

Date/time of Birth: ___ / ___ / ___ _____ Admitted to ☐ Mother/Baby ☐ Holding Nsy ☐ SCN

Sex: M F   NSVD Forcep   Vacuum   C/S: repeat primary   Mother's Blood Type: O A B AB Rh: + -   Breast   Bottle _____

Wt. ___ lbs. ___ oz. ___ gms. Length ___ in. ___ cm.	Group B Strep: NB Sepsis Algorithm Initiated ___ Yes ___ No
Head ___ in. ___ cm. Chest ___ in. ___ cm.	Dr./Office _____ notified @ _____ by _____

Gestational Age Assessment:

GA by dates: _____ weeks

NB age at time of exam: _____ hours of age

Infant is classified as:

☐ Term   ☐ AGA
☐ Preterm ☐ SGA
☐ Postterm ☐ LGA

Ballard if infant <2500 gms, >4082 gms, suspected IUGR, or by MD order

GA by Ballard: _____ weeks (See attached records for details)

Exam by: _____

GBS at one, two and three hours of age on all infants that are:

1. <37 weeks or >42 weeks gestation
2. SGA
3. LGA
4. Infant of a diabetic mother

☐ If result < 40 mgs %, initiate Hypoglycemia Algorithm

(Document on Graphic Record)

Dr. _____ notified of admission

☐ on rounds or @ _____ by _____

Initial Vital Signs: (Record on Graphic Record)

Time: _____ Rectal Temp: _____ Pulse _____ Resp _____ BP ___ / ___

Coombs Positive ☐ MD called with results at _____

RN Signature: _____

Initial Newborn Physical Assessment

✓ = consistent w/parameters   N = See notes   0 = N/A or not assessed

Alert, lusty cry, strong suck		No unusual pigmentation
Moves all extremities well		No skin tags
Good muscle tone, not jittery		No skin lesions
Reflexes WNL, symmetrical		Heart tones normal ∅ murmur
Ant. fontanel flat, sutures open		Regular cardiac rhythm
Molding: ∅. +mild/mod, ↑ marked		Femoral pulses +, equal
No caput		Normal bowel sounds
Eyes clear, not red, ∅ drainage		Abdomen soft, not distended
Ears normal, not low set		External genitalia normal for gestational age/sex
Face, neck normal		Anus patent
Palate intact		Male, both testes ↓ ↓
Breathing easily, rate WNL (30-60/min)		3 vessel cord
Lungs clear		Umbilicus clamped, no bleeding or herniation
Good equal breath sounds		Extremities normal, 5 digits each
Thorax normal		Spine normal, closed without dimples
Skin color appropriate, no jaundice		Joints/range of motion WNL
Skin intact		Neonatal infant pain score
No bruising/hematomas		

Assessment Completed By: _____ Time: _____

Medications:

Erythromycin Ophthalmic Ointment 1% to each eye within one hour of delivery.

Time: _____ RN: _____

Aqua Mephyton 1 mg IM R/L LT Time: _____ RN: _____

Newborn Risk Indicators Observable at Birth

☐ **NO RISK FACTORS NOTED**
☐ Abnormal Presentation   ☐ Mother c̄ + GBS
☐ Multiple birth   ☐ Pallor   ☐ Jaundice
☐ Low birth weight <2500 gms   ☐ Plethora
☐ 1 min APGAR <5   ☐ Seizures
☐ 5 min APGAR <7   ☐ Imperforate anus
☐ Placental abnormalities   ☐ Decreased tone
☐ Two vessel cord   ☐ Congenital malformation
☐ Grunting   ☐ Cephalhematoma
☐ Retractions   ☐ Other: _____
☐ < 37 weeks

INITIAL BATH – Bathe with soap when temp and condition stable

Temp prior to bath: _____ Bath given at: _____

by: _____

Temp 30-60 min post bath: _____ (Document all temps on graphic)

ADMISSION NOTES

NEONATAL INFANT PAIN SCALE (NIPS)

	Cry	Breathing Pattern	Arms	Legs	State of Arousal
0	No Cry	Relaxed	Relaxed/Restrained	Relaxed/Restrained	Sleeping/Awake
1	Whimper	Change in Pattern	Flexed/Extended Flexion	Flexed/Extended Flexion	Fussy
2	Vigorous Cry				

NORTHEAST
MEDICAL CENTER
Concord, NC

NEWBORN RECORD

7602279 (5/01)

TAB 12

Source: Courtesy of Northeast Medical Center, Concord, North Carolina. Reproduced with permission.

EXHIBIT 5–12   Daily Shift Assessment Form

NEWBORN ASSESSMENTS

SHIFT ASSESSMENTS	✓ = consistent w/parameters N = See notes 0 = N/A or not assessed									
	Date →									
	Time →									
Assessment	Alert, lusty cry, strong suck									
	Good muscle tone, not jittery									
	Eyes clear, not red, Ø drainage									
	Breathing easily, rate WNL (30-60/min)									
	Lungs clear, good equal breath sounds									
	Jaundice: Ø = none, sl = slight, mod = moderate									
	Skin intact, Ø bruises, or skin lesions									
	Heart tones normal, Ø murmur									
	Regular cardiac rhythm, rate WNL (110-160)									
	Abdomen soft, not distended									
	Anterior fontanel flat									
	Umbilical cord drying: Ø drainage, odor, redness									
	Neonatal infant pain score									
Bonding	M = Mother F = Father O = Other Family Members	Cuddles baby								
		Talks softly to baby								
		Participates in baby care								
Safety	ID bracelets x 2 / Security bracelet intact									
	Bulb syringe in crib									
	RN Initials →									

FEEDING OBSERVATIONS

	Date →											
	Time →											
Breast	Breast Feeding Rooting, latched on with flanged lips											
	Rhythmical suck, few pauses											
	Some audible swallows											
	Mother needs assistance											
	0 = None ✓ = 10-15 minutes ✓+ = 16-30 minutes ✓++ = > 30 minutes											
	Feeding not observed											
Bottle	Bottle Feeding Formula _____											
	Amount taken in ccs.											
	Fed by: M = Mother, N = Nurse, O = Other											
	Spitting, emesis, feeding problem = N											
	RN/CP Initials →											

Source: Courtesy of Northeast Medical Center, Concord, North Carolina. Reproduced with permission.

THE NEWBORN'S ADAPTATION

The newborn emerges from a warm, dark, liquid environment to a cool, bright, dry environment filled with noise. Establishing and maintaining an open airway for unobstructed breathing and maintaining a normal body temperature are immediate needs of the newborn.

Physical Restoration

Apgar scoring at 1 and 5 minutes is essential, as are initial physical and gestational age assessments in order to recognize any problems immediately. With parents holding the baby, the care provider can make these initial observations without disturbing the parent–infant interaction (Phillips, 1996).

According to the World Health Organization (WHO), in the postpartum period, newborn infants need easy access to the mother, appropriate feeding, adequate environmental temperature, a safe environment, cleanliness, nurturing, cuddling and stimulation, and protection from disease, harmful practices, and abuse/violence. In addition newborns need observation of body signs and access to health care for suspected or manifest complications (WHO, 1998).

Parent–Infant Interaction

How well and rapidly parents go through the postpartum phases is influenced greatly by their interactions with the new baby. The baby's response to the parents' attempts at communication is very important. New parents first touch their babies with fingertips, then palms of the hands, then total hands, and then total body in hand to arm embrace. They frequently hold the infant on the left side close to the chest, near the parents' heart. Eye-to-eye contact is important in this "en face" positioning. Parents talk instinctively to their babies in high-pitched voices, cooing and oohing. Rhythm-reciprocity patterns are often developed: the parent "oohs" and the baby "oohs"; the parent smiles and the baby smiles. When parental–infant bonding is occurring the behaviors just identified are observable.

The nurse can help the parents in the bonding process by explaining to them that their infant is a unique, distinct individual with a separate personality. Many parents do not understand that their infant can see, hear, and respond to stimuli and is not as fragile as they may believe. The infant's ability to exhibit purposeful movements and to imitate more adult movements never fails to amaze new parents. The nurse can also help parents to understand the phases a newborn goes through and the newborn's states of awareness so that they can see their baby as an individual, unlike any other baby.

State Cycles

Each baby has an individual pattern of reactivity in which separate states of awareness can be identified. These are:

Quiet sleep state—Respirations are slow and regular, and the infant rarely moves.

REM sleep state—Rapid eye movements can be seen through the eyelids. Respirations are irregular and grimaces and other facial expressions are frequent.

Active alert state—There is diffuse motor activity involving the whole body. The face may be relaxed or in a cry expression.

Quiet alert state—The infant is alert and relaxed, and the eyes are open wide and focusing. It is in this state that the infant is most apt to mimic facial expressions.

Crying state—Vigorous diffuse motor activity accompanies crying.

Transitional state—In this state the infant may be between any of the preceding states (moving from one to the other).

It is important for new parents to know about these phases and states of awareness so that they can understand their own babies. Each baby is a separate individual and responds in a unique way. Parents are usually fascinated to learn this because they may have grown up with the myths that babies cannot see or smile or react to stimuli. Meaningful interaction between infants and parents helps to facilitate bonding and attachment.

FAMILY EDUCATION

In FCMC all healthcare providers are teachers. Education in the postpartum period is essential to help new mothers and their families adapt to their new roles and care for themselves and their newborns. Family education helps family members feel comfortable caring for the new baby and ensures that the mother understands the changes in her body and practices self-care.

In 1995 the Committee on Fetus and Newborn of the American Academy of Pediatrics (1995) published 16 criteria that should be met before discharge of a newborn from the hospital. These criteria include that the mother's knowledge, ability, and confidence to provide adequate care for her newborn be documented before her discharge from the hospital. This is a formidable task to accomplish in the first day or two post birth, when new mothers are fatigued from the stress effect of labor and birth and may be having difficulty concentrating (Stark, 2000; Ruchala, 2000; Eidelman et al. 1993).

Individualized Teaching

The essence of mother–baby care is teaching by demonstration and role modeling while providing bedside care for the mother and baby. When one nurse cares for both mother and baby, the mother's level of fatigue can be determined over the course of a shift. Thus, the nurse can teach when the mother appears rested and ready. (See Figure 5-3.)

By caring for the mother and baby together, the nurse can observe how the mother interacts with her baby and pick up cues about what she needs to learn. In this way teaching is personalized. Also, by praising how well the mother repeats

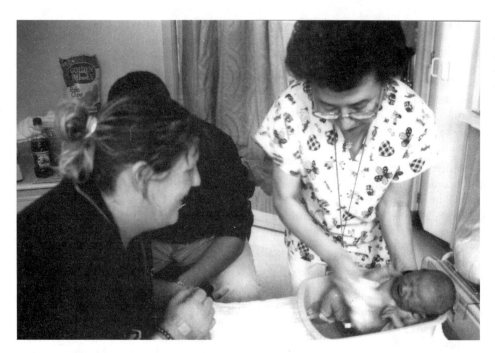

FIGURE 5–3 Nurse bathing baby while parents watch. *Source: Photo by Emily Pascoe courtesy of Boston Medical Center, Boston, Massachusetts.*

infant care demonstrations that the nurse has given, the mother receives reinforcement that she is performing capably as a mother.

When the physician examines the newborn at the mother's bedside, there is an opportunity for the mother to ask questions about her baby. The physician can teach by responding to her questions, which are specific to her baby and her immediate concerns.

Mother–baby care establishes an environment in which the care providers can prioritize to the new mother's learning needs, preferences, and readiness. In this way, the focus is on the "essentials" as determined by each new mother and her family.

Assessing Learning Needs

There is often incongruity between what nurses believe postpartum women want to know and what new mothers say they want to know (Beger and Cook, 1996; Ruchala, 2000). Consequently, the emphasis has to be on assessing each woman's need for information and prioritizing the teaching on an individual basis. In some situations women need to focus on their own needs before they can learn about babies (Ruchala, 2000). In other care settings, women may rate more infant care topics as very important than maternal topics (Davis et al., 1988; Beger and Cook, 1996). Parental self-assessment using a postpartum teaching checklist can begin a dialogue about what information is important to the family.

Gaston Memorial Hospital uses a maternal self-assessment sheet to help mothers identify their learning needs. The form (shown in Exhibit 5-13) is completed by the new mother and discussed with nursing staff. In this way, patient education is individualized.

Depending on their education level, mothers themselves are a great resource for learning, with many independently

reading about topics of interest and concern to them. Thus, careful selection of reading materials to distribute in the hospital is important. Loading down women with numerous pamphlets and booklets supplied as a courtesy to the hospital by various companies may only serve to confuse women and their families. Overload of conflicting information can be very frustrating for new mothers and may quickly lead to "burn out." As a result, the woman will turn away from reading about post-birth issues.

All printed material must be in the language of the patient and be written in a culturally sensitive manner. Also, it is possible that some written material is not adapted to the literacy level of many mothers (DiFlorio, 1991). When distributing reading material it is important to recognize that women with several children at home may not have time to devote to reading.

Learning Content

The challenge in postpartum education is identifying those things that each family is most likely to encounter and organize information that is pertinent, practical, and helpful. In the first hours and days after birth, women often want information on how to care for their own personal needs and those of their babies. Although these needs vary from family to family, high priority infant teaching often includes feeding, cord, circumcision care, infant illness, and elimination patterns. The important maternal needs are often identification of postpartum complications, episiotomy/incision care, medications, afterbirth pains, and breast care (Beger and Cook, 1996; Ruchala, 2000).

At Gaston Memorial Hospital a newborn 24-hour flowsheet is used (see Exhibit 5-14). This flowsheet is organized by systems and coordinated with the clinical paths described in Chapter 2.

EXHIBIT 5–13   Maternal Self-Assessment Form

The Birthplace
Gaston Memorial Hospital

Maternal Self Assessment

The Patient Care Team at *The Birthplace* want you to know how to take care of yourself and your baby after you go home. We would like for you to take a few moments to tell us more about what you want to learn about self and baby care during your hospitalization.

**Please check YES for all areas you want more information
and NO for areas you are already comfortable with.**

M.S.A. explained to patient by:

_____RN/LPN   Date/Time:_____.

Self Care - Postpartum Care

YES	NO		Taught by/Date/Time
☐	☐	Postpartum Care ▪ return of period ▪ signs of infection	_____
☐	☐	Daily care / personal hygiene	_____
☐	☐	Rest / exercise	_____
☐	☐	Nutrition	_____
☐	☐	Breastfeeding Breast Care ▪ mastitis ▪ engorgement ▪ pumping	_____
☐	☐	Formula Feeding Breast Care ▪ engorgement ▪ comfort	_____
☐	☐	Emotional changes ▪ postpartum blues	_____
☐	☐	Birth control methods	_____
☐	☐	Elimination ▪ bladder and bowel	_____

⇨   ⇨   **Baby Care on Back of Page**   ⇨   ⇨

EXHIBIT 5–13   Maternal Self-Assessment Form *(continued)*

Baby Care

YES	NO		Taught by/Date/Time
☐	☐	Safety measures ▪ CPR ▪ home safety	_____
☐	☐	Breastfeeding ▪ positioning ▪ latch-on ▪ frequency ▪ growth spurts	_____
☐	☐	Bottle-feeding ▪ types ▪ preparation ▪ amount ▪ bottle/nipple selection	_____
☐	☐	Bathing ▪ sponge/tub bath ▪ diapering ▪ cord care ▪ bowel/bladder habits	_____
☐	☐	Temperature taking	_____
☐	☐	Immunizations	_____
☐	☐	Comfort measures ▪ swaddling ▪ sleep patterns ▪ burping ▪ holding position ▪ clothing	_____
☐	☐	I wish to attend Baby Care Basics Class	_____

I understand what I have been taught and feel that I can take care of myself and my baby.

_____   _____   _____

Patient signature   **Nurse signature**   **Date**

ESI#

Source: Courtesy of Gaston Memorial Hospital, Gastonia, North Carolina. Reproduced with permission.

EXHIBIT 5–14   Newborn 24-Hour Flowsheet

The Birthplace
Gaston Memorial Hospital

Newborn 24 Hour Flowsheet

Daily weight/date/time:_____

DATE:	TIME:								
VITAL SIGNS	TEMPERATURE								
	PULSE								
	RESPIRATIONS								
	DEXTROSTIX								
RESPIRATORY	UNLABORED								
	LABORED								
	CHEST SYMMETRICAL								
CIRCULATORY	HEART RHYTHM REG								
	BRISK CAP REFILL								
INTEGUMENTARY	PINK								
	PALE								
	JAUNDICE								
	CLEAR								
	RASH								
	PETECHIAE								
	ACROCYANOTIC								
	UMB CORD:MOIST/DRY								
NEURO-MUSCULAR	SYMMETRY IN MOTION								
	REFLEXES: MORO								
	SUCK								
	ROOTING								
	CRY LUSTY								
	WEAK								
	MUSCLE TONE FLEXED								
	OPEN EXTENDED POS.								
	ACTIVITY:ALERT/QUIET								
	ACTIVE WITH STIM								
	CRYING								
	DROWSY								
	SLEEPY								
	FONTANELS FLAT								
	FULL								
G.I.	ABDOMEN SOFT								
	FIRM								
	DISTEND								
G.U.	GENITALIA CLEAR								
IV SITE	NO REDNESS / SWELLIN								
	TENDER								
	REDDENED								
	SWELLING								
	PRN ADAPTER								
PSYCHO-SOCIAL	NORMAL BONDING/ATTACH.								
	INVOLVEMENT S.O.								

SHIFT:	0700-1900			1900-0700		
SAFETY	ACCURATE CRIB CARD					
	2 ACCURATE ID BANDS					
	BULB SYRINGE IN CRIB					
HYGIENE	CORD CARE					
	BATH					
CLINICAL PATH REVIEWED/ REVISED						

CIRCUMCISION CHECK TIMES									
POST CIRC CK. Q 15 X 4, Q 1 X 2, Q 24HR									
CIRC.	NO BLEEDING								
	GAUZE INTACT								
	HEALING/DRY								

EXHIBIT 5–14 **Newborn 24-Hour Flowsheet** *(continued)*

DATE/TIME	FOCUSING/NSG. DX	INTERVENTION/OUTCOME

Breastfeeding Descriptors

Excellent Breastfeeding (EBF)- Baby latches on without difficulty, deep sucks with steady rhythm, freq. swallowing, brief pauses, baby quickly resumes sucking, mother able to position & latch-on baby without assistance, no nipple discomfort.

Good Breastfeeding (GBF)- Baby latches on without difficulty, deep sucks with steady rhythm, some swallowing heard, brief pauses, baby resumes sucking without being moved or prodded, mother requires a little help with positioning or latch-on, no nipple discomfort.

Fair Breastfeeding (FBF)- Baby is able to stay on once he latches on to the breast, sucks are short and quick, occasional deep suck, no steady rhythm, occasional swallow heard, mother has to stroke or prod infant to resume sucking, mother requires a lot of assistance with positioning and latch-on, could be experiencing nipple discomfort.

Poor Breastfeeding (PBF)- Baby roots for breast, licks the nipple, latches on with difficulty, does not maintain latch or maintains latch but doesn't suck, no swallowing heard, mother requires a lot of assistance with positioning and latch-on, could have nipple discomfort or pain.

Attempted Breastfeeding (ABF)- Baby roots and licks at the nipple, unable to latch-on, mother requires a great deal of assistance.

No Breastfeeding (NBF)- No effort at the breast (too sleepy, lethargic), pushes away from the breast, fights and/or cries, unable to accomplish feed despite lots of assistance.

INTAKE TIME:												
BREASTFEEDING ASSESSMENT DESCRIPTOR **EBF**=EXCELLENT BF **GBF**=GOOD BF **FBF**=FAIR BF **PBF**=POOR BF **ABF**=ATTEMPTED BF **NBF**=NO BF												
BREASTFEEDING # OF MINUTES												
BREASTFEEDING OBSERVED												
BREASTFEEDING REPORTED												
FORMULA FEED AMOUNT (TYPE:)												
ROUTE **B**=BOTTLE **C**=CUP **FF**=FINGERFEED **SNS**=SUPP NURSING SYSTEM												
SPITTING												
OUTPUT NUMBER OF VOIDINGS												
NUMBER OF STOOLS												
M=MECONIUM **GR**=GREEN **Y**=YELLOW												
L=LOOSE **S**=SOFT **W**=WATERY												

0700-1900		1900-0700	
INITIAL	SIGNATURE/TITLE	INITIAL	SIGNATURE/TITLE

Source: Courtesy of Gaston Memorial Hospital, Gastonia, North Carolina. Reproduced with permission.

Teaching Methods

In addition to the individualized teaching that occurs with mother–baby care, gathering a group of parents together provides an opportunity for discussion, the exchange of ideas, mutual problem solving, and support. Another teaching strategy that can help parents learn about maternal and infant care is the use of educational TV in the form of videos or in-hospital newborn channels. Videos that are purchased or developed in-house can be loaned to families, given as gifts, or purchased in the hospital gift shop (Simpson, 1996). However, TV is not a substitute for one-on-one teaching. Whenever TV or a video is used, it should be followed by discussion with nursing staff about points of interest as well as question and answer sessions about video content. As with all aspects of family-centered maternity care, flexibility and sensitivity to the family's needs are the key to effective teaching. All videos used for teaching must be culturally sensitive and in the language of the families being served.

Most hospital maternity services have well-developed teaching plans and checklists. The advantage of these plans is that staff members communicate similar information to parents, lessening the confusion that occurs when conflicting information is given.

Evaluation

An important but often neglected part of family education is evaluation. Family education surveys can provide valuable knowledge to assist in prioritizing the learning needs of new mothers and their families. The survey can be reviewed by staff on a regular basis and help them refocus on any areas that need improvement.

VISITATION

In FCMC, the father and other family members are never considered visitors. (See Figure 5-4.) The mother determines which family members and friends will be welcome at her bedside and when.

The baby's father is encouraged to participate in infant care and if the mother chooses, family members may also participate in infant care. They are instructed in handwashing before touching the baby and asked to be responsible for not exposing the newborn to colds or infections. (See Figure 5-5.)

Samples of policy and procedures for visiting in the maternity unit and in the holding nursery are shown in Exhibits 5-15 and 5-16. (See Appendix J for the full-page version of Exhibit 5-16.)

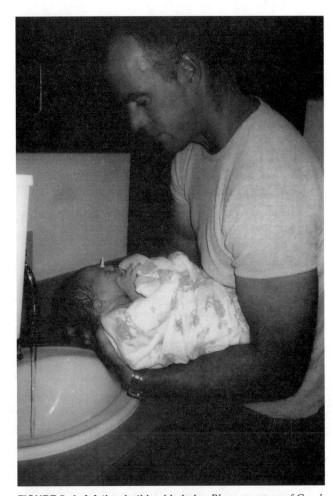

FIGURE 5–4 A father bathing his baby. *Photo courtesy of Good Samaritan Hospital, Lebanon, Pennsylvania.*

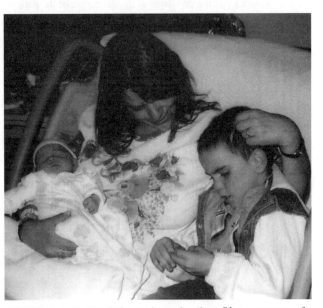

FIGURE 5–5 Mother, baby, and new brother. *Photo courtesy of Good Samaritan Hospital, Lebanon, Pennsylvania.*

EXHIBIT 5–15   Policy and Procedure for Visiting in the Maternity Unit

VISITING IN THE MATERNITY UNIT

Procedure

Welcome visitors while promoting family-centered care.

Policy

Maternity nursing staff will provide support persons and visitors—who are important components of family-centered maternity care—the opportunity to visit with the infant and mother in a safe environment.

Patient Education

Teach the mother to screen visitors for illness and exposure to communicable diseases and to promote hand washing by visitors prior to handling the newborn.

Implementation

I.   The support person(s) present during labor, birth and postpartum period are encouraged to support the woman through the birthing process. The patient's primary support person(s) may benefit from attending childbirth preparation classes.

II.   Do not limit support persons that the childbearing woman chooses to be with her during her birthing and recovery process. Based on the mother's safety, comfort, and desire, formulate visiting policies for fathers that are as flexible and liberal as possible, and follow them consistently.

III.   Screen visiting family and friends for communicable disease or recent exposure. Have them wear unsoiled clothes and wash their hands prior to holding the newborn. If visitors' clothes are soiled, provide them with a cover gown.

IV.   Place the maternity patient's safety and comfort as the first priority. Ask support person(s) to leave the room if their presence distresses the laboring mother or other support person(s) assisting her.

V.   Siblings present for the birth must have been prepared either through sibling preparation classes or by their parents.

VI.   An adult who is not a primary support person for the expectant woman must accompany children under 12 years of age. If the child becomes upset, have the support person leave with the child(ren) if necessary.

VII.   Have parents screen all visiting children for signs of communicable disease or recent exposure. Ask children's parents to do this before they bring their children to the hospital.

VIII.   Have children remain in their mother's hospital room or under supervision in the lounge area.

IX.   Restrict visiting privileges at the discretion of the patient's doctor and/or staff in cooperation with the patient.

X.   During the postpartum period, immediate family members (fathers, siblings, grandparents) will have unrestricted visitation.

XI.   Visitation for the antepartum period will follow the same guidelines as postpartum visitation.

_____

VP Nursing

_____

Department Chair

EXHIBIT 5–16   Policy and Procedure for Visiting in the Holding Nursery

VISITING IN THE HOLDING NURSERY

Procedure

Provide an opportunity for visitation with the infant in a safe and supervised environment.

Policy

Maternity nursing staff will ensure that parents or designated significant others may visit the newborn in the holding nursery anytime.

Implementation

1. Have the mother approve all visitors.
2. Screen visitors for communicable disease and exposure prior to the visit (e.g., upper respiratory, chicken pox, or influenza). Instruct visitors to wash their hands thoroughly with a hospital-approved soap.
3. Encourage and answer all questions.
4. Promote quiet time for visitors with the infant.
5. Plan on no more than 2 visitors at one time due to the need to maintain a restful environment in the holding nursery.

VP Nursing

Department Chair

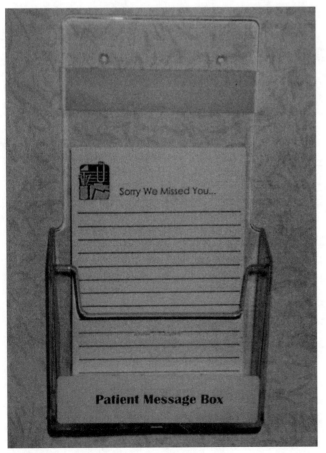

FIGURE 5–6 A patient message box.

When the mother wants private time with her baby, or time to sleep without being disturbed, there can be signs available for her door that read "Quiet Family Time" or "Mother Sleeping, Please Do Not Disturb." There is space on the signs for the mother's signature and she can place the appropriate sign where it will be visible on the door, or ask the nurse to do this whenever the mother needs privacy or rest. A note pad and pen outside her door is convenient for family and friends to leave a message for a mother who is sleeping. (See Figure 5-6.)

Also useful are printed materials welcoming family members but also raising their awareness of the mother's need for rest. This material can be given to each person who comes to visit the new mother and baby. Exhibit 5-17 is a sample of a "Welcome Letter" that can be distributed to all those visiting the new mother and baby. (See Appendix J for the full-page version of this exhibit.)

Markham Stouffville Hospital in Markham, Ontario, Canada, reserves 1:00 to 3:00 P.M. each day as a quiet time for the new mother, her baby, and her husband/partner. This time is to allow for the mother's rest and recovery.

EXHIBIT 5–17   Sample of a Welcome Letter That Can Be Distributed to Visitors

A WELCOME LETTER TO THE NEW FAMILY'S VISITORS

Dear friends of the new family:

Welcome! Your visit reflects a loving community of support, which is important to every new family. We would like to offer some ideas on ways that you can help the new family.

At the hospital:

- Consider keeping your visit brief, about 15 minutes. This has several benefits: new parents will be less exhausted, nurses can spend more time teaching infant care, and babies can be fed when hungry. Feeding is a learning experience for both baby and mother and can be difficult in a room full of people.

- Ask the new family how you can help when they return home. Parents have told us that the following things really helped them in the first month:
  - Bring over a few meals that can go from freezer to oven.
  - Offer to drop by to do a few household tasks, such as laundry, grocery shopping, lawn mowing, or housecleaning.
  - If there are other children in the family, offer to take care of the other children for a few hours.
  - After a few weeks, offer to come over to watch the baby for an hour or two while the new parents go out.

At home, when you call or visit:

- Ask how the parents are doing, as well as how the new baby is doing.
- Offer lots of words of praise for the good job they are doing. All new parents need support in the hard work of taking care of their baby.
- Stress to parents that this is their special time to "be taken care of" by others; they should not have to care for anyone but the baby.
- It is usually best to offer advice only when asked for advice. New parents get so much advice they often feel overwhelmed. Support them as they learn about their role and this new and unique baby. They will really appreciate knowing you support their decisions about how they care for their baby.
- If concerns are expressed about the health of mom or baby, encourage the parents to call their doctor or midwife for guidance.

We hope these suggestions have been helpful to you. We are glad you came to visit! All new parents need to know others care about their new family.

The Staff

Source: Adapted from Fairview Riverside Medical Center, Minneapolis, Minnesota.

BREASTFEEDING

Unrestricted breastfeeding has been found to be a beneficial form of care, with effectiveness demonstrated by clear evidence from controlled trials (Enkin et al., 2000). The World Health Organization (WHO), the American Academy of Pediatrics (AAP), the American College of Obstetricians and Gynecologists (ACOG), and the Association of Women's Health, Obstetrics and Neonatal Nurses (AWHONN) all have endorsed breastfeeding as the preferred method of feeding in the first year of life (American Academy of Pediatrics, 1997; Kyenkya-Isabirye, 1992; Saadeh and Akre, 1996). Time and again the experts have proven that breastfeeding is best—both for moms and for babies.

Establishing Lactation

Early suckling has been shown to be associated with prolonged nursing. Early feeding also decreases the likelihood of low blood sugar in the newborn (DiGirolamo, Grummer-Strawn, and Fein, 2001; Canadian Institute of Child Health, 1996; Health Canada, 2000). To establish breastfeeding immediately after birth the baby is held by the mother, skin to skin, so that the baby can start suckling as soon as he or she shows signs of readiness (WHO, 1998). The mother's body keeps the infant warm and the mother offers her breast to the infant on the infant's cue. It is a finely tuned interactive system at work. Because early contact and early breastfeeding enhance the rate and duration of breastfeeding (Lawrence, 1995), the infant remains with the mother and is not sent to a transition or well baby nursery.

Maintaining Lactation

Once begun, breastfeeding is maintained by the infant's ongoing communication with the mother's breasts (Mulford, 1995; Yamauchi and Yamanouchi, 1990). The infant signals, "I am hungry or I need comforting," and the mother responds. Newborns should be nursed approximately 8 to 12 times every 12 hours until satiety, which is usually 10 to 15 minutes on each breast (American Academy of Pediatrics, 1997). Nonseparation of mothers and babies and breastfeeding guidance throughout the hospital stay support the homeostasis-seeking interaction known as breastfeeding (Perez-Escamilla et al., 1994).

Formal Staff Training

Medical and nursing staffs who work with new mothers need a good understanding of the physiology of breastfeeding, as well as philosophical agreement that successful breastfeeding is beneficial to mother and baby. Hospitals that practice FCMC provide formal in-service education in breastfeeding to enable medical and nursing staff to teach and support breastfeeding. (See Figure 5-7.) An outline of such continuing education is presented on the following page in bulleted list format, courtesy of Barbara Ford, IBCLC.

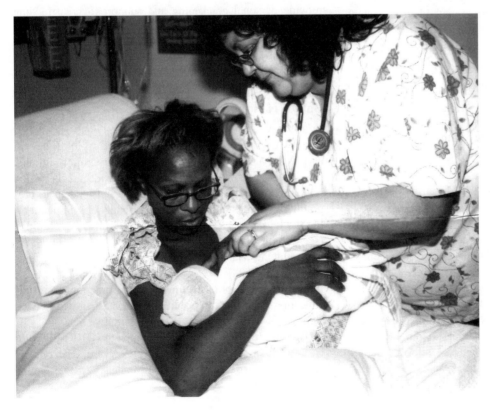

FIGURE 5–7 Nursing support for early breastfeeding. *Source: Photo by Emily Pascoe, courtesy of Boston Medical Center, Boston, Massachusetts.*

Breastfeeding—The Family-Centered Approach

- Review the Ten Step Program promoted by the WHO and UNICEF as part of the Baby-Friendly Hospital Initiative.
- Review and discuss AAP's statement on breastfeeding.
- Review and discuss the hospital's family-centered breastfeeding policy and procedure.
- Review the anatomy and physiology of the breast and of the newborn infant.
- Identify states of behavior in the newborn related to breastfeeding.
- Describe and discuss a breastfeeding timeline of events in both mother and baby in the first 24–48 hours after birth.
- Assess breastfeeding using the LATCH system.
- Identify and demonstrate alternative feeding methods when an infant does not latch-on and breastfeed effectively by the first 24 hours post birth.
- Review and demonstrate ways of collecting and storing mother's breastmilk.
- Review and discuss breast care for the breastfeeding mother during her hospital stay and post discharge.
- Review and discuss discharge planning.

Breastfeeding the High-Risk Newborn in a Family-Centered Setting

- Define ways to offer encouragement and support to the mother who is pumping, collecting, and storing milk for her infant in the NICU setting.
- Identify the need to protect the mother's right to breastfeed her infant by using alternative methods to feed her baby until breastfeeding can be initiated.
- Recognize readiness of the infant to initiate Kangaroo Care (skin-to-skin contact) and to begin breastfeeding.
- Discuss methods of support for the mother and infant post-discharge.
- Review situations and potential problems encountered by or related to the infant and mother both before and after discharge from the NICU.

Education and Support for Mothers

All members of the staff should be capable of helping mothers breastfeed. Lactation specialists serve as resources for the staff and for those mothers and babies who many need additional specialized assistance. There must be consistency in hospital policies and procedures related to breastfeeding, and physicians and nurses must give consistent messages to new mothers (Tiedje et al., 2002).

Breastfeeding Success Centers on hospital campuses often offer many services: prenatal breastfeeding classes, private consultations, pump rentals and breastfeeding aids, support groups, and phone consultations, and will weigh a baby free of charge. Staffed by lactation specialists who

EXHIBIT 5-17 Ten Steps to Successful Breastfeeding

Every facility providing maternity services and care for newborn infants should:

1. Have a written breastfeeding policy that is routinely communicated to all healthcare staff.
2. Train all healthcare staff in skills necessary to implement this policy
3. Inform all pregnant women about the benefits and management of breastfeeding.
4. Help mothers initiate breastfeeding within 30 minutes after birth.
5. Show mothers how to breastfeed and how to maintain lactation even if they should be separated from their infants.
6. Give newborn infants no food or drink other than breastmilk, unless medically indicated.
7. Practice rooming-in—allow mothers and infants to remain together—24 hours a day.
8. Encourage breastfeeding on demand.
9. Give no artificial teats or pacifiers (also called dummies or soothers) to breastfeeding infants.
10. Foster the establishment of breastfeeding support groups and refer mothers to them on discharge from the hospital or clinic.

Source: The Baby-Friendly Hospital Initiative (1991), UNICEF and WHO.

have been certified by the International Board of Lactation Consultant Examiners (IBCLC), these breastfeeding centers provide personal counseling and support to breastfeeding mothers on an ongoing basis. Another service of the center may be employer consultation, to assist community employers in providing an environment that supports breastfeeding mothers who work outside of the home.

Baby-Friendly Initiative

In 1991, the United Nation's Children's Fund (UNICEF) and WHO developed the Baby-Friendly Hospital Initiative as part of a worldwide program. The program's ultimate goal is to ensure that all babies worldwide are breastfed (Kyenkya-Isabirye, 1992). Maternity and pediatric programs can be designated as "baby-friendly" by implementing the Initiative's "Ten Steps to Successful Breastfeeding" (see Exhibit 5-17).

Achieving Baby-Friendly status is not an easy task (Dodgson et al., 1999; Merewood and Philipp, 2001). Improvements in breastfeeding policies, practices, and staff education are needed to provide care consistent with the ten steps of the Baby-Friendly Hospital Initiative.

Boston Medical Center is a recipient of the UNICEF/World Health Organization Baby-Friendly™ Award. The clinical policy for breastfeeding at Boston Medical Center is shown in Exhibit 5-18.

EXHIBIT 5–18   Clinical Policy for Breastfeeding

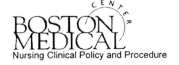

BREASTFEEDING

Nursing Clinical Policy and Procedure

Clinical Policy

The breastfeeding philosophy promoted at Boston Medical Center is the "Ten Steps to Successful Breastfeeding" as documented in the 1989 WHO/UNICEF statement.

Protocols:

1. All pregnant patients will be provided with information on breastfeeding and counseled on the benefits of breastfeeding.
2. The woman's desire to breastfeed will be documented in her medical record.
3. Any infant/child will have his/her method of feeding documented on the medical record. The infant's mother will be encouraged to continue to breastfeed unless medically contraindicated.
4. All newborns, if baby and mother are stable, should be placed skin to skin with the mother and breastfed within one hour of birth.
5. Breastfeeding mothers will be shown how to breastfeed including:
   - Proper position and latch-on.
   - Nutritive suckling and swallowing.
   - Milk production and release.
   - Frequency of feedings/infant feeding cues.
   - Expression of breast milk and use of pump if indicated.
   - How to know if infant is adequately nourished.
   - List reasons for calling the clinician.
   - When to call for breastfeeding help.

   These skills will be taught to primiparous and multiparous women and reviewed before discharge. The baby's position and latch-on will be evaluated on each shift.
6. Breastfeeding mother-infant couples will be encouraged to remain together throughout their hospital stay, including at night.
7. Breastfeeding infants should be put to breast *at least* 8–12 times each 24 hours, including cesarean-birth babies. Infant feeding cues will be used as indicators of the baby's readiness for feeding. Breastfeeding babies should be breastfed at night.
8. Time limits for breastfeeding on each side should be avoided. Infants should be offered both breasts at each feeding, but may only feed on one side at a feeding during the early days.
9. No sterile water, glucose water, or formula will be given unless specifically ordered by a physician or nurse practitioner or by the mother's documented and informed request. In this case, the supplement should be fed to the baby by an alternative feeing method (e.g., cup feeding, Haberman feeder, finger feeding) if possible, Bottles will not be placed in a breastfeeding infant's bassinet. This institution does not give group instruction in the use of formula.

Source: Courtesy of Boston Medical Center, Boston, Massachusetts. Reproduced with permission.

EXHIBIT 5–18   Clinical Policy for Breastfeeding (*continued*)

BOSTON MEDICAL	Breastfeeding	Page 2 of 3

10. Pacifiers will not be given to breastfeeding infants. Preterm infants in the NICU or infants with specific medical conditions may be given pacifiers for non-nutritive sucking. Newborns undergoing painful procedures (for example: circumcision, heel stick) may be given a pacifier as a method of pain management during the procedure. The infant will not return to the mother with a pacifier.

11. Routine use of nipple creams, ointments, or other topical preparations should be avoided unless therapy has been prescribed for a dermatological problem. Mothers with sore nipples will be encouraged to apply expressed colostrum or breastmilk to the areola following each feeding.

12. Anti-lactation drugs will not be given to any postpartum mother.

13. If a baby consistently feeds poorly, consider using a breast-pump to stimulate mother's milk production while continuing to help mother with latch-on. In this case, expressed colostrum/breastmilk should be fed to the baby by an alternative feeding method (not a bottle).

14. Nipple shields or bottle nipples should not be routinely used to cover mother's nipple with the intention of causing latch-on, preventing or managing sore or cracked nipples, or when a mother has flat or inverted nipples.

15. Infants having problems with temperature regulation (axillary temperature <97.6 F) may still go to their mothers to feed in accordance with the Policy and Procedure on Thermoregulation.

16. Healthy, appropriate-for-gestation-age infants who have not successfully fed within 6 hours after birth and those who fit the criteria listed in the Neonatal Blood Glucose Monitoring Policy will have a blood glucose test done and the Policy and Procedure on Hypoglycemia will be followed regarding the management of the results.

17. Breastfeeding assessment, teaching, and documentation will be done on each shift and whenever possible with each contact with the mother. Mothers will be encouraged to attend the breastfeeding classes held on the unit. The clinician or nurse will make a referral to the lactation consultant if clinically indicated.

18. Mothers who are separated from their sick or preterm infants will be:
    - Instructed on how to use and how often to use the double breast pump.
    - Encouraged to breastfeed on demand as soon as the infant's condition permits.
    - Taught proper storage of breastmilk.
    - Provided with information on pump rentals.

19. This institution does not accept free formula or free breastmilk substitutes. Nursery or NICU discharge bags offered to all mothers will not contain any infant formula, coupons for formula, logos of formula companies, or literature with formula company logos.

20. Prior to discharge, mothers will be given the names and telephone numbers of community resources to contact for help with breastfeeding, including the BMC Breastfeeding Center Support Line (617-414-MILK).

21. Before leaving the hospital, breastfeeding mothers should be able to:
    - Position the baby correctly at breast with no pain during the feeding.
    - Latch the baby to breast properly.
    - State when the baby is swallowing milk.
    - State how many times in 24 hours the baby should be fed.
    - Describe feeding cues that indicate when it is time to feed the baby.
    - State how many bowel movements the baby should have each day during the first two weeks home.

Source: Courtesy of Boston Medical Center, Boston, Massachusetts. Reproduced with permission.

EXHIBIT 5–18   Clinical Policy for Breastfeeding (*continued*)

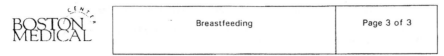

BOSTON MEDICAL	Breastfeeding	Page 3 of 3

- List indications for calling a pediatrician, nurse practitioner, midwife, or family physician.
- State when and who to call for help with breastfeeding.

22. All breastfeeding mothers will be given a follow-up appointment or will be advised to make an appointment for their baby's first check-up within one week of discharge.

23. BMC health professionals will attend ongoing education on lactation to ensure that correct, current, and consistent information is provided to all mothers wishing to breastfeed.

Contraindications:

- Breastfeeding is contraindicated in the following situations:
- If a mother is taking certain medications that are essential for her well-being, but may be harmful to her infant (Medications and Mothers' Milk by Thomas Hale, 2000).
- If a mother is a know user of cocaine, heroin, or other "street drug."
- If a mother has active tuberculosis. (She may breastfeed only after she has received adequate drug therapy and is considered by her physician to be noninfectious.)
- If a mother is HIV positive.
- If there are active herpes lesions on a mother's breast.
- If a mother has varicella that is determined to be infectious to her infant.
- If an infant has galactosemia.
- If a mother is identified with primary cytomegalovirus infection (should not breastfeed during the acute phase of the illness).

References:

American Academy of Pediatrics. Pickering LK, ed. *2000 Red Book: Report of the Committee on Infectious Diseases*, 25th Ed. American Academy of Pediatrics: Elkgrove, Illinois.

American College of Obstetricians and Gynecologists. (July 2000) *Educational Bulletin*, ACOG: Washington, D.C.

Hale, Thomas. (2000) *Medications and Mothers' Milk*, 9th Ed. Pharmasoft Medical Publishing: Amarillo, Texas.

U.S. Dept. HHS. (2000) *HHS Blueprint for Action on Breastfeeding*. U.S. Dept. of HHS, Office on Women's Health: Washington, D.C.

Work Group on Breastfeeding. (1997) American Academy of Pediatrics. Breastfeeding and the Use of Human Milk. *Pediatrics*. 100:1024–39.

Prepared and Issued by:	Approved by:
Breastfeeding Task Force	Perinatal Committee Infection Control 7/99
Issue Date: 4/97	Revision Dates: 3/99, 7/99, 12/01
Next Review.	Review Dates:

Source: Courtesy of Boston Medical Center, Boston, Massachusetts. Reproduced with permission.

FOLLOW-UP

Going home from the hospital following labor and birth can be a time of joy, but at the same time it can be a time of fear and anxiety. Many women talk about the fatigue and exhaustion that result from sleep deprivation for the first weeks post birth (Lee et al., 2000). Resuming normal activities, such as driving a car and taking a shower, can be major accomplishments for a new mother.

Because of the short timeframe of hospitalization for childbirth, teaching has to focus on the specific information a mother will need when going home, such as feeding the baby and maternal self-care. The amount of anticipatory guidance given is often limited. Many breastfeeding mothers do not encounter problems until their breasts become engorged three days postpartum (72 hours), after they've returned home. Also, postpartum "blues" and the peak of newborn hyperbilirubinemia may not occur until the third postpartum day.

Even though the new mother was given information on community resources and breastfeeding support groups such as the LaLeche League, she may be reluctant to call for help. Thus, follow-up care is very important.

Telephone Follow-Up

Some hospitals use telephone interviews of all new mothers within two days of discharge. A hospital maternity nurse inquires about any problems the mother may be having with aspects of infant feeding or care, as well as problems the mother may be having with her own physiologic and emotional transition. The nurse responds to any questions the mother may have and makes referrals as appropriate. Phone call assessment is documented on a hospital postpartum follow-up log, with copies sent to care providers for mother and baby and referrals made as deemed necessary.

Ideally, all new mothers receive at least one phone call after discharge. However, if that is not possible calls can be made to selected women with special needs (Simpson, 1996).

The postpartum phone call policy and follow-up form used at the Good Samaritan Hospital in Lebanon, Pennsylvania, is shown in Exhibits 5-19 and 5-20.

Hospital-Based Clinic

In response to a need for postpartum follow-up, some hospitals have developed postpartum care centers (PCC) on the hospital campus. The new mother and baby return to the PCC clinic for a follow-up assessment.

An innovative PCC has been in operation at Evergreen Hospital Medical Center in Kirkland, Washington, since 1991 (Keppler, 1995). The PCC's mission is to provide assessment, care, and education to mothers, infants, and families three to four days after birth in a nurse-run clinic (Keppler, 1995; Keppler and Roudebush, 1999). The hospital nurse makes clinic appointments as part of the discharge

---

EXHIBIT 5–19   The Postpartum Phone Call Policy

Section: **Maternal Care**

Title: **Postpartum Follow-Up Phone Call**

Policy:

It is the policy of The Maternity Unit to provide a follow-up phone call to all postpartum mothers who have a phone and who speak English.

Purpose:

To provide an opportunity for mothers to ask questions about normal postpartum and newborn care after discharge.

Instructions:

1. Each patient who delivers will have a Phone Call Follow-up sheet stamped and the upper portion filled out by the unit secretary or admitting nurse.

2. Upon discharge, the date of discharge will be written at the top of the form and the form will be placed in the designated binder.

3. Phone calls will be made within one week of the patient's discharge whenever possible and as early as two days after discharge. Three attempts will be made to reach the patient unless the phone has been disconnected or does not belong to them. In the latter cases, only one attempt will be made to reach the patient. The calls will be listed by date and recorded in the PP Phone Call Log Book. If unable to reach a patient on a given day, the date and the reason is written at the top of the form in order to keep track of the number of attempts that have been made (i.e., 5-30-03, line busy). After the third attempt or if the patient has a disconnected number or does not reside at the location of the phone, a large "X" is marked over the form and the form is forwarded as noted in #5.

4. All calls will be documented on the Phone Call Follow-up sheet. Calls may be made by any RN on the maternity staff. Teaching and any referrals must be noted on the form. All referrals to physicians' offices must be made by the nurse completing the phone call.

5. The white Phone Call Follow-up sheet will be sent to Medical Records when completed and will be kept as a permanent part of the patient's record. The pink copy is sent to the mailbox of the physician who delivered the patient and the yellow copy is sent to the mailbox of the baby's physician.

6. Whenever possible, the phone call will be made by the same staff member who may be following the patient at home via the VNA.

7. The hospital reserves the right to temporarily suspend this practice at any time it deems necessary.

Source: Courtesy of Good Samaritan Hospital, Lebanon, Pennsylvania.

---

process, the clinic visit is discussed in prenatal classes, and providers are all extremely supportive of the PCC. In addition, a reminder call is made to the family the day before the visit to confirm the appointment.

EXHIBIT 5–20   Follow-up Form for the Postpartum Phone Call

The Good Samaritan Hospital

Phone Call Follow-Up

Attempt to Reach

Date 1._____ 2._____ 3._____

Name of patient:_____ Phone number_____

Date of delivery:_____ First baby (circle one) Yes No

Physician who delivered infant:_____

Type of delivery:_____

Male/Female:_____ Infant's Physician:_____

Discharge date:_____

1.   How are you feeling?

2.   What are you doing to take good care of yourself?

3.   Do you have any questions related to breast care or postpartum care?

4.   How are you feeding your baby?

      Have you changed any aspect of feeding since you were discharged?

      How did you decide to make those changes?

Breastfeeding	**Bottle Feeding**
5. How often is the baby nursing?	5. How much formula is the baby taking/how often?

6.   How many wet diapers does baby have in 1 day?

7.   Any problems with feedings or baby sleeping?

8.   Do you have any questions or concerns regarding yourself or the baby?

<u>"Thank you for choosing to have your baby at the Maternity Center."</u>

Referrals made:_____ Physician's office notified:_____

Nurse's signatue/Title:_____

Nurse's name (print):_____

Date of phone call:_____

Source: Courtesy of Good Samaritan Hospital, Lebanon, Pennsylvania. Reproduced with permission.

The cost of a clinic visit is estimated to be about $50 and is included in the education fee for all families attending prenatal classes (about half of all families). For families who do not attend prenatal classes, third-party payers, including Medicaid, are billed for the PCC visit. Individual payment plans or scholarships cover those families without insurance (Keppler and Roudebush, 1999).

Program outcomes of the PCC at Evergreen Hospital Medical Center include high patient and provider satisfaction, significant program growth, and hospital re-admission rates that have not increased despite shorter maternity stays and increasing births. An unexpected benefit has been that the follow-up clinic established a "postpartum place" within the hospital (Keppler and Roudebush, 1999). Families feel safe in returning to the clinic for all kinds of help and sometimes simply to show off their babies.

Postpartum Support Groups

Evergreen Hospital Medical Center also conducts "Baby Parent Time" groups to support new parents as they grow into their new roles. Weekly meetings are free until the infant is 12 weeks old. From that time on there is a small fee for continuing weekly support through the first year (Keppler and Roudebush, 1999).

Home Care

Home visits offer a unique chance to instruct the whole family. Visiting in the home, the nurse can assess the home environment and the support available (Williams and Cooper, 1996). Assessment of mother–baby interaction, the home environment, and psychological support will help the nurse determine the level of family functioning.

Malnory (1997) described a post-discharge perinatal program consisting of two post-discharge contacts—either two phone calls or a home visit and a phone call. Because each family is unique, decisions about which follow-up option to use must be made in consultation with families.

Rockingham Memorial Hospital in Harrisonburg, Virginia, has had a home visitation program since 1988. The program began as a service for those families who made a prearrangement to stay in the hospital for less than 24 hours after the delivery of their infant. It was therefore limited to healthy moms and babies. There was no extra charge for this visit. A predelivery preparation class was mandatory and the visits were made within 1–3 days after discharge. The visits included a history/physical on both the mother and the baby and the PKU was drawn at that time.

In 1994 the program was extended to *every* woman who delivers (approximately 1,800 babies a year) at Rockingham Memorial Hospital. (The only exception is the woman who is traveling and just "happens" to deliver at their hospital.) There are currently six nurses who participate in the program. Two of those nurses see the Hispanic population. There is still no added cost for the visit, and the mission/objectives of the visits continue to be the same. Approximately 79 percent of the families who give birth at Rockingham Memorial Hospital accept the home visit.

The mission of the Family Care Nurse Program follows:

The Family Care Nurse program encompasses a continuum of care that includes prenatal education, care during hospitalization, and postpartum assessment and intervention. A holistic approach comprised of psychosocial, economic, spiritual, and physical needs assessment is the basis of our practice.

Protocol and maternal and infant record forms for the home visit follow in Exhibits 5-21, 5-22, and 5-23.

EXHIBIT 5–21   Protocol for Home Visits

Rockingham Memorial Hospital— Family Birthplace

Protocol for Home Visits of Family Care Nurse (FCN)

1. All clients are eligible for home visits if they received their prenatal care at the offices of our hospital physicians.
2. All first time moms will be encouraged to accept a follow-up home visit.
3. All moms and infants discharged in less than 24 hours will have a home visit within 1 to 3 days and a physical exam will be done. Blood will be drawn for a PKU test and brought to the nursery. Exception: Those declining a home visit will need to make alternate arrangements for the PKU test with their physicians.
4. All moms staying more than 24 hours including Cesarean Births may choose to receive a home visit in 1 to 5 days of discharge. All moms and infants will have a complete physical exam. Exception: Visit may be made in 6–14 days after discharge due to inclement weather or at the discretion of the nurse.
5. When mother and infant are not discharged together, each family unit will be entitled to one visit if discharged within 2 weeks of delivery. Infants on extended antibiotic therapy who need a PKU test may be seen at the nurse's discretion. For other discharges greater than 2 weeks post delivery, if a visit is indicated, the home visit may be done either by the Family Care Nurse at her discretion or visit may be done through a home health consult.
6. Verbal contact with the patient after delivery will be made by the Family Care Nurse either in the hospital or after discharge to coordinate follow-up care.
7. For a mother placing the infant for adoption, a visit will be offered the mother. A visit may be offered to the adoptive parents of the infant at the discretion of nurse. If both the birth mother and the adoptive parents want a home visit, a different nurse will do each visit.
8. Families who experience the death of their infant at Rockingham Memorial Hospital will be offered a follow-up visit as desired.
9. If the visit is cancelled prior to the appointment—document the refusal on the Family Care Nurse direction paper.
10. If the client is not at home at the scheduled visit—a follow-up call is made but no additional visit is scheduled except for extenuating circumstances.

Source: Courtesy of Rockingham Memorial Hospital, Harrisonburg, Virginia. Reproduced with permission.

EXHIBIT 5–22   Maternal Home Visit Record

RMH
Rockingham Memorial Hospital

FAMILY BIRTHPLACE
Family Care Nurse Home Visit - Maternal Record

Name_____ Age_____   Delivery Date____/____/____

MR#_____ OB_____   Parity_____

If indicated by a check mark (√), interventions taught according to protocols based on assessment. Additional needs and interventions are addressed in this column.

Level of Understanding:
B = Basic   D=Demonstrated
G=Good   V=Verbalized

Visit Date_____ Arrival_____ Departure_____

I. ASSESSMENT

A. Vital Signs: T_____   P_____   R_____   BP_____/_____

Comments: _____

A. Vital Signs
☐ Normal/abnormal   B G D V

Comments:_____

B. Breasts
1. Tension   Soft_____   Firm_____   Engorged_____   Nodules_____
2. Color   WNL_____   Reddened_____
3. Lactation   Nursing? *Circle one:*   Yes   No
 a. Nipples   Erect_____   Inverted_____   Flat_____
 b. Discharge Colostrum_____   Milk_____   None_____
 c. Nipple Condition   Normal_____   Tender_____   Cracked_____
 d. Cleansing Soap_____   Water only_____   Air dry_____
 e. Breast Shells_____   Nipple Shield_____   Evert-it_____   Pump_____
   Hydrogel_____   Lanolin_____   Periodontal Syringe_____

Comments:_____

B. Breasts
☐ Breast Pain R/T Engorgement   B G D V
☐ Breast Pain, Pain R/T Mastitis   B G D V
☐ Flat, inverted or retracted nipples B G D V
☐ Colostrum/Milk   B G D V
☐ Nipple Pain   B G D V
☐ Latch ons/Positioning   B G D V
☐ Breast shells, Nipple shields   B G D V
☐ Evert-it/Hydrogel   B G D V
☐ Periodontal Syringe   B G D V
☐ Pump   B G D V
☐ Lanolin   B G D V

Comments:_____
_____
_____

C. Reproductive Tract
1. Lochia
 a. Amount   Small_____   Moderate_____   Heavy_____
 b. Color   Rubra_____   Serosa_____   Alba_____
 c. Clots   No_____   WNL_____   Excessive_____
 d. Odor   Fleshy_____   Foul_____
 e. Peri-care   Appropriate_____   Inappropriate_____

Comments:_____
2. Uterus
 a. Condition   Non-Tender_____   Tender_____
 b. Firm   Y_____   N_____   Describe_____
 c. Position   Midline_____   Displaced_____   Level_____

Comments:_____

C. Reproductive Tract
☐ Normal process of involution/
   hemorrhages or uterine infection B G D V

Comments:_____
_____

3. Perineum
 a. Laceration/Episiotomy   Y____ N____   Declined Physical/NA _____
   Tender_____   Painful_____   Throbbing_____
 b. Condition   Reddened   Y____ N____   Describe_____
   Eccymosis   Y____ N____   Describe_____
   Edema   Y____ N____   Describe_____
   Discharge   Y____ N____   Describe_____
   Approximated   Y____ N____   Describe_____
 c. Sitz Bath _____   Tucks_____   Spray/Foam_____

Comments:_____

☐ Perineal discomfort/infection
   epis./laceration   B G D V

Comments:_____
_____
_____

4. ABD Incision: C-Birth_____   BPS_____
 a. Clips   In_____   Out_____   Removed_____   NA_____
 b. Condition   Reddened   Y____ N____   Describe:_____
   Eccymosis   Y____ N____   Describe:_____
   Edema   Y____ N____   Describe:_____
   Discharge   Y____ N____   Describe:_____
   Approximated Y____ N____   Describe:_____

Comments:_____

☐ Incisional pain/infection   B G D V

Comments:_____
_____

D. Elimination
1. Urinary Tract
 a. Emptying Bladder   Y____ N____
 b. Signs of UTI   Y____ N____
 c. Comments_____
2. GI Tract
 a. BM   Y_____   N_____
 b. Problems None_____   Constipation_____   Diarrhea_____
 c. Hemmorhoids   Y___   N___   Non-painful___   Painful___
 d. Treatment Tucks_____   Ointment_____   Suppository_____   Sitz_____

Comments:_____

D. Elimination
☐ Bladder function/infection   B G D V
☐ Bowel function/diarrhea/
   constipation   B G D V
☐ Hemorrhoids   B G D V

Comments:_____

Courtesy of Rockingham Memorial Hospital, Harrisonburg, Virginia. Reproduced with permission.

EXHIBIT 5–22   Maternal Home Visit Record (*continued*)

E. Extremities
1. Varicosities   Absent_____   Present_____   Location_____
2. Homan's Sign   Right/Positive_____   Negative_____
    Left/Positive_____   Negative_____
3. Redness   Y_____   N_____   Describe_____
4. Pain   Y_____   N_____   Describe_____
5. Edema   Y_____   N_____   Describe_____

F. Pain   (0 = None / 10 = Intense)
1. Headache   Levels 0 1 2 3 4 5 6 7 8 9 10 Describe_____
2. Back   Levels 0 1 2 3 4 5 6 7 8 9 10 Describe_____
3. Abd. Cramp/Pain Levels 0 1 2 3 4 5 6 7 8 9 10 Describe_____
4. Perineal   Levels 0 1 2 3 4 5 6 7 8 9 10 Describe_____
5. Breast   Levels 0 1 2 3 4 5 6 7 8 9 10 Describe_____
6. Other _____
7. Use of Medication(s)
    a. Pain   N____   Type: Ibup./APAP   Tabs _____   Frequency_____
    b. RX   N____   Type: Docusate Na   Tabs _____   Frequency_____
    c. RX   N____   Type: _____   Tabs _____   Frequency_____
    d. Other   N____   Type: _____   Tabs _____   Frequency_____
    Comments_____
    e. Vitamin Supplements   Y_____   N_____   Instructed to resume_____

II. PSYCHOLOGICAL ASSESSMENT/ACTIVITIES OF DAILY LIVING
A. Nutrition
    1. Appetite   Good_____   Fair_____   Poor_____
    2. 24 Hour Diet History
        a. Breakfast:_____
        b. Lunch:_____
        c. Dinner:_____
        d. Snacks:_____
    3. Fluid Intake:_____ adequate_____
    4. Comments:_____
B. Sleep/Activity
    1. Sleep Hours   2   3   4   5   6   +
    2. Sleep Interruptions   0   1   2   3   4   +
    3. Naps/Rest Periods   0   1   2   3   4
    4. Energy Level (*0=none; 4=high*)   0   1   2   3   4
C. Infant Care Abilities (*Check appropriate box*)
    ☐ 0--Lack of interest/ability   ☐ 3--Growing competence; verbalizes understanding
    ☐ 1--Seems overwhelmed   ☐ 4--Confident, seems relaxed
    ☐ 2--Asks many questions   ☐ 5--Highly confident, comfortable
D. Responds to Infant Cues
    (*0=none; 4=high*)   0   1   2   3   4
E. General Hygiene   Adequate_____   Inadequate_____
E. Mother's General Comments (*feelings, body image, self-respect, PP blues*)
    1. Emotional Status   WNL_____   Altered_____
    2. Body Image   WNL_____   Altered_____
    4. Comments_____
G. Missing pieces of Labor & Delivery   Y____   N____
    1. Birthing experience as expected?   Y____   N____
    2. Comments_____
H. Control of Environment
    1. Home Environment (*safety, cleanliness*)   Adequate_____   Inadequate_____
    2. Modifications
        a. Stairs   Y____   Describe _____   N____
        b. Organizes home and activities to conserve energy   Y____   N____
        c. Support person's involvement_____
    3. Environment conducive to stimulating infant development   Y_____   N_____
    4. Siblings   Y____   N_____   Comment:_____
    5. Aware of birth control options   Y____   N____ Discussed_____
    6. Aware of community resources & support systems Y____ N____ Discussed_____
REFERRALS (*CODES: AI=Already involved; S=Suggested; RM=Referral made*)
A. Agencies   Healthy Families_____   PHD_____   WIC_____   Medicaid_____
    Hand-in-Hand_____   LC_____   New Moms_____   Behavioral Medicine_____
B. Other identified needs:_____

E. Extremities
☐ Varicosities   B   G   D   V
☐ Edema in legs   B   G   D   V
Comments:_____

F. Pain
☐ General Discomfort/Medications   B   G   D   V
Comments:_____

A. Nutrition
☐ Amount of calories from fat   B   G   D   V
☐ Appetite   B   G   D   V
☐ Nutritional requirements   B   G   D   V
Comments:_____

B. Sleep/Activity
☐ Sleep/activity/fatigue   B   G   D   V
Comments:_____

C. Infant Care Abilities
☐ Care abilities   B   G   D   V
Comments:_____

D. Responds to Infant Cues
☐ Cues   B   G   D   V
Comments:_____

E. General Hygiene
☐ Hygiene   B   G   D   V
Comments:_____

F. Mother's General Comments
☐ PP Blues, Depression/Body Image   B   G   D   V
Comments:_____

G. Missing Pieces of Labor & Delivery
☐ Concerns   B   G   D   V
Comments:_____

H. Control of Environment
☐ Appropriateness of environment
    for safety & infant stimulation   B   G   D   V
☐ Sibling   B   G   D   V
☐ Birth Control   B   G   D   V
☐ Community resources &
    support systems   B   G   D   V
Comments:_____

Patient ID Label

Nurse's Signature: _____

EXHIBIT 5–23   Infant Home Visit Record

RMH
Rockingham Memorial Hospital

FAMILY BIRTHPLACE
Family Care Nurse Home Visit - Infant Record

Name _____   Sex _____   DOB _____

Parent(s) _____   MR# _____

Visit Date _____   Peds _____

I.   PHYSICAL ASSESSMENT

A.   Vital Signs: T _____   AP _____   R _____
        Wt. _____   Length _____   head circumference _____

B.   Head
    1.   Fontanels: Level   Y ____   N ____   Describe: _____
    2.   Sutures: WNL   Y ____   N ____   Describe: _____
    3.   Molding: Y ____   N ____   Describe: _____
    4.   Cephalhematoma: Y ____   N ____   Left _____ Right _____ Occipital _____
    5.   Bruising: Y ____   N ____   Describe: _____
    6.   Abrasions: Y ____   N ____   Describe: _____
    7.   Eyes: Drainage   Y ____   N ____   Left ____ Right ____ Describe _____
            Sclera Jaundiced   Y ____   N ____
            Reacts to light   Y ____   N ____   Observed by parents: Yes _____ No ____
            Subconj. Hem.   Y ____   N ____   L _____ R _____
    8.   Ears: (shape, size, position)
            WNL   Y ____   N ____   Describe: _____
            Auditory Response   Y ____   N ____   Noted by parents: Yes _____ No ____
    9.   Nose: (patency)
            WNL   Y ____   N ____   Describe: _____
    10.   Mouth: (mucous membranes, tongue, palate, frenulum)
            WNL   Y ____   N ____   Describe: _____

C.   Chest
    1.   Breath Sounds:
            WNL   Y ____   N ____   Describe: _____

D.   Abdoment
    1.   Soft, Symmetrical
            WNL   Y ____   N ____   Describe: _____
    2.   Cord: Shedding Process
            WNL   Y ____   N ____   Describe: _____
            Cord   Dry _____   Moist _____   Off _____
            Cord clamp off   Y ____   N ____   Removed: _____
            Cord care   Y ____   N ____   Describe: _____

E.   Genitalia
    1.   Male:
            a.   Scrotum: (testicles descended, no bruising, normal appearance, normal scrotal edema)
                    WNL   Y ____   N ____   Describe: _____
            b.   Penis:
                    WNL   Y ____   N ____   Describe: _____
            c.   Circumcision: Y ____   N ____   Plastibell Y ____ Off ____
                    WNL   Y ____   N ____
                    Healing _____ Edematous _____ Bleeding _____ Drainage _____
                    Comments: _____
    2.   Female: (labia, introitus, normal appearance including hormonal swelling)
            WNL   Y ____   N ____   Describe: _____

F.   Skeletal
    1.   Extremities symmetry: Y ____   N ____   Describe: _____
    2.   Back (alignment):   Y ____   N ____   Describe: _____
    3.   Hands: WNL   Y ____   N ____   Describe: _____
    4.   Feet: WNL   Y ____   N ____   Describe: _____

G.   Elimination
    1.   Stools: #/24_: _____   Color _____   WNL: _____
    2.   Voiding: #/24_: _____   Concentrated _____   WNL: _____
    3.   Comments: _____

If indicated by a check mark (√), interventions taught according to protocols based on assessment. Additional needs and interventions are addressed in this column.
Level of Understanding:
B - Basic   D = Demonstrated
G = Good   V = Verbalized

A.   Vital Signs
☐   Temperature   B   G   D   V

Comments: _____

B.   Head
☐   Molding   B   G   D   V
☐   Cephalhematoma   B   G   D   V
☐   Eye drainage   B   G   D   V
☐   Subconj. Hemorrhage   B   G   D   V
☐   Congested nose   B   G   D   V
☐   Cleft lips or palate   B   G   D   V

Comments: _____

D.   Abdomen
☐   Umbilical Cord   B   G   D   V

Comments: _____

E.   Gentalia
☐   Mom's hormonal effect on
        baby girls and boys   B   G   D   V

Comments: _____

☐   Circumcision   B   G   D   V

Comments: _____

G.   Elimination
☐   Normal progression of stools
        after birth   B   G   D   V
☐   Gas retention   B   G   D   V
☐   Fluid imbalance/wt. Gain   B   G   D   V

Courtesy of Rockingham Memorial Hospital, Harrisonburg, Virginia. Reproduced with permission.

EXHIBIT 5–23   Infant Home Visit Record (*continued*)

H. Skin
    1. Condition: WNL_____   Dry_____   Cracked_____   Peeling_____
    2. Color: Pink_____   Pale_____   Jaundice_____
        Describe: _____
    3. Rash: None_____   Newborn_____   Diaper_____
        Describe:_____
    4. Bruises: Y _____   N _____   Describe: _____
    5. Variations: Mongolian Spots _____   "Stork Bites" _____   Birth Marks _____
        Describe: _____
    6. Pilonidal Dimple/Crease: Y _____   N _____

I. Neurological
    1. Muscle Tone: WNL _____   Describe: _____
    2. Reflexes: *(pressure, symmetry)*
        a. Moro: Y _____   N _____   Observed by Parents   Y_____   N _____
        b. Grasp: Y _____   N _____
        c. Babinski: Y _____   N _____
    3. Behavior Observed: Asleep _____   Awake_____   Fussy_____
    4. Cry: None during visit _____   Strong _____   Weak _____   Shrill_____

J. Nutritional Assessment
    1. Feeding
        a. Types: Breast _____   Formula (type) _____   Combination _____
        b. Frequency:
            Schedule_____   Demand _____
            Times per 24 hrs._____
            Length each nursing_____   PC feeding _____
            Amt. of formula _____
        c. Reflexes: Root _____   Suck _____   Swallow _____
        d. Vomiting: Y _____   N _____   Describe: _____
        e. Formula Preparation: Aseptic _____   Clean _____
        f. Bottle Preparation: Aseptic _____   Clean _____
    2. Pacifier: Y _____   N ____   Comments: _____

K. Neonatal Infant Pain Scale (NIPS) 0 1 2 3 4 5 6 7

	0	1	2
Facial expression	Relaxed muscles	Grimace	
Cry	No Cry	Whimper	Vigorous Cry
Breathing Patterns	Relaxed	Change in breathing	
Arms	Relaxed/Restrained	Flexed/Extended	
Legs	Relaxed/Restrained	Flexed/Extended	
State of Arousal	Sleeping/Awake	Fussy	

Comments: _____

L. Behavioral Assessment
    1. Sleep Activity: *(past 24 hours)*   Contented _____   Sleepy _____   Fussy _____
        Comments: _____
    2. Consolability: *(0=low / 4=high)*   0   1   2   3   4
    3. Techniques used: _____

M. REFERRALS *(CODES: AI=Already involved; S=Suggested; RM=Referral made)*
        Healthy Families_____   WIC _____   Lactation Consultant _____
        Medicaid _____   Public Health ____   Other _____

N. Additional written or verbal information given: _____
    _____
    _____
    _____
    _____

O. Follow-up call: Date_____   No questions/concerns: _____
    Issues addressed: _____
    _____
    _____
    _____

    1. PKU Drawn: Hospital _____   Home ___   Time _____
    2. Billirubin Drawn: _____   To Hospital _____
    3. Infant Appointment Scheduled:_____(Mom To Call)
    4. Ped notified: _____

H. Skin
☐ Skin care   B   G   D   V
☐ Baby bath   B   G   D   V
☐ Jaundice   B   G   D   V
☐ Diaper rash   B   G   D   V
☐ Care of pilonidal
    dimple/crease   B   G   D   V

Comments: _____
_____

I. Neurological

☐ Normal infant reflexes   B   G   D   V

Comments: _____
_____

☐ Infant temperament   B   G   D   V

J. Nutritional Assessment

☐ Breast Feeding   B   G   D   V
☐ Bottle Feeding   B   G   D   V
☐ How to burp baby   B   G   D   V

Comments: _____
_____
_____
_____

K. Pain

☐ Normal/Abnormal   B   G   D   V

Comments: _____
_____
_____

L. Behavioral Assessment

☐ Consoling techniques   B   G   D   V
☐ Safety   B   G   D   V
☐ First Steps Brochure   B   G   D   V

Comments: _____
_____
_____
_____
_____
_____

Comments: _____
_____
_____
_____
_____
_____

Patient ID Label	Nurse's Signature: _____

CHAPTER SUMMARY

Family-centered maternity care recognizes the importance of the postpartum period for family formation. All care concentrates on nonseparation of mothers and babies in order to promote attachment and successful breastfeeding.

Family-centered maternity care supports the developmental tasks of postpartum, which include physical restoration, emotional exploration of pregnancy, birth and role change, attachment work, assumption of the care-taking role, and redefinition of relationships within the family.

The model of care provided combines postpartum and nursery care into mother–baby care. In order to provide this care, postpartum and nursery nurses are cross-trained to become mother–baby nurses. One nurse cares for the mother and her baby as an interdependent couplet. Physicians examine newborns in the mother's room and teach the mother at the same time.

Mother–baby nurses help parents in the bonding process by explaining that their infant is a unique, distinct individual. The nurse teaches the parents about the newborn's states of awareness and personality, and demonstrates and role models infant care at the mother's bedside.

In FCMC, the father and other family members are never considered visitors. The mother determines which family members and friends will be welcome at her bedside and when.

Continuity of care is assured with postpartum follow-up services in the form of telephone calls, postpartum support groups, home care, and hospital-based clinics.

FACILITY FEATURES FOR FAMILY-CENTERED MOTHER–BABY CARE

Facility design for mother–baby care provides an environment that facilitates nonseparation of mothers and babies.

1. Privacy:

   If the facility design is LDR and a mother–baby unit:

   Private rooms with private baths are available for all women postpartum

   • These rooms are comparable in size and design to the LDRs.

   • There are an adequate number of these rooms to accommodate birth volume.

   If the facility design is LDRPs:

   • There are an adequate number of these rooms to accommodate birth volume.

   Private areas exist for:

   • Nursing report.

   • Staff consultation.

   • Counseling or comfort for the mother, baby, family, and visitors.

2. Mother–baby care space

   • Lighting and space are adequate in the mother's room to facilitate complete physical examination by an infant care provider.

   • Infant exam area is next to mother's bed.

3. Holding nursery/respite area

   • A holding nursery or respite area is adjacent to the nursing control and communication area.

   • A holding nursery allows ease of infant transfer (in cribs) by mothers and/or family members from the mother's room back to the nursery for brief periods of time.

4. Family space

   • There is adequate space for waiting family and visitors with toilet and kitchen or food services nearby.

   • There is adequate space, comfortable furniture, and bathrooms available for the father or other family member to remain overnight in the mother's room.

   • There is a sibling play area.

   • Space is provided for families to eat together during the postpartum stay.

5. Environment

   • Signs reflect the philosophy of FCMC.

   • Walls and furniture are clean and attractive.

   • There is individual control of temperature and light in each room.

   • Décor is appropriate for a mother–baby unit.

   • Décor diminishes the hospital environment.

6. Breastfeeding consultation rooms

   • There are private rooms for breastfeeding consultation and breast pump storage.

7. Staff and family education rooms

   • There is a large, home-like, comfortable room for family education.

   • There is adequate space for staff education, reporting, and conferencing.

COMPONENTS OF FAMILY-CENTERED MOTHER–BABY CARE

The following components of family-centered maternity care are emphasized in the postpartum period:

1. Promotion of mother's physical restoration

   • Assessment, prevention, detection and early treatment of complications.

   • Calm environment, rest, nourishment, and "mothering" of the mother.

2. Promotion of attachment
   - Nonseparation of mother and baby.
   - Early breastfeeding encouraged.
   - Support through emotional exploration of pregnancy and birth.
   - Social support.
   - Family cared for as a unit.
3. Provision of mother–baby care
   - One nurse cares for both mother and baby in couplet care.
   - Care is done at the mother's bedside in full view of the mother.
   - Newborn transitional care is provided at the mother's bedside in the LDR or LDRP.
   - Mothers and babies are separated only upon mother's request.
   - The mother–baby nurse role-models and demonstrates infant care and teaches parents about the state-related behavior of their unique baby.
   - Care is flexible and appropriate to physiologic needs as well as social and cultural needs of each family.
   - Newborn baths and weighing are done at the mother's bedside while teaching the mother.
4. Promotion of newborn's adaptation
   - Unobstructed breathing.
   - Maintenance of body temperature.
   - Assessment, prevention, detection, and early treatment of complications.
   - A safe environment.
5. Support for breastfeeding
   - Breastfeeding initiation within one hour of birth.
   - Breastfed babies are not fed formula or glucose water.
   - No formula gift packs for breastfeeding mothers.
   - Breastfeeding success center staffed with Certified Lactation Specialists.
6. Family education
   - One-to-one education is provided at the mother's bedside.

- Physicians examine babies at the mother's bedside and teach parents about their baby at the same time.
- Teaching is individualized.
- Mothers self-assess learning needs.
- Staff also does learning needs assessment.
- Teaching is attuned to individual learning styles.
- Parents are given written discharge instructions that include parenting issues/skills.
- Videos and printed instructional materials are available and distributed as appropriate.
- Videos and printed instructional materials are in the language(s) of the population served and are culturally appropriate.
- The mother is assessed prior to discharge for necessary infant care skills and satisfactory initiation of breastfeeding (if applicable).
- Mother–baby teaching and discharge planning includes parenting skills, community resources, and family adaptations and adjustments.

7. Visitation
   - The father and family members are not considered visitors.
   - The mother determines which family members and friends will be welcome at her bedside and when.
   - The baby's father and/or family members of the mother's choice are encouraged to participate in infant care.
8. Follow-up
   - Parents are given the birth facility phone number and told they may call on a 24-hour basis.
   - Referral to community sources of assistance is initiated when appropriate.
   - A nurse makes a follow-up phone call and/or home visit within one week of discharge to assess status of mother and baby.
   - Outpatient in-hospital follow-up care is available when appropriate.
   - Referrals to physicians, mid-level providers, or community agencies and support groups are made when appropriate.

BIBLIOGRAPHY

Ament, L. 1990. Maternal tasks of the puerperium reidentified. *Journal of Obstetrics, Gynecologic, and Neonatal Nursing* 19, no. 4, 330–335.

American Academy of Pediatrics. 1997. Work group on breastfeeding and the use of human milk. *Pediatrics* 100, no. 6: 1035–1039.

American Academy of Pediatrics, Committee on Fetus and Newborn. 1995. Hospital stay for healthy term newborns. *Pediatrics* 96, 788–790.

Association of Women's Health, Obstetric, and Neonatal Nurses (AWHONN). 1986. *Postpartum Follow-Up: A Nursing Practice Guide*. Washington, DC: Author.

———. 1989. *Mother Baby Care*. Washington, DC: Author.

———. 1991. *Postpartum Nursing Care: Vaginal Delivery*. Washington, DC: Author.

———. 1996. *Compendium of Postpartum Care*. Washington, DC: Author.

————. 1997. *Standards and Guidelines*. 5th ed. Washington, DC: Author.

Beckett, P., Wynn, B., and Redmond, S. 1996. Mother-baby nursing: A road map for success: Changing traditional delivery system to a single-room service. *Mother-Baby Journal* 1, no. 1: 7–13.

Beger, D., and Cook, C. 1996. Maternal postpartum learning needs. *International Journal of Childbirth Education* 11, no. 1: 23–26.

Blank, D., et al. 1995. Major influences on maternal responsiveness to infants. *Applied Nursing Research* 8, no. 1: 34–38.

Brazelton, T., and Cramer, B. 1990. *The Earliest Relationships: Parents, Infants and the Drama of Early Attachment*. Reading, MA: Addison-Wesley Publishing Company.

Canadian Institute of Child Health. 1996. *National Breastfeeding Guidelines for Health Care Providers*. Ottawa: Author.

Davis, J. H., Brucker, M. C., and MacMullen, N. J. 1988. A study of mothers' postpartum teaching priorities. *Maternal-Child Nursing Journal* 17, 41–50.

DiFlorio, I. 1991. Mother's comprehension of terminology associated with the care of the newborn baby. *Pediatric Nursing* 17, no. 2: 193–196.

DiGirolamo, A., Grummer-Strawn, L., and Fein, S. 2001. Maternity care practices: Implications for breastfeeding. *Birth* 28, no. 2: 94–100.

Dodgson, J., et al. 1999. Adherence to the ten steps of the baby-friendly hospital initiative in Minnesota hospitals. *Birth* 26, no. 4: 239–247.

Eidelman, A., et al. 1993. Cognitive deficits in women after childbirth. *Obstetrics and Gynecology* 81, no. 5: 764–767.

Enkin, M., et al. 2000. *A Guide to Effective Care in Pregnancy and Childbirth*. 3rd ed. New York: Oxford University Press.

Field, P. A., and Renfrew, M. 1991. Teaching and support: Nursing input in the postpartum period. *International Journal of Nursing Studies* 48, no. 2, 131–144.

Harvey, K. 1982. Mother-baby nursing. *Nursing Management* 13, no. 7: 22–23.

Health Canada. 2000. Family-centered maternity and newborn care: National guidelines. Ottawa: Minister of Public Works and Government Services.

Keefe, M. R. 1987. The impact of infant rooming-in on maternal sleep at night. *Journal of Obstetric, Gynecologic, and Neonatal Nursing* 17, no. 2: 122–126.

Keppler, A. 1995. Postpartum care center: Follow-up care in a hospital-based clinic. *Journal of Obstetric, Gynecologic, and Neonatal Nursing* 24, no. 1: 17–21.

Keppler, A., and Roudebush, J. 1999. Postpartum follow-up care in a hospital-based clinic: An update on an expanded program. *Journal of Perinatal Neonatal Nursing* 13, no. 1: 1–14.

Kyenkya-Isabirye, M. 1992. UNICEF launches the baby-friendly hospital initiative. *Maternal Child Nursing Journal* 17: 177–179.

Lawrence, R. 1995. The clinician's role in teaching proper infant feeding techniques. *The Journal of Pediatrics* 126, no. 6: S112–S117.

Lee, K., et al. 2000. Parity and sleep patterns during and after pregnancy. *Obstetrics and Gynecology* 95, no. 1: 14–18.

Lentz, M., and Killien, M. 1991. Are you sleeping? Sleep patterns during postpartum hospitalization. *Journal of Perinatal and Neonatal Nursing* 4, no. 4: 30–38.

Malnory, M. 1997. Mother-infant home care drives quality in a managed care environment. *Journal of Nursing Care Quality* 11, no. 4: 9–26.

Mansell, K. Mother–Baby Units: the concept works. *American Journal of Maternal Child Nursing* 9: 132–133.

McVeigh, C. 2000. Investigating the relationship between satisfaction with social support and functional status after childbirth. *American Journal of Maternal-Child Nursing* 25, no. 1: 25–30.

Mercer, R. 1986. *First-Time Motherhood: Experiences from Teens to Forties*. New York: Springer.

Merewood, A., and Philipp, B. 2001. Implementing change: Becoming baby-friendly in an inner city hospital. *Birth* 28, no. 1: 36–40.

Mulford, C. 1995. Swimming upstream: Breastfeeding care in a nonbreastfeeding culture. *Journal of Obstetric, Gynecologic, and Neonatal Nursing* 24, no. 5: 464–474.

Norr, K. F., Roberts, J. E., and Freese, U. 1989. Early postpartum rooming-in and maternal attachment behaviors in a group of medically indigent primiparas. *Journal of Nurse-Midwifery* 34, 85–91.

Panwar, S. 1986. Introducing family-centered care for mothers and newborns. *Nursing Management* 17, no. 11: 45–47.

Perez-Escamilla, R., Politt, E., Lonnerdal, B., and Dewey, K. 1994. Infant feeding policies in maternity wards and their effect on breastfeeding success: An analytic overview. *American Journal of Public Health* 84, no. 1: 89–95.

Phillips, C. 1996. *Family-Centered Maternity Newborn Care: A Basic Text*. 4th ed. St. Louis: Mosby–Yearbook.

Phillips, C. R. 1997. *Mother-Baby Nursing*. Washington, DC: Association of Women's Health, Obstetric and Neonatal Nurses.

Phillips, C., and Fenwick, L. 2000. *Single-Room Maternity Care*. Philadelphia: Lippincott.

Pridham, K., et al. 1991. Early postpartum transition: Progress in maternal identity and role attainment. *Research in Nursing and Health* 14: 21–31.

Rubin, R. 1961. Puerperal change. *Nursing Outlook* 9, no. 12: 753–755.

————. 1975. Maternity nursing stops too soon. *American Journal of Nursing* 75, 10: 1680–1685.

————. 1984. *Maternal Identity and the Maternal Experience*. New York: Springer.

Ruchala, P. 2000. Teaching new mothers: Priorities of nurses and postpartum women. *Journal of Obstetric, Gynecologic, and Neonatal Nursing* 29, no. 3: 265–273.

Saadeh, R., and Akre, T. 1996. Ten steps to successful breastfeeding: A summary of the rationale and scientific evidence. *Birth* 23, no. 3: 154–160.

Simpson, K. 1996. *Easing the Transition from Hospital to Home: Postpartum Discharge Planning and Homecare Services*. White Plains: March of Dimes Birth Defects Foundation.

Stark, M. 2000. Is it difficult to concentrate during the 3rd trimester and postpartum? *Journal of Obstetric, Gynecologic, and Neonatal Nursing* 29, no. 4: 378–389.

Symanski, M. 1992. Maternal-infant bonding: Practice issues for the 1990s. *Journal of Nurse-Midwifery* 37, no. 2: 675–735.

Tiedje, L. B., et al. 2002. An ecological approach to breastfeeding. *American Journal of Maternal Child Nursing* 27, no. 3: 154–161.

Todd, L. 1996. *ICEA Postnatal Education Certification Program Study Guides*. Minneapolis: ICEA.

———. 1998. Reciprocal interactions as the foundation for parent-infant attachment. *International Journal of Childbirth Education* 13, no. 4: 5–8.

———. 2001. *Postpartum: The Making of a Family*. Minneapolis: The International Childbirth Education Association.

Vestal, K. 1982. A proposal: Primary nursing for the mother-baby dyad. *Nursing Clinics of North America* 17, no. 3: 3–9.

Watters, N.E. 1985. Combined mother-infant nursing care. *Journal of Obstetric, Gynecologic, and Neonatal Nursing* 14: 478–483.

Watters, N. E., and Kristiansen, C. M. 1995. Two evaluations of combined mother-infant versus separate postnatal nursing care. *Research in Nursing and Health* 18, no. 1: 17–26.

White, M. B. 2002. Becoming a father: The postpartum man. *International Journal of Childbirth Education* 17, no. 3: 4–6.

Wilkerson, N. N., and Barrow, T. L. 1988. Reuniting mothers and babies: Synchronizing care with mother-baby rhythms. *The American Journal of Maternal Child Nursing* 13: 264–268.

Williams, L., and Cooper. M. 1996. A new paradigm for postpartum care. *Journal of Obstetric, Gynecologic, and Neonatal Nursing* 25, no. 9: 745–749.

World Health Organization. 1998. *Postpartum Care of the Mother and Newborn: A Practical Guide*. Report of a technical working group. Publication no. WHO/RHT/MSM/ 98.3. Geneva: Author.

Yamauchi, Y., and Yamanouchi, I. 1990. Breastfeeding frequency during the first 24 hours after birth in full-term neonates. *Pediatrics* 86, no. 2: 171–175.

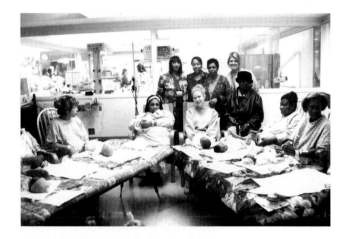

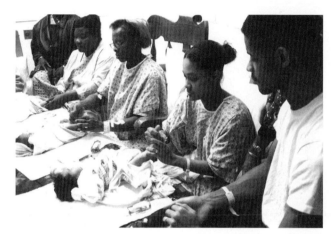

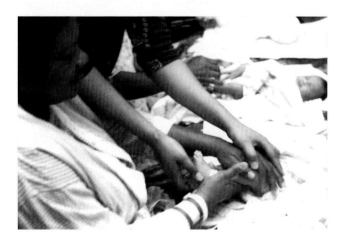

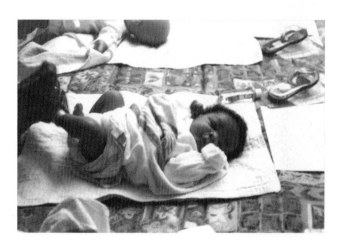

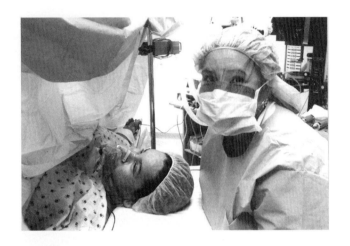
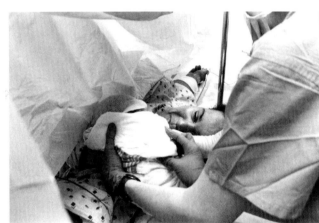
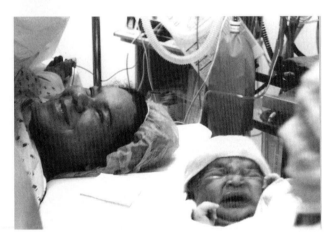
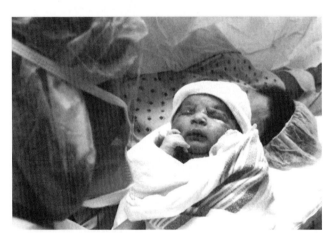

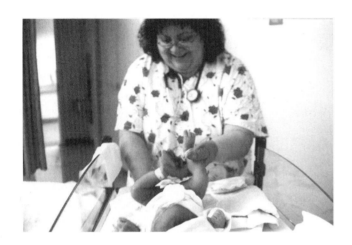

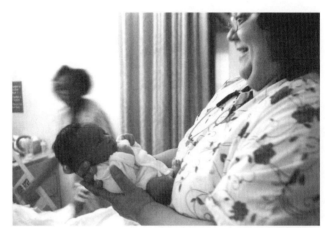

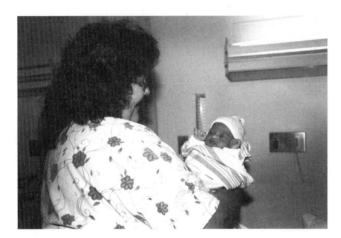

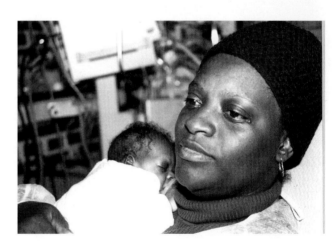

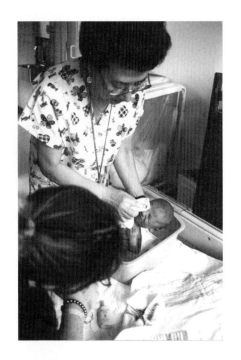

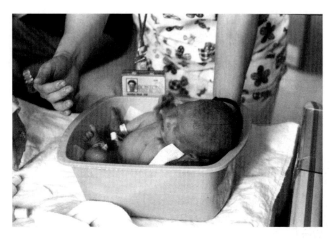

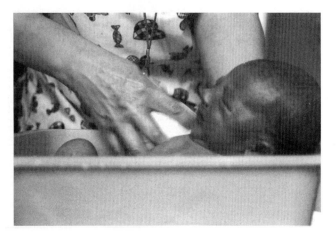

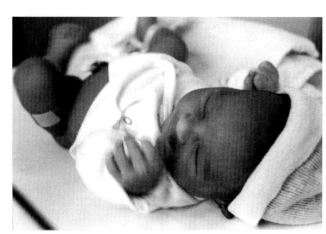

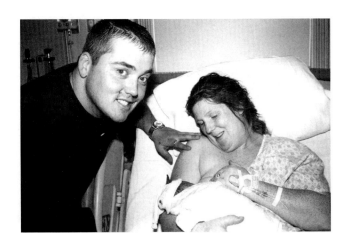

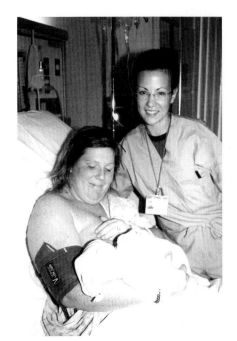

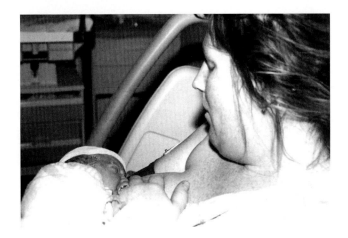

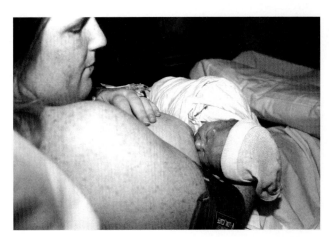

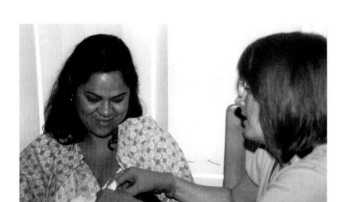
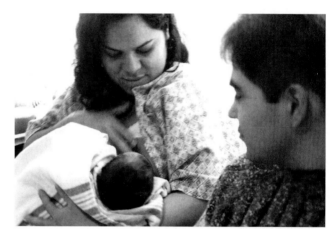
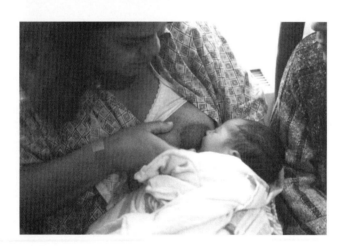
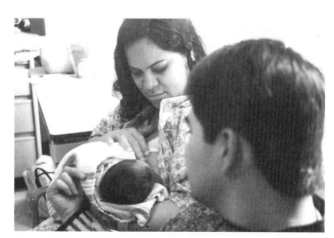

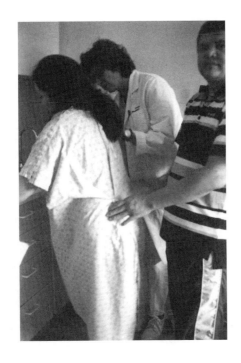

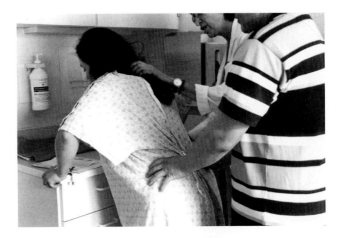

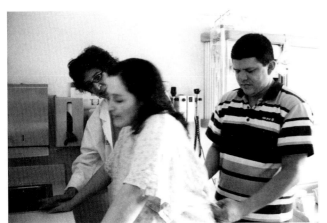

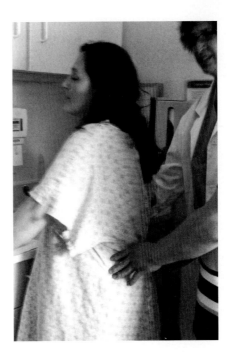

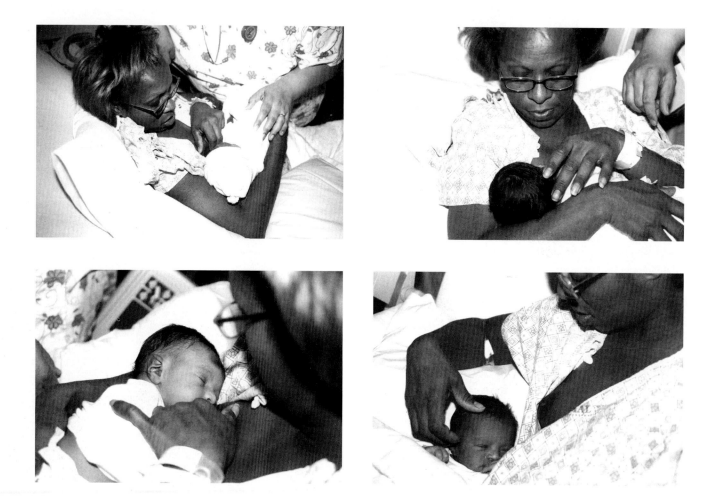

Marketing Family-Centered Maternity Care

by Elizabeth Hamilton, PhD

INTRODUCTION

Developing a family-centered maternity care (FCMC) program does not end with the implementation of mother–baby nursing care and the adaptation of a mission, vision, and philosophy of care suitable for the care model. Integrating the clinical program and marketing is also necessary for success. Many hospitals forget this critical step in the process and do not achieve the success that might have been attained had they developed a well thought-out strategic marketing plan.

WHAT IS MARKETING?

Marketing is a puzzling and misunderstood concept to many people, both inside and outside of hospitals. Some people believe that marketing and advertising are synonymous; the author has frequently heard caregivers state, "If they would just run an ad, we would increase our volume." There are others who believe that placing an article about a hospital service in the newspaper satisfies the need for marketing. This is consistent with the "tell them about it and they'll come" philosophy. Neither viewpoint is true.

Marketing, at the most fundamental level, can be defined as: *the total of all activities and strategies that result in offering a product that satisfies customers while increasing profitability for the organization that offers the product.* It really is no more difficult than that! The American Marketing Association, an international professional organization for marketing professionals, presents a more formal definition:

> *Marketing is the process of planning and executing the conception, pricing, promotion and distribution of ideas, goods and services to create exchanges that satisfy individual and organizational objectives. (Bennett, 1995)*

Whether you prefer the simple or the formal definition, each one points to three key marketing mandates:

- Marketing involves some type of product.
- Marketing focuses on customer need.
- Marketing satisfies organizational objectives.

The first mandate is that *there must be a real product to market*. Contrary to popular belief, large rooms, wallpaper borders, and mauve or teal paint and bedspreads do not constitute a product! Many hospitals across the country have marketed pretty rooms for labor and birth only to find that the women who chose them for their first births based on the rooms did not remain loyal to them for future events. The end result was that the bottom line did not improve as anticipated. In order to be a product, a philosophy of care that appeals to consumers must be integrated into daily operations in that beautiful facility. It is not the rooms that sell the service; it is informing women how they will be treated in the rooms, and then carrying through on that promise, that creates the marketing opportunity.

The second mandate of marketing is that *marketing focuses on what the customer wants or needs*. This means that in order to be successful, it is necessary to determine what consumers want or need *before* the product (or program) is created and marketed. If a decision is made to provide a product that administrators, nurses, or physicians perceive as best, and attempts are then made to convince the consumer to want that product, a very steep uphill climb will be experienced. Few people will purchase and be loyal to a product that they really do not want. Gravett (1989) dramatically demonstrated the disparity between what women want and what administrators *think* women want when she asked both groups the same set of questions and found their responses "alarmingly dissimilar."

The definition of marketing includes a third directive. It is the mandate that ensures that *organizational objectives (for profitability or market share, for example) are enhanced* through the marketing effort.

Based on these definitions, it can be seen that marketing is not a static, one-time activity. It is a fluid and creative blending of the many activities that are required to meet *all* of the objectives of marketing. It is important that all the objectives are met, for when marketing is managed well, it results in a win-win situation for both consumers and hospitals—consumers get the product or service they want, and the hospital gains increased market share, profitability, and loyalty share.

FINDING OUT WHAT THE CONSUMER WANTS

So how does one determine what the female consumer wants? There are myriad national studies that attempt to determine what women want. Although national research is acceptable about 70 percent of the time, regional variation or community-based differences should not be overlooked. Before finalizing the planning process, it is important to find out what women in your own community or region want in addition to noting what women across the nation desire. Finding out what women in the area want is best accomplished by primary marketing research.

The most common research techniques include focus groups, telephone and mail survey research, and personal interviews. Each technique gathers different types of information and each has advantages and limitations.

Focus Groups

Focus groups rely on data that is unstructured and first person in nature. These data are termed "qualitative" or "soft science" because they are expressed by words and ideas rather than by numbers. A focus group is a small number of interacting individuals focusing on a limited number of issues or topics. Focus groups are typically limited to between 8 and 12 people per group and last one and one-half to two hours. This method is particularly useful in exploratory research where little is known about the topic of interest. Focus groups are often used very early in the research process and then are followed with large-sample research to validate findings. On the other hand, focus groups may follow a quantitative survey as a means of adding depth to the findings. Focus groups are also preeminent in research where you wish consumers to look at some feature in several formats and decide which format is most appealing (as in room décor or layout, or an ad campaign that is in the formative stages). For a more in-depth discussion of focus groups in a marketing context, the reader is referred to Bellenger, Bernhardt, and Goldstucker (1976) and Higgenbotham and Cox (1979).

Designing Focus Groups The first step in the focus group research process is consistent with other type of research—it must begin with a problem to which answers are required. Steps in the process then proceed as follows:

- The problem or issue of interest must be clearly defined before the research commences.

- Next you must determine how many groups to hold. For example, you might want to hold two groups of women from the same general service area. One group would comprise women who delivered at your hospital and the other group would comprise women who did not. Or you might want to hold four groups, splitting them on insurance provider and the hospital where they delivered. Decisions about the many ways to configure groups are ultimately based on the issues of interest and your budget.

- The next decision in the process is where to hold the groups. Is there a focus group facility nearby? If not, what other location would be private, quiet, and appropriate? This will also depend on whether you wish to videotape and audiotape the proceedings and whether you would like observers from the hospital to be able to watch the proceedings. In a focus group facility, a two-way mirror facilitates observation of the groups as they are in process. Short of this type of facility, remote video can be arranged between, for example, two hotel meeting rooms.

- You must decide what honorarium to offer those who are being recruited. In some areas, only money talks. If that is the case, you probably already know what amount is optimally persuasive for your region. In other locales, coupons for dinner or a movie are incentive enough to persuade people to participate. You must decide for yourself what will work for your consumers.

- The next step is to define the characteristics of those who will be group members. For example, you may want females between the ages of 18 and 39 who live in particular zip codes or who have particular types of insurance. You might also want women who have had a baby in the last two years or plan to have another child. Many characteristics could be included, but it is key that they are consistent with the problem that is being investigated. In addition, group characteristics should not be too many layers deep. Each additional layer means that more and more people will not qualify for inclusion.

- Now you must decide whether you wish the groups to be "blind." In a blind study, group members will not know who is sponsoring the groups. For example, if your purpose in holding the groups is to find out what people know about your obstetrical program, you may not want them to know who is asking their opinion. That knowledge might bias responses of women who delivered at your hospital and who might be eager to please you or, alternatively, those who came to your hospital and want to let the world know that they did not have a good experience.

- After the criteria for recruiting have been defined and you have decided whether the groups will be blind or open, recruiting resources must be decided upon. How will group members be recruited? Where will you find the names of people to contact? Be very careful with this step. HIPAA regulations (Health Insurance Portability and Accountability Act of 1996) make it very clear that relying on computer records of hospital discharges for names is inappropriate and unacceptable. If you live in a relatively large area and have marketing or focus groups firms nearby, you may wish to hire them to do your recruiting based on a recruiting script that defines the criteria for inclusion in each group. If you do not have this option, you must be creative in coming up with other options. Sometimes, placing a blind ad works to recruit people. You must have a non-hospital phone number for them to respond to, however, if you wish the survey to remain blind.

- Next it is time to find a moderator for your groups. If the area has a focus group facility, they may have a moderator who can assist you. You may also wish to contact a consulting firm or research firm that moderates focus groups. Rarely, you can find someone in your hospital that is qualified to lead the groups. Moderating looks easy, but it is really an art, and it is not for the faint of heart. The moderator must be able to tap dance along with the group, changing subjects and adapting as events occur. In addition, the moderator must be very familiar with the topic(s) that the discussion will focus on and be capable of guiding the group and keeping it on track.

- At this juncture the topical script is written. This is the moderator's guide for conducting the groups. It typically contains five or six subtopics, all aimed at answering the question set forth in the statement of the problem in step one. The moderator's script highlights areas to probe, questions to ask, and so forth. This script details what the groups will accomplish.

- Finally, the groups are held, and the detailed report on the findings is produced.

Advantages of Focus Groups
- Results can be obtained in less time than it would take to interview people individually or assemble and conduct a large-scale quantitative survey.

- Focus groups are less expensive than a large quantitative survey.

- The moderator can interact directly with the group and is able to clarify responses on the spot.

- Group members can respond to one another and build on ideas expressed by other group members. This interaction may lead to new ideas that had not been considered previously.

- Nonverbal group cues are apparent, and the moderator can respond to them as appropriate.

- Data are in the participant's own words so local nuances and colloquialisms can be factored into findings.

- Data are rich and in-depth.

- Focus group results are easily understood. No statistical terminology is required to comprehend their meaning.

- All participants, from the most literate to the least, can participate.

Limitations of Focus Groups
- The moderator can easily bias the outcome by intentionally or unintentionally providing cues about desirable responses.

- Results cannot be generalized to the larger population, even if several focus groups on the same topic are held. This is due to the convenience nature of the recruiting methods used. Additionally, there may be differences of opinion and character between people who would voluntarily drive to a location to participate in up to two hours of research for some type of payment and those who would not.

- Responses are not independent. One person's response may be affected by the response of some other group member.

- A particularly forceful member of the group may bias results by intimidating other group members.

- Summarization of qualitative findings is difficult.

- A transcript is typically required to interpret the findings. Transcription of focus group tapes is an art form requiring a great deal of patience and time. Consequently, transcription is quite expensive.

Survey Research

Survey research is typically termed "quantitative" research because results are generated through structured measures and are communicated using a variety of numbers, graphics, and statistical measures. These are typically termed "hard data," and because they are generated through large-sample methodology, they are given greater validity than focus groups. This is so because findings are most typically based on random selection of participants.

At one time or another many of us have been called on the telephone and asked to participate in a survey. Frequently, we have no idea how our name was obtained for this call. Most likely it was not our name at all that produced the call. Rather, it was our phone number that came up as a result of random digit dialing (RDD), a technique in which a computer generates a phone number. This is one means of random sampling a population of interest. There are others, such as using a table of random numbers that can be obtained from a computer programmed to generate them.

The way in which randomness is attained has been the subject of many research projects, some more clarifying than others. The *importance* of randomness in daily life tends to be overlooked. An example that illustrates the importance of the random process will serve to verify the significance of random selection.

The event occurred in 1969 shortly after the first draft lottery was held for the war in Vietnam. The lottery used birthdays encased in capsules and placed in a bowl. John Ware, a statistician, conducted an analysis of the order in which birth dates were selected and arrived at the conclusion that the process for selecting young men for service was not random. He found that the birth dates in the last six months of the year were more likely to be drawn than were birth dates in the first six months of the year. In reporting the finding, he stated:

> *I would guess that they probably placed the capsules containing the numbers into the bowl in a chronological order.... In the course of shuffling the capsules, the months tended to stay together. The first six months may have been placed in the bowl first, and they tended to stay together and be drawn last.... The cards were stacked against its being fair.... It wasn't the best procedure with our current knowledge of probability. (Berman, 1969)*

Random sampling is important in survey research because it is only through such sampling of a population that results can be generalized to those who did not participate. This is because random sampling requires every person, technically, to have an equal opportunity to be included in the sample. It is assumed that if a sample is randomly generated, it will be representative of the population from which it was drawn, and that the opinions expressed by the sample to research questions will also be true of the population.

There are many ways to gather data from a population. Three to be discussed in this chapter are mail surveys, telephone surveys, and personal interviews.

Designing a Survey As was true in the focus group example, the first step in the survey research process is careful definition of the research question or questions that need to be answered. Once that decision is made, a series of questions about the research must be answered. Entire methodology books have been written about survey research. This chapter is not an attempt to compete with those lofty tomes. The list that follows is a short one, pointing out only the most important points to be answered in the process:

- Will the survey be telephone, mail, or personal interview? Personal interviews are the most expensive but also tend to have the highest response rate because they are one on one. Telephone surveys typically cost more than mail surveys, but the response rate is higher in the former than in the latter. More surveys will need to be mailed than phone calls made because response rates differ dramatically. A 50 percent return would be considered excellent for a mailed survey. More typically the response can be 11–50 percent depending on the questionnaire content and length. Telephone compliance rates on the other hand are routinely in the 90 percent range, and personal interviews are even higher in compliance.

- How will random sampling be achieved? The most reliable methods include a random number generator or random digit dialing (so unlisted telephones also have the potential to be included).

- What size sample is required? This depends on the answers to three questions:

  - What error rate is acceptable? The larger the sample size, the lower the error rate.

  - What response rate is acceptable? Suppose a sample of 300 people is desired and a 75 percent response is anticipated to a telephone survey. In this event, 400 people would actually have to be contacted to compensate for the 25 percent who will either be unable or unwilling to participate. The same is true for mailed surveys. If a 15 percent return is anticipated and a sample of 300 is desired, then 2,000 questionnaires would need to be mailed.

  - What confidence level is acceptable? The confidence level indicates the level of error that the researcher is willing to accept and is based on the normal curve and probabilities. It refers to the degree of certainty needed to be sure that the sample response (or value) reflects that of the total population. The researcher assigns confidence levels before data collection, and the levels are usually set at 90 percent, 95 percent, or 99.9 percent, depending on the issue being studied. For highly critical research potentially involving people's lives, researchers would wish to be 99.9 percent certain that sample results were representative of the population. For survey research, the most typical value is 95 percent. The greater the certainty desired, the larger the sample size necessary.

- Will there be subpopulations or criteria for inclusion? The more screening questions, the greater the cost of the survey. As the pool of eligible people becomes smaller and smaller, the number of calls required to connect with a qualified respondent increases. For example, if you wanted to contact only childbearing women who had a baby in the past two years, you would need to contact many more households to find those women than you would need to call if just any household would do. Stratifying samples to be sure that they are representative of minority populations also adds to the cost of a survey.

- How long will the questionnaire be? In a telephone survey, interview length refers both to time and to the number of questions. The longer the interview, the more the survey will cost. In a mailed survey, a complex, multi-paged questionnaire may result in few people being willing to complete it.

- What indicators will be used? Creating indicators and response categories that deliver the information that is desired is a serious endeavor requiring a great deal of time. There are "canned" questions that are frequently used in market surveys, but these may not be suitable for all research questions. Sometimes, new specific questions must be created.

- Who will make the telephone calls? Performing this kind of research in-house is very difficult. It is recommended that you contract with a qualified research or consulting company with access to a phone bank for this type of research.

- Who will do the personal interviews? If this is someone from in-house, this person's primary job must be put on hold for the duration of the survey, and he or she should receive training in appropriate interviewing technique.

- Pretest or not? Pretesting prevents misleading or ambiguous questions from being used in the final survey and increases the instrument's reliability. Pretesting costs money, so its value may be underestimated and not considered worth the dollars. Pretesting ultimately saves money, however, because questions that are likely to cause problems can be identified and changed prior to field interviewing.

- How will results be analyzed? Hand tabulation is not the best choice! Assuming a research firm was hired to do the survey, the analysis will be part of the package. If you did not hire a research firm, purchasing and using a statistical analysis software program or contracting out the analysis is frequently the best option.

Advantages of Telephone Survey Research
- Results from the sample can be generalized to a larger population.
- Structured questions make analysis easier than unstructured format and open-ended questions.
- Random sample findings have greater validity than those generated by research methods that do not use random methodology.
- Almost all homes in the United States have a telephone so access is easy.
- Large sample coverage is simplified.
- Overall reliability and validity of the findings is maximized.

Limitations of Telephone Survey Research
- Expensive due to the large sample requirement.
- Time consuming; from start to finish a survey can take six to eight weeks or longer.
- Requires a random sample for validity.
- Difficult to obtain sensitive or attitudinal information.
- Increasing number of unlisted telephones.
- Survey response rates have been negatively impacted by consumer aversion to telemarketers.

- If the questionnaire is too long, the subject may hang up in the middle of the survey.

- Interviewers must be trained and must be qualified to speak to others on the phone. Poor readers, those who do not speak English well, and so forth, will not be successful telephone survey interviewers.

- Structured questions prevent probing for clarification of responses.

Advantages of Mail Questionnaires
- Minimally expensive both in dollars and in effort.
- Permit wide geographic coverage.
- Reach people who are difficult to locate and otherwise reach.
- Questions can be presented uniformly.
- Respondent answers questions in private.
- There is no interviewer so the impact of an interviewer's voice or appearance is not an issue.
- Respondent answers questions in his or her own time frame.

Limitations of Mail Questionnaires
- Non-returns are problematic and must be addressed. Intensive follow-up with postcards and/or telephone calls may be required to generate an acceptable response rate, thus adding cost to the research effort.
- The person to whom the questionnaire was mailed may not be the one who is actually answering it.
- Talking to friends or neighbors about the questionnaire may bias responses.
- Those who respond may be significantly different from those who do not, leaving you with a group of people about whom nothing is known.
- Return postage must be included or response will be very low.
- Some type of incentive for response is almost mandatory. This inevitably adds cost.

Advantages of Personal Interviews
- People are willing to cooperate in most instances, and the response rate is high.
- The interviewer can interact with the respondent to clarify meaning.
- The respondent can be shown visual material to which he or she may be asked to respond.
- The interviewer can get spontaneous responses from the respondent who has not had prior notification of the questions to be asked.
- The interview can take longer than in a telephone survey. Once the interview begins, most respondents will complete it.

- Groups who are rarely included in research can be included (such as the homeless, the poor, or those who do not attend school).

Limitations of Personal Interviews

- Higher costs are involved in all aspects of the survey. Many times, this involves travel costs for interviewers to get to the interview location.

- People in urban areas are reluctant to open the door to a stranger. More buildings in urban areas have locked central entrances preventing access to the building.

- Interviewers must be particularly well trained and astute or data may be inaccurate or incomplete.

- The interviewers' unintentional bias may lead them to unconsciously ask questions with a particular inflection in order to validate their own views.

- Personal interviews take a great deal of time.

In addition to the methods discussed above, convenience samples can also be used to take the pulse of your consumer base. These are not random and cannot be generalized to the population at large, but they can give you insight into a program's appeal. For example, if you have a perinatology clinic as part of your obstetrical program, periodically give women a five- to seven-item questionnaire while they are sitting in the waiting room. Ask what they think of the service and solicit ideas about what else might be helpful. Over time, some patterns might emerge that will evoke new ideas. Patient satisfaction tools typically work on this principle, although some are not as specific as might be desirable.

Asking consumers what they want is both a device for acquiring information and a smart marketing tool. If you ask consumers their preferences, you are sending a message that you value their opinions and want to know what will make them happy. As a result, they perceive that you care about them. And caring is one of the things that hospitals do best!

WHAT WOMEN SAY THEY WANT

When women are directly asked what kinds of things are important to them when they are having a baby, some of their responses are amazingly similar. Responses tend not to depend on region, level of education or income, race, type of insurance, or marital status. In other words, for the big things, women speak with one voice. In the following paragraphs, key components of a satisfactory maternity program are presented. These are derived from a number of research sources.

Research about Maternity Care

Between 1992 and 2001, the author conducted national primary research, including focus groups and phone surveys, about women's healthcare in general as well as specific to

maternity care choices. With regard to maternity care choices, focus groups included approximately 1,500 women, and phone surveys added another 7,500 women, for a grand total of 9,000 respondents. In addition, secondary data illuminates women's comments about maternity care, particularly data from birth stories (Simpkin, 1991, 1992), and *Parent* magazine's poll of 72,000 women (1992).

When data from focus groups and surveys conducted by the author are analyzed for consistencies, some significant patterns and preferences emerge. The following bullet points list the percentage of women who desire each program characteristic and a brief explanation for each. Percentages are based on 9,000 cases.

- 100% **Private room and bath.** Having a baby is an intimate experience, and most women wish to have complete privacy. Since childbirth involves bleeding, women are quite opposed to sharing a bathroom with another woman who is also bleeding, as they fear contact with AIDS, HIV, and Hepatitis C through blood-borne pathogens.

- 95% **Special care nursery.** While the majority of newborns are well, many mothers prefer to deliver in a hospital that has a special care nursery "just in case." When asked how many of their newborns required the special care nursery, about 15% responded in the affirmative. This figure is consistent with the percentage of newborns nationally who require special care. In short, 80% of women who feel that this option is critically important are being influenced by perceived rather than real need.

- 95% **Place for my partner to sleep.** This is not an unreasonable request. New dads do not want to miss out on the joys of this intimate family event. Having a place for the partner to sleep makes it possible for full participation of all members of the new family. Some hospitals have a lounge chair for dads, others provide a sleeper sofa in the mother's room, and some bring in a double or queen-sized bed following birth. Whatever the furniture arrangement, this is very high on the list of consumer satisfiers.

- 85% **No moving.** The majority of women would prefer to stay in one room from admission to discharge. About 15% of women, however, feel that they would like to move to a new room following delivery because it feels like "a graduation." Clearly, there is an interaction between staying in the same room for labor, delivery, recovery, and postpartum and having a private room, however. When the 15% who want to move to another room are asked whether they would mind being moved to a semiprivate postpartum room, they are adamant that they would mind a great deal. Those who wish to move to another room following recovery prefer that option *only* if they can move to a private postpartum room.

- 80% **Same nurse for mother and baby.** Eight in ten women prefer having the same nurse for themselves and their newborn, citing better communication and educational opportunities. The 20% who prefer the more traditional model believe that newborns require a specialized nurse and do not feel comfortable having care provided to their baby by a nurse who is cross trained.

- 80% **Baby in the room (with baby lounge option).** The vast majority of women would like to have their newborn in the room with them as much as possible if they have an option to send their baby to a holding nursery or baby lounge should they feel the need to do so and *if* there is a nurse available to assist them when their baby is in the room. They are completely opposed to the old rooming-in model in which the new mother and family members were responsible for all newborn care and the baby was *required* to stay in the room all the time. The 20% of mothers who do not want their baby in the room with them feel that they "need rest" and "have plenty of time to get to know the baby in the next eighteen years." Not coincidentally, women who do not want their baby in the room are frequently the same ones who want a specialized nursery nurse for their newborn.

Notice that none of these research findings mention room size, wall color, or matching curtains and bedspreads. All are program-based rather than facility-based issues.

WHY MARKET YOUR MATERNITY SERVICE?

To some people, the good old days were those decades when hospitals did not market. In fact, it was considered undignified and unprofessional to tell people about one's services, and neither hospitals nor doctors engaged in marketing. Those were the days when the hospital had a service to provide, the patient came to the hospital to get that service, and everybody was happy with the result. Patients were treated, doctors were paid, hospitals made money. Word of mouth was sufficient marketing.

Times have changed!

In contrast to those good old days, patients have become consumers, and many of the services that hospitals offer have become commodities. Packaged goods such as soap, toilet tissue, and cereal typically fall into the commodity category of commerce, not hospital services. This transition in focus has created a need for a very different kind of marketing in the healthcare sector. The goal of commodity marketing is to differentiate one's product and gain consumer loyalty so a competitor's product will not even be considered, let alone purchased. Differentiation in the commodities marketplace frequently relies on branding.

Branding

The term *branding* derives from the brand symbol that is used to distinguish livestock owned by one party from that owned by another. It is a permanent "mark" that makes the ownership visible (McStravic, 2001). Branding has frequently been translated into a distinctive logo for an organization or a service. Branding is much more than its graphic representation, however. The brand indicates what it is about the organization or the service that makes it deserving of admiration, preference, and loyalty. In a sense, the brand becomes the shorthand for consumers to use when deciding between two products. For example, when faced with the choice between a brand-name product and a store-brand product, many consumers will select the brand name because they feel they will reduce their risk in doing so. In other words, they trust the brand name on the basis of prior experience or prior knowledge about that product. If the product is consistently good, that is the one that will be chosen rather than one that is unknown.

Branding is considered somewhat new with respect to marketing strategy, coming to the forefront of attention only in the last decade or so. But as Sam Hill, president and CEO of Helios Consulting, reported in a speech to library directors recently, "Branding is nothing new in the marketplace" (Hill, 2001). In his talk, Mr. Hill traced the history of branding, suggesting that it started in 200 B.C. as a maker's mark on the bottom of a sandal in Syria. The mark brought recognition of the maker then, just as it does today.

Most of us can list several brands off the top of our heads. The most powerful brands are known for superiority in one area even though they may be excellent overall. In the retail industry, "First in customer service" evokes the Nordstrom name. Where automobiles are concerned, BMW is branded as "the ultimate driving machine." The soup in the red, white, black, and yellow can has long been Campbell's. Branding, however, is more than just a logo or a gimmick. The brand has to be backed with action that proves that the customer is correct in trusting the company that has the familiar brand. Customer emotion, what David Shore (2001), dean of the Harvard School of Public Health, calls "top of heart," only comes about when the promise is met consistently.

Branding is tricky in the healthcare sector. The key concepts for healthcare tend to be intangibles such as quality, trust, and caring. Virtually every hospital in the nation claims to be best at each of these. Of all healthcare institutions, the Mayo Clinic may be the most successful at expanding its brand image for high quality care from expert providers whom you can trust from Rochester, Minnesota, all the way across the nation.

How is brand identity based on intangibles developed? Shore (2001) says that the simple formula for brand value is "strategic awareness + perceived quality + singular distinction." Let's look at each of the three components in the brand value formula and see how they can be broken down into workable units.

Strategic awareness derives from the marketing tools that the hospital uses. These are the ways in which the hospital gets it message out to the woman that the hospital is trying to attract. So the first step must be increasing her awareness, but doing so in a way that is consistent with the hospital's overall strategy.

Perceived quality, the second variable in the formula, has many components. Quality is a difficult concept to measure and means different things to different constituencies. For example, if physicians are asked what they think quality means to patients, they will invariably point to physician credentials as key. Yet research that asks women to state what signifies that a hospital is a quality place records an entirely different response. Focus group research moderated by the author has demonstrated time and again that women take it for granted that physician credentials are a given and that *all* doctors are qualified or they would not be in practice. Instead, women cite such things as "They treat me like an individual," "They respect me," "There are enough nurses," and "The place is clean." Most of the *perceived* factors that point to quality, then, are those that speak to how a woman is treated by caregivers rather than what academic degrees they have and what initials follow their names.

The final element in the formula, *singular distinction*, refers to that aspect of the service that makes it unique and unlike anything that competitors offer.

Hatch and Schultz (2001) point out that a strong brand is the result of three interdependent elements that they call "strategic stars." These include vision (top management's aspirations), culture (organizational values, behaviors, and attitudes), and image (the world's impression of the place of interest). All three must be in alignment for the brand to be effective.

Once the brand is built, the goal is to create brand loyalty. The brand is communicated via all of the tools that marketing has at its disposal, including advertising, public relations, a web site, signage, and, most important, actually *living the brand*. The brand is the face of the relationship that exists between the service provider and its consumers. Remember, as discussed above, branding aims first of all to create awareness, then a positive perception, and finally a singular distinction that will lead consumers to prefer the hospital that created the brand. The brand promises consumers that they can expect experiences that will meet their needs and expectations each and every time they interact with that hospital.

Family-centered maternity care (FCMC) is an example of a brand. Most hospitals in the nation claim to practice FCMC but few really manage to incorporate all ten principles of FCMC into daily practice. Hospitals that actually do incorporate the principles are inundated with patients, primarily through word of mouth. Not all of these facilities have beautiful rooms, but the care that women receive there brands those hospitals as the place to go for the best birthing experience in the area. It is a brand that women trust, it is a brand that their family members trust, and it is a brand that the physicians and nurses who work there trust. This is true because the brand is working holistically. The brand is not all marketing; marketing puts the face on the brand, certainly, but it does not train housekeeping, or billing, or the people who manage the web site and answer the phone. This is the cultural part of FCMC that must be communicated to every person who has contact with a consumer in day-to-day moments of truth. Everyone must live the same story for the FCMC brand to be successful.

Loyalty

The goal of marketing, of course, is to build loyalty. Nowhere in the healthcare arena does the impact of branding and subsequent loyalty have more potential than in maternity care where the typical mother-to-be is young and healthy. She no longer comes to the hospital simply to have a baby; she comes to have an experience. And not just *any* experience; this is an experience that she will remember her entire lifetime (Simpkin, 1991, 1992). It is the experience that she will tell her friends about, for good or for ill. Since the majority of births continue to occur in a hospital setting, and maternity services represent the first inpatient hospital experience for most women, competitive pressures make it imperative that hospitals capture the hearts of patients so they will return for their next birth. Peltier, Boyt, and Schibrosky (1999a and 1999b) studied obstetrical patients to determine the roots of loyalty. Initially, they hypothesized that either patient satisfaction or quality of care would be predictive of patient loyalty or could be proxies for loyalty. Their findings, however, did not corroborate that assumption. The researchers were surprised to find that the correlation between the performance of caregivers and the intention of the patient to return to the hospital for a future birth was low. Instead, relationship-building activities, social bonding, and the degree of communication with patients were much better predictors of loyalty to the maternity program and an intention to return next time.

Forging loyalty in the hearts of patients, and differentiating your program in the minds of potential customers from that of other hospitals in the area, requires savvy marketing knowledge and an in-depth understanding of the product being marketed. This understanding can be developed only through an intense collaboration between marketing and clinical providers.

CLINICAL AND MARKETING COLLABORATION

Marketing a product that you do not have, or incorrectly marketing a service that you do not understand, are unacceptable practices. In fact, the former is fraudulent. The marketer simply cannot do his or her job without complete knowledge of the product. When the product is a multidimensional healthcare product, such as maternity care, it is critical that clinical providers and marketers work collaboratively and harmoniously, even to the point of having the marketer shadow caregivers so he or she can see the philosophy of care in operation. The marketing person might also plan to attend some childbirth education classes so what is promised in marketing materials is consistent with what is taught and practiced on the unit. There should be consistent communication between clinical leaders and marketing so that changes in practice will not be a surprise. By the same token, marketing tactics and the need for all marketing materials to originate in the marketing department will be more understandable to clinical staff if there is an open relationship between the two departments.

FACTORS AFFECTING MARKETING

Marketing does not occur in a vacuum. Larger forces in society affect it in myriad ways. Some of these include changes in the target audience based on demographics and generational characteristics.

Changing Demographics

The U.S. Census Bureau defines the childbearing population as "female, between the ages of 15 and 44." In practical terms, this means that maternity units today are serving women who are the youngest of the Baby Boomers and the entirety of Gen-X. The youngest boomers are now 37 years of age, rapidly approaching the most mature end of the childbearing continuum. They will join their sisters in the midlife cohort in a relatively short time. Gen-Xers ranges from 17 to 36 years of age (U.S. Bureau of the Census, 2000).

Baby Boomers were the largest and most dominant generation ever (almost 85 million strong). Gen-X is a much smaller group, numbering about 57.4 million in number in year 2000 with a male to female ratio of 50:50 (U.S. Bureau of the Census, 2000). Because there are fewer of them, they will produce fewer babies, making the size of the market smaller than it has been in past decades. A smaller market size means that hospitals must capture share from competitors in order to simply maintain volumes.

The educational level of women has increased considerably from what it was in the past. The percentage of women with four-year college degrees was 23% in 2000, up from 18% in 1990 and 12.8% in 1980. In other words, the percentage of women graduating from college almost doubled in twenty years. Comparison of characteristics of women who had a child in the past year for 1995 and 2000 reveal that the percentages of women with a graduate or professional degree increased from 26.8% to 36.6% (U.S. Bureau of the Census, 2000). Greater education has created consumers who ask more questions and who are better informed overall. It has created a generation of women who know what they want and know how to research where to find it. They are not meek about stating their desires, particularly in terms of their childbirth experience. Data on prenatal care in the first trimester is indicative of the greater educational level of consumers. In 1990, 74% of women sought prenatal care in the first trimester; by 1997 (the most current data available) that percentage had increased to 82.5%.

The labor force has also been impacted. Overall, about 60% of the entire female population of the United States was employed in the civilian labor force in 1999; 66% of Gen-X women were employed. These numbers will grow as the youngest end of the cohort graduates from college and enters the job market (U.S. Bureau of the Census, 2000). For hospitals that wish to attract these women, issues of access and convenience will be critically important and will need to be addressed in the marketing strategy. Since time will be at a premium, access to services via the Internet will also be important. Anything that optimizes the ability to obtain services quickly and easily will put your service ahead of those of competitors who have not availed themselves of twenty-first century tools.

Changing Generational Imperatives

In 2000, there were approximately 4 million babies delivered in this nation, 75% of them to women in the Gen-X age range (U.S. Bureau of the Census, 2000). Because this group will be the dominant one giving birth in the next ten years or so, it is important to know something about them, for these women will be today's target market. They are a complex generation, and this small chapter cannot do justice to a complete overview. We will look at only the facets of the generation that are most important to perinatal program development and marketing.

Some Background on Gen-X Gen-Xers were the first generation to come home after school to an empty house while both parents were at work. They acquired the name "latchkey kids" due to the door key they wore on a chain around their neck so they could get into the house after school. During their formative years, the divorce rate peaked in this country, resulting in a generation of children who moved between two homes on a regular basis, sometimes in a car, sometimes in a plane. They became cynical and sophisticated at a young age. Their childhood and adolescence was a time in which they were molded by issues of drug addiction, AIDS, sexual freedom, violence, and environmental and world problems. Hungry for parental companionship and some sense of structure, and growing up in either unhappy or broken families, the idea of the traditional family is preeminent for them as adults. They are starving for stable relationships.

Relationships Are Everything This young generation is determined to have happy, long-lasting marriages in which they can be available to their children as they are growing up. Thus, while they value interesting and challenging work, they want to be able to accommodate the needs of both family and career. They do not live to work; they work to live (Strauss and Howe, 1993). If relationships matter the most, then family and other people who validate them are vital.

The idea that having a baby is equivalent to beginning a family will ring true to them. They are the ideal target audience for a true family-centered maternity program that features supportive, caring staff members operating in a mother–baby model of care. FCMC is relationship marketing in action!

Self-Sufficient and Lacking in Trust Having grown up in a world in which they were alone much of the time, Gen-Xers became very self-sufficient. This self-sufficiency and sense of independence is carried into adulthood. Strauss and Howe report, "They trust hard green because their earliest life experiences taught them that you can't trust anything else" (1993). The task of marketers will be to establish trust between the Gen-X consumer, her family, and the maternity program. The task of clinical staff will be to capitalize on her self-sufficiency to educate herself and family members about newborn care and parenting. These women will appreciate opportunities to "learn to do it myself" with the assistance of a mother–baby nurse who teaches at the bedside.

Skeptical of Institutions This generation has been disappointed by choices made by government, industry, education, and family. They tend to distrust organizations and institutions, including healthcare systems. The task at hand will be to make the hospital appear less of a system and more of a home; a place that can be trusted to help, not hinder, one's choices. Generation X women will reject institutional rules and the explanation that "this is the way we do things here." The individualized care and emphasis on choices that FCMC offers should be well suited to women in this age group.

A Unique Style of Learning and Communicating This is the first generation to feel completely at home with technology and telecommunications. Consequently, they are impatient for answers and are avid consumers of information. Rushkoff (1996) argues that they learn in a "mosaic fashion" rather than linearly. He feels that many of the things for which the generation is criticized, such as short attention spans and lack of ability to concentrate on one task, are coping mechanisms for a world overloaded with information. "The skill to be valued in the twenty-first century is not the length of attention span, but the ability to multitask—to do many things at once . . . [and] the ability to process visual information very rapidly (Rushkoff, 1996). This aspect of the Gen-X character has implications for inpatient and outpatient education as well as for marketing tactics that will grab and hold their attention.

Media Savvy This generation is very dubious about what they see on TV, realizing that the media can both distort and manipulate reality. They know this because Gen-X has produced some of the first and best spin doctors. To Generation X, everything is image. They do not simply receive and digest media; they manipulate and play with it as well. They are in a living relationship with the media (Rushkoff 1996). The tools used in a marketing campaign will need to be web-based and multimedia, as well as print-based, if this generation is to be wooed and convinced to enter the door of your facility.

A Love of Stories "Stories are intensely important to Generation X. We're not big on descriptions and adjectives. We want the feelings, the action, and the story. Our stories give us identity" (Ford 1996). This generation is tailor-made for the recommendations of Lavendar and Walkinshaw (1998). These researchers found in their study of postpartum psychological morbidity that psychological well-being was significantly enhanced and anxiety and depression decreased in postnatal women if they had an opportunity to "tell their story" to a compassionate caregiver. They recommended that maternity units develop a service that offers women the option of attending a debriefing session to discuss their labor process.

In summing up this very interesting and distinctive generation, it is apparent that they will be a unique group to target for maternity care. This is particularly true when we recognize that the common theme of Generation X with their almost fanatical level of individualism is: "I am not a target market" (Coupland, 1992).

THE MARKETING PLAN: WHY BOTHER?

A marketing plan coordinates and directs marketing efforts. It contains an assessment of where things are today and also provides a benchmark for measurement in the future. Although marketing plans sometimes stand alone, they are most typically a chapter in a business plan. As stated in the beginning of this chapter, the marketing plan supports the business objectives of the service (or hospital). The plan is a roadmap for those who must implement it, keeping them on track and reminding them of the goals that were set for the program.

It is important to remember in writing the plan that *every patient contact point* must be considered in writing the plan. For example, the consumer's first impression of the hospital and every service in it is initiated when the telephone is answered. The voice on the answering end of the telephone makes an immediate impression on the consumer. If the person answering the phone does not project friendliness, helpfulness, and caring, a negative feeling may be established momentarily in that potential consumer's mind. If she is transferred to the Maternity Unit and receives the same type of telephone response, you may have lost her forever. Telephone skills are an extremely important but often neglected part of marketing. The pitch and volume of the voice, the speed at which words are spoken, the quality of the voice, and enunciation are all important marketing tools.

So, too, are encounters with people not connected to the maternity program—the admitting clerk, the janitor in the hallway, the lab technician, and the person who delivers the food from Dietary. In fact, every point at which the consumer interacts with an employee is an opportunity for that consumer to be positively or negatively influenced. Every one of these people is a marketer, whether they realize it or not. Consequently, the marketing plan must incorporate an internal marketing strategy to educate those who are not direct participants in the family-centered program. Internal tools may be as simple as a periodic newsletter or as complex as in-depth training for all those who will interact with childbearing families.

Marketing plans have relatively static chapters, but it is the process of writing the plan more than the form that it takes that is most important. Some key chapters for a marketing plan are as follows:

Executive Summary—Introduces the major points of the plan.

Current Situation—Provides information about the target market, demographics, competitive situation, and key issues faced.

Marketing Objectives—States what will be accomplished through marketing efforts and the timeframe in which it will be accomplished. Some goals may be to increase birth volume, increase market share, or meet some financial target.

Marketing Strategy—This section presents the plan for achieving marketing objectives. It is the meat of the marketing plan and should include product features and benefits, promotional tools, and tactics that will accomplish marketing objectives both internally and externally, pricing goals if price is a competitive challenge in the area, how the product will be positioned, and a description of the way in which potential consumers will access the product (in this case, the FCMC program at your hospital).

Action Plan—This is a description of what tasks will be done, when they will be started and completed, and who will accomplish each task.

Budget—States the cost of the marketing activities that have been outlined in the plan.

Evaluation—Statement of numeric, measurable targets that will document the marketing plan's success. Time limits should be included. For example, "Increase market share by 5 percent within 12 months."

Supporting Documentation—This might include the results of any marketing research, spreadsheets projecting utilization or demographic changes, and so on.

SOME THOUGHTS ON INTERNET MARKETING

The web presence that is directed to consumers is as critical an interaction today as those that are live. Simply having a presence in cyberspace is not good enough. The web site is as much a reflection of the program's image as are print media. Therefore, an Internet strategy is an important part of the overall marketing plan for the maternity service. A good starting point is to determine how consumers will use the web site. Some examples to consider include:

- Will the site be a tool for acquiring information only, or will it be interactive? An example of interactive use in maternity care is putting baby photos online. Today, many hospitals post picture of newborns online almost immediately after delivery so family and friends from all over the world can view the photo. Some hospitals also have baby conference calls, where the new parents can present the newborn to friends and family online through video conferencing.

- Will the web site serve as a *replacement* for some interactions, or will it add to them? For example, registration for classes can typically be accomplished through the mail, via telephone, via fax, and in person. If consumers can now also register on the web, the potential for interactions will have been expanded. On the other hand, if the web becomes the sole point for class registration, then some potential attendees might be left out if they do not have web access or are not computer literate.

- Will the web site accommodate administrative and/or clinical functions? Such functions may include completion of admitting documents, advance directives (such as a Living Will), possibly even medical history in advance, checking one's bill online, or getting test results.

- Will the web site be used to capture data about those who visit it? Doing so may increase the potential for consumer encounters, enhance the mailing list for direct mail pieces, and ultimately broaden the consumer base so the cachement area can be redefined.

There are many other ways in which your web presence can be used as a marketing tactic:

- Let people know your web address by including it on *all* printed materials (press materials, business cards, brochures, stationery, yellow pages listing, and newsletters). In short, anything that will be seen and read by the public should have your web address on it.

- Create a distinctive email signature file to be used on all emails that you send. Include your email and web addresses in the signature file.

- Since the goal is to have consumers visit your web site often, update your site on a regular basis. Include what's new at your hospital and what is coming in the future. Have a wide assortment of links for topics that are discussed on your site (e.g., doulas, birth plans, or hydrotherapy). Consider a message board for consumer comments and suggestions. Target your audience with the web site just as you do with print materials, and tailor messages to the audience that you wish to attract.

- Test your web site on a variety of computers (including both Mac and PC) and browsers (and versions of browsers; be aware that not everyone updates software the minute the new version is available!). Be sure that your web site looks as good in Netscape as it does in Internet Explorer, for instance. Also try finding your site using a variety of search engines to determine how easily consumers can find you.

- Check out competitor web sites regularly.

- Use your web site to your full advantage. Give consumers an opportunity to ask questions and be sure to respond to their questions within 24 hours. Provide a variety of ways in which consumers can reach you (an 800 number, a local phone number, a fax number, an email address, a mailing address), and also put a map of your location on your web site so the potential consumer can print it out.

- Provide an easy way to contact you on every page of your web site so the consumer can do so the moment something on the page sparks an interest.

- Put a copy of your newsletter online in Adobe™ PDF format so consumers who are not on your mailing list can download a copy.

- Pay attention to the web site's search log. Many sites have a search box so those who visit the site can easily find what they are seeking. The search log can provide information about those who visit your site, so remember to analyze that data. For example, the search log can reveal unmet customer demand, can validate the efficacy of an advertising campaign, or can allow you to anticipate consumer concerns just by assessing the search terms that are typed into the search box.

Regardless of what you do with your site and what you hope to accomplish with it, there are a few rules that should be kept in mind:

- Above all, web marketing is relationship marketing. The goal of the web site is to get people to come back time and time again. In order to make them feel welcome and comfortable on your site, the language with which you communicate should be neither too lofty nor too dumbed down. Aim for the average reader and write in a manner that suggests a conversational and friendly tone.

- The web site does not "flow"; it is actually somewhat disjointed. The message that you want the visitor to your site to grasp must be repeated several times in different ways. If the goal is to tell the world that you are the only family-centered maternity care program in town, then tell your site visitors on every page of your web site to be sure that they get it. Otherwise, they may log in, follow a link to someplace else, come back around to another topic, and never get back to your home page to see how you are different from the competitor.

- If you have a feedback mechanism of some type on your site (such as an email address to a marketing person), it is courteous to include the original message to you in your response so the reader will know to what you are referring. People do not always remember what they said in an email and may not even recall what question they asked you.

These are just a few of the points that could be considered in developing an Internet strategy as a subset of your overall marketing strategy. Others will come to mind as you ponder your own web site. The key is to be sure to include the web in your strategy and to remember that the generation for which you are competing will eventually expect that you will have an interactive, and possibly multimedia, web presence.

EXAMPLES OF MARKETING TOOLS FOR FCMC

Family-centered maternity care is really a marketer's dream product. It is a philosophy of care, it is a brand, and it is a complete product. It has been demonstrated to produce loyal clientele. Plus, once they are accustomed to working within the model, nurses love it, too, and nursing job satisfaction increases (Janssen et al., 2001). Physicians enjoy it as well. Even though it tends to sell itself once women start talking about it, a more effective strategy is to implement a full complement of marketing tactics and tools. Some ideas are presented in the following paragraphs.

Advertising

The purpose of advertising is twofold: to get people to notice you and to persuade them to act in some way. Each ad typically includes a call to action. You may want those viewing the ad to call you, to come in and see you, or to write to you. Whatever the call to action might be, when the consumers act, you know that your advertisement has reached them. Advertising can be used to promote some event, persuade potential consumers that your product is best, develop a need for your product or service, or establish your brand in the community. In all cases, you are establishing awareness among consumers and presenting a positive image to them.

Advertising can take many forms, including billboards; taxi, train, and bus ads; the Internet; radio, broadcast television, or public television ads; or newspaper, magazine, or other print media ads. Whatever form you select, it is imperative that you have a message. The message should address what makes you special, why you are better than the competitor, and why your product should be selected. The newspaper ad shown in Exhibit 6-1 speaks to the benefits of mother–baby nursing, emphasizing the uniqueness of each baby and the importance of learning all about the infant through one nurse for both mom and baby.

Choosing the right medium for your advertising depends on your budget, but it also depends on your target

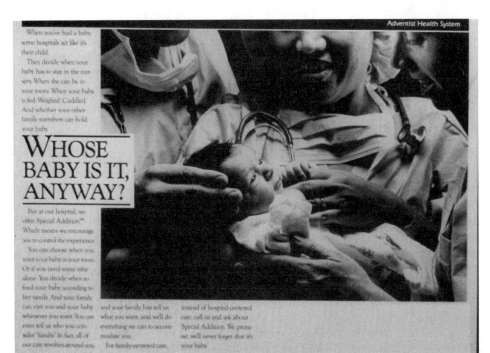

EXHIBIT 6–1 Newspaper Ad

audience. If, for example, your target consumer is today's typical woman, she works all day, comes home, fixes dinner, takes care of children, does laundry, plans and creates lunches for the next day, possibly attends to work she has brought home with her, and falls into bed. Using your marketing budget on television ads probably will not be the wisest way to target this woman! Hopefully, you have done marketing research in your area, and you know what medium works best for your target audience. The key to successful advertising is to use your head. If you have a lot to say, don't try to cram it all into a 30-second radio ad. If you have an event coming up in three or four days and want to remind people about it, don't put it in a weekly paper that will be published after the event has been held. And remember that repetition is mandatory with advertising. An ad that runs once is not going to be fruitful and will not be worth the money you spend on it; consumers must see an ad several times before they respond to your call to action. Exhibit 6-2 shows a print ad emphasizing the family-centered care model. The call to action is the phrase "For more information on Special Additions, just call our hospital."

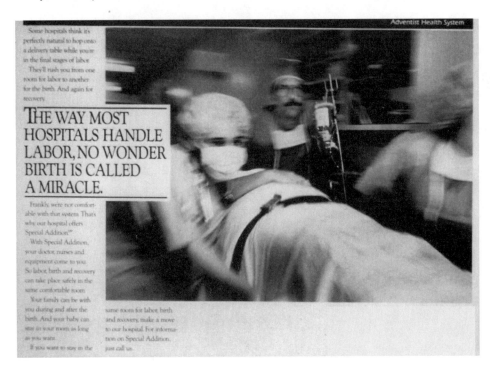

EXHIBIT 6–2 Print Ad

Direct Mail

Direct mail is actually a form of advertising, but it is a unique enough form that it is being presented in this chapter as a separate category. Direct mail allows you to expand your traditional geographic reach and inform an audience who might not otherwise know about you.

Direct mail provides you with an opportunity to communicate directly with the consumer; in effect, you are entering her home. The materials that you mail to her must be meaningful and informative regardless of the form that they take. Your direct mail piece must be written to the educational level of your audience, and it must focus immediately upon consumer benefits. Direct mail pieces can include newsletters, articles, books, class listings, brochures, fliers, and/or slip sheets (small fliers suitable to use as mailing inserts). In contrast to, for example, a newspaper ad, direct mail allows you to get your message to a specifically targeted audience, the childbearing woman. The materials can even be personalized for each reader. Thus, although direct mail can be expensive, it permits you to maximize the potential to capture each consumer. When people open their mail, they tend to focus on it for a few seconds; they are actively involved in the activity rather than simply flipping through the newspaper, for example. So your message will be given undivided attention at least for a few seconds. Busy people frequently throw away unopened those pieces of mail that they view as junk mail. In order to merit attention, the direct mail piece must be compelling to the reader, either through a catchy phrase or a striking photo or graphic. The reader's attention must be captured immediately or the moment will be lost. Always put a call to action statement in your direct mail medium (for example, "Call today" or "Fill in the card and mail it today"). It is always a good idea to include a postage-paid reply card so the reader can get more information if she so desires. Exhibit 6-3 is an example of a brochure that explains mother–baby nursing and gives women a checklist of features to seek for an authentic family-centered care experience.

Media Relations

Planning an effective media campaign is a lot of work, but it is an excellent way to get exposure in the community. This is assuming, of course, that the reason you are being mentioned is something positive about your program! Newspaper columns and radio and television interviews are excellent exposure and help to establish the "expert" status of caregivers. Establishing a relationship with reporters is one of the most important things that you can do. Journalists are much too busy to seek out a variety of experts. Instead, they focus on a few very obvious ones, especially the ones they have used in the past. The goal is for you to be one of the experts that they seek out. You do that by developing a relationship with reporters who write for publications in which you would like to be quoted. Do not call reporters simply to talk. Call when you have important news about your program. Call for a specific reason, and be prepared to offer information that is not widely known—to explain the philosophy of family-centered care, for example. The newspaper column in Exhibit 6-4 would serve that purpose and could be bylined by one of the physicians at your hospital.

Press releases are also an important part of media relations; they are used to announce your news to journalists in the hope that they will publish your information. Press releases are sent to print, radio, and television reporters and

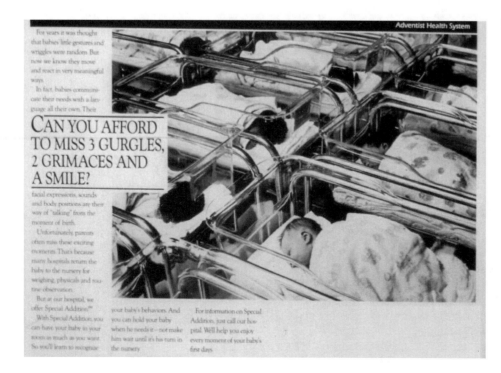

EXHIBIT 6–3 Brochure

Adventist Health System

CAN YOU AFFORD TO MISS 3 GURGLES, 2 GRIMACES AND A SMILE?

EXHIBIT 6–4   The Advantages of Mother–Baby Nursing for Your Family

THE ADVANTAGES OF MOTHER–BABY NURSING FOR YOUR FAMILY BY YOUR PHYSICIAN(S)

In mother–baby nursing, one nurse cares for mother and baby together. This might sound simple and logical, but many hospitals do not have mother–baby nursing. Instead they have "mother nurses" who take care of women after they've had a baby and "baby nurses" who take care of newborns—usually in a nursery. While having different nurses for mother and baby may sound like specialized care, it can actually be an exercise in confusion, missed opportunities, and inflexibility. You see, when more than one nurse is involved in caregiving, signals can get crossed. Messages can get lost or confused.

Mother–baby nursing is not the same as rooming-in, where the mother is expected to care for her baby when the infant is with her. Mother–baby nurses care for both mother and baby, and they nurture bonding and attachment in the new family.

In fact, with mother–baby nursing, the nurse cares for the whole family. Dad and other family members are included—whomever the new mother calls "family." The daily schedule is adjusted to family needs. Each morning the mother–baby nurse helps the new mother plan her day. Care is flexible for each family according to their needs—not according to some rigid hospital schedule.

There are many benefits for the family with mother–baby nursing:

- There is better communication. Because there is only one nurse on each shift for both mother and baby, communication is improved.

- If there is an obstetrician and a pediatrician, they both work with the same nurse rather than with two separate nurses. At shift change the needs and wants of each mother–baby couplet are easily passed on to the next nurse.

- Questions are answered more quickly. In most hospitals, if a mother has a question about her baby and she asks them of the postpartum nurse, she's likely to hear, "I don't know. You'll have to ask the nursery nurse." Or perhaps the mother's nurse will go to the nursery nurse and find out the answer. With mother–baby nursing, one nurse doesn't have to ask another nurse. One nurse knows the answer and can tell the mother right away. She knows because she is taking care of both mother and baby.

- Families have a closer relationship with the nurse. Because there are fewer nurses to relate to, the mother and nurse are more likely to develop a feeling of trust, caring, and comfort.

- Families receive more education. The mother–baby nurse demonstrates baby care as she takes care of the infant at the mother's bedside.

- Mothers don't miss special moments with their baby. When the baby spends most of its time in the nursery, mothers miss lots of gurgles and coos. With mother–baby nursing, most infant care takes place in the mother's room so the mother can share those special moments.

- Families know their baby is receiving good care. Because the nurse cares for the baby in the mother's room, families see the care their babies receive. No one has to wonder whether their baby is the one they hear crying in the nursery.

- There is increased security. Nobody likes to think about it, but mother–baby nursing increases security. There are fewer opportunities for someone to kidnap a baby, as infants are not constantly traveling between the mother's room and the nursery. Having a mother–baby nurse reduces the number of people caring for a family and makes the appearance of strangers more obvious.

Mother–baby nursing makes sense for new families. Parents have greater involvement with their baby's care, their bonding and attachment with their newborn are strengthened, and they leave the hospital more confident in their parenting skills. In our next column, we will talk about the special benefits of mother–baby nursing for the newborn.

HOSPITAL NAME, CITY, publishes this column as a public service. For a free reprint of this column and the four others in this series, call (XXX) XXX-XXXX.

journalists. Press releases are written for an audience that is in a hurry and does not have time to read everything that passes before them; thus important information should be summarized at the beginning of the press release. Journalism stresses "who, what, when, where, and why," and these points should be included in the first part of a press release. When written well, the first sentence will provide the reader with enough information to understand the reason for the release. Details that authenticate the lead paragraph come next. The final section contains information that is relevant but not critical. If your press release is published, the newspaper editor typically will cut it from the bottom first if space is limited. That is another compelling reason to put the most important information right up front!

It is important to have a well-prepared press kit that contains your business card, your press release about the new program, reprints of articles that help back up the novelty and appropriateness of your story, copies of any presentations given in association with your program, photographs, a profile about your hospital, testimonials if you have some, profiles of yourself and key employees involved in the program, copies of your brochures, newsletters, and mail pieces, and graphics or art that illustrates facts about your FCMC program.

Another form of media presentation is the public service announcement (PSA). A PSA is a short, noncommercial announcement designed to inform the public. Although they are typically associated with nonprofit organizations, there is no reason why for-profit concerns cannot use them to promote activities and events that are being offered for public well-being (preconception counseling, for example). Public service announcements offer free air time on radio and/or TV for between 10 and 60 seconds. You can use PSAs effectively to inform and influence public opinion about FCMC, assist in raising funds for the program, provide information about the health and safety benefits of FCMC, and publicize any community events that will educate women.

Special Events

Special events can take many forms. Typical ones for hospitals include health fairs; "lunch with the doctor," in which a different physician specialist speaks every other month or once a quarter; grand opening events; and maternity unit tours.

CHAPTER SUMMARY

In summary, there are any number of tools that can be used both internally and externally to tell the story of family-centered maternity care. It is up to you to determine which are most appropriate for your program. And never forget the most important marketing tool of all—word of mouth! If everyone does the job right, if all participants understand and embrace the philosophical underpinnings of the care model, FCMC practically sells itself!

BIBLIOGRAPHY

Bellenger, D., et al. 1976. *Qualitative Research in Marketing*. Chicago: American Marketing Association.

Bennett, P., ed. 1995. *Dictionary of Marketing Terms*, 2nd ed. Chicago: American Marketing Association.

Berman, A. 1969. Statistician brands draft lottery unfair. *Los Angeles Times*, December 3, part 1: 13.

Coupland, D. 1992. *Generation X*. British Edition. London: Abacus.

Ford, K. 1996. *Jesus for a New Generation*. London: Hodder and Stoughton.

Gravett, W. S. 1989. Women's centers: 10 common misconceptions. *Hospitals*, July 20: 10.

Hatch, M., and Schultz, M. 2001. Are the strategic stars aligned for your corporate brand? *Harvard Business Review*, February: 129–134.

Higgenbotham, J. B., and Cox, K. K., eds. 1979. *Focus Group Interviews: A Reader*. Chicago: American Marketing Association.

Hill, S. 2001. Branding the library and the university in an online world. Paper presented at the 19th annual Online Computer Library Center International Conference of Research Library Directors. Dublin, OH. March 26.

Janssen, P., et al. 2001. Single-room maternity care: The nursing response. *Birth* 28, no. 3: 173–179.

Lavender, T., and Walkinshaw, S. A. 1998. Can midwives reduce postpartum psychological morbidity? A randomized trial. *Birth* 25, no. 4: 220–221.

McStravic, S. 2001. Brand, position or identity in healthcare marketing. *COR Healthcare Market Strategist* 2, no. 7: 1–4.

Peltier, J. W., et al. 1999a. Obstetrical care and patient loyalty. *Marketing Health Services* 19(3): 5–14.

Peltier, J. W., et al. 1999. Obstetrical care and patient loyalty: Part 2. *Marketing Health Services* 19, no. 4: 13–20.

Rushkoff, D. 1996. *Playing the Future*. New York: Harper Collins.

Shore, D. 2001. The essence of brand trust in healthcare. *COR Healthcare Market Strategist* 2, no. 6: 1–3.

Simpkin, P. 1991. Just another day in a woman's life? I. Women's long-term perceptions of their first birth experience. *Birth* no. 18: 203–210.

Simpkin, P., 1992. Just another day in a woman's life? II. Nature and consistency of women's long-term memories of their first birth experiences. *Birth* no. 19: 64–81.

Strauss, W., and Howe, N. 1993. *13th Gen: Abort, Retry, Ignore, Fail?* New York: Vintage Books.

U. S. Bureau of the Census. 2000. *Statistical Abstract of the United States*. 120th ed. Washington, DC: Author.

Yarrow, L. 1992. Giving birth: 72,000 moms tell all. *Parents*, November, 149–159.

Family-Centered Hospital Care: The Core Concepts

Family-centered maternity care has set an example of patient-centered care for the rest of our traditional healthcare system. It is becoming clear that a family-centered approach is applicable to patients of all ages.

Family-centered care promotes meaning and joy in the everyday work of patient care and builds a culture of community in the workplace. For the staff, the result is increased job satisfaction and the sense of belonging and commitment. For the patient, satisfaction improves. For the hospital, dollar savings accrue as staff are cross-trained and families are involved in care.

DEFINITION

Family-centered care *for the entire hospital* is a healthcare delivery model that places the patient at the center of the care given. In this model, the emphasis changes from focusing on the provider or institution to focusing on the patient and family, with the concentration on collaboration, empowerment, and education.

VALUES

The values of the family-centered care model are:

- Respect for patients' values, preferences, and expressed needs
- Multidisciplinary care coordination
- Open communication and information shared between providers and patients
- Involvement of families in patient care
- Multiskilled, flexible, and empowered employees
- A warm, friendly, and healing environment

GOALS

The goals of a family-centered care model are to:

- provide a hospital program and environment that jointly promote healing and restoration of physical and emotional well-being.
- build a hospital culture that people in the caring professions can be proud to call their workplace.

THE FAMILY-CENTERED CARE MODEL

The family-centered care model promotes the following concepts:

- A registered nurse coordinates and manages care of each patient from admission to discharge.
- Care of patients is multidisciplinary in approach.
- Patients and families are advisors in policy and program planning, implementation, and evaluation.
- The program of care is built on the cornerstones of the hospital's family-centered vision, mission, and philosophy, and the principles of family-centered care.
- Patient care is coordinated and integrated with ancillary and support services.
- All patient care teams are self-directed and accountable, solving problems at the group level.
- Cross-trained, multifunctional teams are formed and educated to provide nonfragmented care to meet patients' needs.
- Provider education and performance evaluation are ongoing to ensure quality family-centered care.

PRINCIPLES OF FAMILY-CENTERED HOSPITAL CARE

The principles of family-centered care represent a change in culture for most hospitals and healthcare organizations. The principles that follow are the foundation for family-centered program development for the entire hospital:

- *Practice:* A knowledgeable interdisciplinary team collaborates with the patient and family unit in the shared goals of achieving and promoting health.

- *Quality:* The interdisciplinary approach provides patients and their families with meaningful information on services, outcomes, and costs, and strives to continuously improve the value of services.

- *Decision making:* Patients and families have the right to participate in decisions concerning the patient's care and are encouraged to be active and involved in the decision-making process.

- *Communication:* Family-centered care recognizes and values open, honest communication between patients and families and all members of the healthcare team.

- *Patient education:* Continual patient and family education assists patients in achieving a high level of self-care, autonomy, and health promotion.

- *Individualized care:* Each patient and family has a unique set of needs, values, fears, and intentions that guide the nature, course, and duration of their healthcare. Thus, each encounter with the patient and family is made with respect, empathy, and a "go the extra mile" attitude.

- *Staff motivation:* Healthcare providers are valued for their compassionate and caring interactions with patients and families, and are rewarded for continuous improvement of what they do.

- *Staff education:* Continual staff education is provided so staff can expand knowledge and skills to be skillful, knowledgeable, and competent caregivers.

- *Facility:* A healing environment that provides both comfort and safety helps to promote wellness and physical and emotional well being for the patient and family. The flexible, universal care room fosters nursing efficiency and increased patient satisfaction.

- *Value:* The value of service is defined through assessing patient and family satisfaction, program reputation, and other qualitative factors along with clinical and financial measurements.

EXAMPLE OF A FAMILY-CENTERED HOSPITAL

Some hospitals place importance not only on treating illness, but also on meeting the needs of the whole person within the context of the family. These hospitals are changing their cultures to focus on the patient first through innovative programs and facility design.

An excellent example of a family-centered hospital is the Woodwinds Health Campus in Woodbury, Minnesota. This 70-bed community hospital southeast of the Twin Cities was created in 2000 through a partnership between HealthEast Care System and Children's Hospitals and Clinics. All patient rooms are private and include a couch for family members' comfort during the day. This couch pulls out to make a comfortable bed for family members to sleep on at night. A table and chairs at the nurses' station provide a place for patients and families to sit and talk with staff. In this welcoming environment patients, families, and care providers have ample opportunities to interact as a community, informing and supporting one another.

The Woodwinds care model is delivered in a healing environment and culture that fosters partnership with patients and families. Traditional and complementary therapies are integrated into care at the Woodwinds. There is a Natural Care Center on the campus; services include chiropractic, naturopathy, health and wellness assessments, acupuncture, therapeutic massage, and natural healthcare products along with expert advice and guidance.

The Woodwinds vision is: To be the innovative, unique, and preferred resource for health by fundamentally creating the healthcare experience in a way that has not been done before.

The Woodwinds purpose is to promote health and healing of body, mind, and spirit for all—through relationships, choices, and learning.

The Woodwinds values are:

- *Compassionate Service:* Placing the needs of those we serve above our own; treating individuals with dignity, respect, and empathy.

- *Ethical Practice:* Demonstrating the highest standards of integrity, honesty, and loyalty.

- *Meaningful Collaboration:* Working together with patients, families, coworkers, and outside partners to strengthen mutually beneficial collaborative relationships.

- *Human Potential:* Growing through personal development, fulfilling work, and continual teaming while encouraging growth in others.

The culture at Woodwinds Health Campus promotes individual well-being for patients, families, staff, and physicians. To staff the hospital, administrators sought out qualified, dedicated people with a belief in caring for the whole person. Believe it or not, in a very tight job market 2,500 job seekers applied for 400 available positions.

When the culture supports a healing environment for patients and staff and innovative thinking is celebrated and rewarded, a hospital can be an exciting place to work. The evidence can be found at the Woodwinds Health Campus.

CULTURE CHANGE

As with family-centered maternity care, the most radical change necessary to create a family-centered hospital is the shift to new attitudes of the caregivers. In a family-centered hospital, staff will no longer treat families as visitors, but as valued members of the healthcare team.

Times have changed and healthcare consumers—patients and families—are asking for family involvement in care. It is time to make this culture change not just for maternity care, but for the entire hospital.

Family-centered care is an evolving masterpiece; still under development, it is far from finished. Together, families and healthcare providers will eventually complete the work. But doing so will require constant attention to the dream of what could be.

Perhaps Don Quixote said it best:

Oh my friends, I have lived almost 50 years, and I have seen life as it is: pain, misery, hunger, cruelty beyond belief. I have heard the singing from taverns and the moans from bundles of filth in the street. I've been a soldier and I've seen my comrades fall in battle or die more slowly under the last.... I've held them in my arms at the final moment. No glory. No gallant last words. Only their eyes filled with confusion. Whimpering the question: "Why?" I don't think they asked why they were dying, but why they had lived...too much sanity may be madness. And maddest of all is to see life as it is and not as it ought to be.*

---

* Wasserman, D. *Man of La Mancha*. In Guernsey, O. L., Jr. *The Best Plays of 1965–66*, New York: Dodd, Mead, 1996.

REFERENCES

Gerteis, M., et al. 1993. *Through the Patient's Eyes*. San Francisco: Jossey-Bass, Inc.

Moore, N., and Komras, H. 1993. *Patient-Focused Healing*. San Francisco: Jossey-Bass, Inc.

Phillips, C., and Fenwick, L. 2000. *Single-Room Maternity Care: Planning, Developing, and Operating the 21st Century Maternity System*. Philadelphia: Lippincott Williams and Wilkins.

Scheller, M. D. 1990. *Building Partnerships in Hospital Care*. Palo Alto, CA: Bull Publishing Co.

Internet Resources for Developing Evidence-Based Practices

- Agency for Healthcare Research and Quality—www.ahrq.gov
- American Academy of Pediatrics—www.aap.org
- American Association of Critical Care Nurses—www.aacn.org
- American College of Nurse–Midwives—www.acnm.org
- American College of Obstetricians and Gynecologists—www.acog.org
- American Nurses Association—www.ana.org
- American Society of Anesthesiologists—www.asahq.org
- American Society of Perianesthesia Nurses—www.aspan.org
- Association of PeriOperative Registered Nurses—www.aorn.org
- Association of Women's Health, Obstetric and Neonatal Nurses—www.awhonn.org
- Best Practice Network—www.best4health.org
- Centre for Evidence-Based Child Health—www.ich.bpmf.ac.uk/ebm/ebm.htm
- Centre for Evidence-Based Nursing—www.york.ac.uk/healthsciences/centres/evidence/cebn.htm
- Centers for Disease Control and Prevention—www.cdc.gov
- CenterWatch Clinical Trials Listing Service—www.centerwatch.com
- Cochrane Library—www.update-software.com/cochrane/
- Evidence-Based Medicine Journal—www.ebm.bmjjournals.com
- March of Dimes—www.modimes.org
- National Association of Neonatal Nurses—www.nann.org
- National Guideline Clearinghouse—www.guideline.gov
- United States Food and Drug Administration—www.fda.gov
- United States Preventive Services Task Force—www.ahcpr.gov/clinic/uspstfix.htm

Adapted from Simpson, K. R., and Knox, G. E. (1999). Strategies for developing an evidence-based approach to perinatal care. MCN The American Journal of Maternal Child Nursing, 24(3), 122–132.

Effective Care in Pregnancy and Childbirth: A Synopsis

Murray Enkin, MD, FRCS(C), LLD, Marc J. N. C. Keirse, MD, Dphil, DPH, FRANZCOG, FRCOG, James Neilson, BSc, MD, MSc(Epid), MRCOG, Ellen Hodnett, RN, PhD, and G. Justus Hofmeyr, MBBCH, MRCOG.

The following tables are from the new third edition of *A Guide to Effective Care in Pregnancy and Childbirth*, as reproduced in *Birth* 28:1 March 2001, 41–51. Reproduced with permission.

TABLE B-1 Beneficial Forms of Care

Effectiveness demonstrated by clear evidence from controlled trials		*Chapter*
Basic care	Women carrying their pregnancy record to enhance their feeling of being in control	3
	Pre- and peri-conceptional folic acid supplementation to prevent recurrent neural tube defects	5, 6
	Folic acid supplementation (or high folate diet) for all women envisaging pregnancy	5, 6
	Assistance (especially behavioral strategies) to stop smoking during pregnancy	5
	Balanced energy and protein supplementation when dietary supplementation is required	6
	Vitamin D supplementation for women with inadequate exposure to sunlight	6
	Iodine supplementation in populations with high incidence of endemic cretinism	6
Screening and diagnosis	Doppler ultrasound in pregnancies at high risk of fetal compromise	12
Pregnancy problems	Antihistamines for nausea and vomiting of pregnancy that is resistant to simple measures	13
	Local imidazoles for vaginal candida infection (thrush)	13
	Local imidazoles instead of nystatin for vaginal candida infection (thrush)	13
	Magnesium sulphate rather than other anticonvulsants for treatment of eclampsia	15
	Administration of anti-D immunoglobulin to Rh-negative women whose newborn baby is not Rh-negative	18
	Administration of anti-D immunoglobulin to Rh-negative women at 28 weeks of pregnancy	18
	Antiretroviral treatment of HIV-infected pregnant women to prevent transmission to fetus	19
	Antibiotic treatment of asymptomatic bacteriuria	19
	Antibiotics during labor for women known to be colonized with group B streptococcus	19
	Tight as opposed to too strict or loose control of blood sugar levels in pregnant diabetic women	20
	External cephalic version at term to avoid breech birth	22
	Corticosteroids to promote fetal maturity before preterm birth	25
	Offering induction of labor after 41 completed weeks of gestation	26
Childbirth	Physical, emotional, and psychological support during labor and birth	28, 25, 41
	Continuous support for women during labor and childbirth	28
	Agents to reduce acidity of stomach contents before general anesthesia	29
	Complementing fetal heart rate monitoring in labor with fetal acid-base assessment	30
	Oxytocics to treat postpartum hemorrhage	33
	Prophylactic oxytocics in the third stage of labor	33
	Active versus expectant management of third stage of labor	33
Problems during childbirth	Absorbable instead of non-absorbable sutures for skin repair of perineal trauma	36
	Polyglycolic acid sutures instead of chromic catgut for repair of perineal trauma	36
Techniques of induction and operative delivery	Prostaglandins to increase cervical readiness for induction of labor	39
	Amniotomy plus oxytocin for induction of labor instead of either amniotomy alone or oxytocin alone	40
	Vacuum extraction instead of forceps when operative vaginal delivery is required	41
	Antibiotic prophylaxis (short course or intraperitoneal lavage) with cesarean section	43
Care after childbirth	Use of surfactant for very preterm infants to prevent respiratory distress syndrome	44
	Support for socially disadvantaged mothers to improve parenting	45
	Consistent support for breastfeeding mothers	46
	Personal support from a knowledgeable individual for breastfeeding mothers	46
	Unrestricted breastfeeding	46
	Local anesthetic sprays for relief of perineal pain postpartum	47
	Cabergoline instead of bromocriptine for relief of breast symptoms in non-breastfeeding mothers	48

TABLE B-2   Forms of Care Likely to Be Beneficial

The evidence in favor of these forms of care is strong, although not established by randomized trials		*Chapter*
Basic care	Adequate access to care for all childbearing women	3
	Social support for childbearing women	3
	Financial support for childbearing women in need	3
	Legislation on paid leave and income maintenance during maternity or parental leave	3
	Midwifery care for women with no serious risk factors	3
	Continuity of care for childbearing women	3
	Antenatal classes for women and their partners who want them	4
	Advice to avoid excessive alcohol consumption during pregnancy	5
	Avoidance of heavy physical work during pregnancy	5
Screening and diagnosis	Ultrasound to resolve questions about fetal size, structure, or position	8
	Selective use of ultrasound to assess amniotic fluid volume	8
	Selective use of ultrasound to estimate gestational age in first and early second trimester	8, 9
	Ultrasound to determine whether the embryo is alive in threatened miscarriage	8, 14
	Ultrasound to confirm suspected multiple pregnancy	8, 17
	Ultrasound for placental location in suspected placenta previa	8, 21
	Second trimester amniocentesis to identify chromosomal abnormalities in pregnancies at risk	9
	Transabdominal instead of transcervical chorionic villus sampling	9
	Genetic counseling before prenatal diagnosis	9
	Clinical history to assess risk of pre-eclampsia	10
	Regular monitoring of blood pressure during pregnancy	10
	Uric acid levels for following the course of pre-eclampsia	10
	Fundal height measurements during pregnancy	12
Pregnancy problems	Ultrasound to facilitate intrauterine interventions	8, 9
	Antacids for heartburn of pregnancy if simple measures are ineffective	13
	Bulking agents for constipation if simple measures are ineffective	13
	Local metronidazole for symptomatic trichomonal vaginitis after the first trimester	13
	Antibiotics for symptomatic bacterial vaginosis	13
	Antiplatelet agents to prevent pre-eclampsia	15
	Antihypertensive agents to control serious hypertension in pregnancy	15
	Calcium to prevent pre-eclampsia, for women at high risk or with low calcium in diet	6, 15
	Balanced protein/energy supplementation for impaired fetal growth	6, 16
	Ultrasound surveillance of fetal growth in multiple pregnancies	17
	Screening all pregnant women for blood group isoimmunization	18
	Anti-D immunoglobulin to Rh-negative women after any uterine bleeding, intrauterine procedure, or abdominal trauma during pregnancy	18, 21
	Intra-uterine transfusion for a severely affected iso-immunized fetus	18
	Advice to not breastfeed for HIV-infected women to prevent transmission to baby	19, 46
	Routine screening for, and treatment of, syphilis in pregnancy	19
	Rubella vaccination of seronegative women postpartum	19
	Screening for and treatment of chlamydia in high prevalence populations	19
	Cesarean section for active herpes (with visible lesion) in labor with intact membranes	19
	Prepregnancy counseling for women with diabetes	20
	Specialist care for pregnant women with diabetes	20
	Home instead of hospital glucose monitoring for pregnant women with diabetes	20

TABLE B-2 Forms of Care Likely to Be Beneficial (continued)

The evidence in favor of these forms of care is strong, although not established by randomized trials

Pregnancy problems (*continued*)	Ultrasound surveillance of fetal growth for pregnant women with diabetes	20
	Allowing pregnancy to continue to term in otherwise uncomplicated diabetic pregnancies	20
	Careful attention to insulin requirements postpartum	20
	Encouraging diabetic women to breastfeed	20
	Checking for clotting disorders with severe placental abruption	21
	Vaginal instead of cesarean delivery for placental abruption in the absence of fetal distress	21
	Vaginal instead of cesarean birth for a dead fetus after placental abruption	21
	Repeat ultrasound scanning of a low-lying placenta in late pregnancy	21
	Delaying planned cesarean section for placenta previa until term	21
	Cesarean section for placenta previa covering any portion of the cervical os	21
	Ultrasound examination for vaginal bleeding of undetermined origin	21
	External cephalic version for transverse or oblique lie at term	22
	Tocolysis for external cephalic version of breech, particularly if unsuccessful otherwise	22
	External cephalic version for breech in early labor if the membranes are intact	22
	Corticosteroid administration after prelabor rupture of the membranes preterm	23
	Vaginal culture after prelabor rupture of the membranes preterm	23
	Antibiotics for prelabor rupture of the membranes with suspected intrauterine infection	23
	Not stopping spontaneous labor after prelabor rupture of the membranes preterm	23
	Elective delivery for prelabor rupture of the membranes preterm with signs of infection	23
	Amnioinfusion for fetal distress thought to be due to oligohydramnios in labor	23, 30
	Betamimetic tocolysis to allow effective preparation for preterm birth	24
	Short-term indomethacin to stop preterm labor	24
	Offering induction of labor as an option after fetal death	27
	Prostaglandin or prostaglandin analogs for induction of labor after fetal death	27
Childbirth	Respecting women's choice of companions during labor and birth	28
	Respecting women's choice of place of birth	28
	Presence of a companion on admission to hospital	29
	Giving women as much information as they desire	29
	Freedom of movement and choice of position in labor	29
	Change of mother's position for fetal distress in labor	30
	Intravenous betamimetics for fetal distress in labor to "buy time"	30
	Respecting women's choice of position for the second stage of labor and giving birth	32
	Guarding the perineum versus watchful waiting during birth	32
	Intramyometrial prostaglandins for severe postpartum hemorrhage	33
Problems during childbirth	Regular top-ups of epidural analgesia instead of top-ups on maternal demand	34
	Maternal movement and position changes to relieve pain in labor	34
	Counter-pressure to relieve pain in labor	34
	Superficial heat or cold to relieve pain in labor	34
	Touch and massage to relieve pain in labor	34
	Attention focusing and distraction to relieve pain in labor	34

TABLE B-2 Forms of Care Likely to Be Beneficial (continued)

The evidence in favor of these forms of care is strong, although not established by randomized trials

Problems during childbirth (continued)	Music and audio-analgesia to relieve pain in labor	34
	Epidural instead of narcotic analgesia for preterm labor and birth	34, 37
	Amniotomy to augment slow or prolonged labor	35
	Continuous subcuticular suture for perineal skin repair	36
	Primary rather than delayed repair of episiotomy breakdown	36
	Delivery of a very preterm baby in a center with adequate perinatal facilities	37, 44
	Presence of a pediatrician at a very preterm birth	37, 44
	Trial of labor after previous lower segment cesarean section	38
	Trial of labor after more than one previous lower segment cesarean section	38
	Use of oxytocic agents when indicated for labor after a previous cesarean section	38
	Use of epidural analgesia in labor when need after previous cesarean section	38
Techniques of induction and operative delivery	Assessing the state of the cervix before induction of labor	39
	Transverse instead of vertical skin incision for cesarean section	42
	Low-dose heparin with cesarean section to prevent thrombo-embolism	42
	Transverse lower segment uterine incision for cesarean section	42
Care after birth	Keeping newborn babies warm	44
	Prophylactic vitamin K to the baby to prevent hemorrhagic disease of the newborn	44
	Nasopharyngeal suctioning of babies who have passed meconium before birth	44
	Presence of someone skilled in neonatal resuscitation at birth of all infants likely to be at risk	44
	Oxygen for resuscitation of distressed newborn infants	44
	Cardiac massage for infants born with absent heartbeat	44
	Naloxone for infants with respiratory depression due to narcotic administration before birth	44
	Encouraging early mother-infant contact	45
	Allowing mothers access to their own supply of symptom-relieving drugs in hospital	45
	Consistent advice to new mothers	45
	Offering choice in the length of hospital stay after childbirth	45
	Telephone service of advice and information after women go home from hospital after birth	45
	Psychological support for women depressed after childbirth	45
	Encouraging early breastfeeding when mother and baby are ready	46
	Skilled help with first breastfeed	46
	Flexibility in breastfeeding practices	46
	Antibiotics for infectious mastitis in breastfeeding women	46
	Breast binding and fluid restriction for suppression of lactation	48
	Support and care programs for bereaved parents	49
	Encouraging parental contact with a dying or dead baby	49
	Providing parents with prompt, accurate information about a severely ill baby	49
	Encouraging autopsy for a dead baby and discussing the results with the parents	49
	Help with funeral arrangements for a dead baby	49
	Self-help groups for bereaved parents	49

TABLE B-3   Forms of Care with a Trade-off Between Beneficial and Adverse Effects

Women and caregivers should weigh these effects according to circumstances, priorities, and preferences		*Chapter*
Basic care	Continuity of caregiver for childbearing women	3
	Legislation restricting type of employment for pregnant women	3
Screening and diagnosis	Formal systems of risk scoring	7
	Routine ultrasound in early pregnancy	8
	Chorionic villus sampling versus amniocentesis for diagnosis of chromosomal abnormalities	9
	Serum alpha-fetoprotein screening for neural tube defects	9
	Triple-test screening for Down syndrome and neural tube defects	9
Pregnancy problems	Corticosteroids to promote fetal maturity before preterm birth in diabetic pregnancy	20, 25
	Routine elective cesarean for breech presentation	22
	Induction of labor for prelabor rupture of the membranes at term	23
	Oral betamimetics to maintain uterine quiescence after arrest of preterm labor	24
	Cervical cerclage for women at risk of preterm birth	24
	Betamimetic drugs to stop preterm labor	24
	Induction instead of surveillance for pregnancy after 41 weeks gestation	26
	Expectant care versus induction of labor after fetal death	27
Childbirth	Continuous electronic monitoring (with scalp sampling) versus intermittent auscultation during labor	30
	Midline versus mediolateral episiotomy, when episiotomy is necessary	32
	Prophylactic ergometrine/oxytocin (syntometrine) versus oxytocin alone in the third stage of labor	33
Problems during childbirth	Routine preloading with intravenous fluids before epidural analgesia	34
	Narcotics to relieve pain in labor	34
	Inhalation analgesia to relieve pain in labor	34
	Epidural analgesia to relieve pain in labor	34
	Epidural administration of opiates to relieve pain in labor	34
	Early amniotomy in spontaneous labor	35
Techniques of induction and operative delivery	Mechanical methods for cervical ripening or induction of labor	39, 40
	Endocervical versus vaginal prostaglandin for cervical ripening before induction of labor	39
	Oral prostaglandin E_2 for induction of labor with a ripe cervix	40
	Natural prostaglandins versus oxytocin for induction of labor	40
	Soft versus rigid vacuum cups	41
	Regional versus general anesthesia for cesarean section	42
	Epidural versus spinal anesthesia for cesarean section	42
	Ampicillin versus broader spectrum antibiotics for cesarean section	43
Care after childbirth	Prophylactic antibiotic eye ointments to prevent eye infection in the newborn	44
	Prophylactic versus "rescue" surfactant for very preterm infants	44

TABLE B-4   Forms of Care of Unknown Effectiveness

There are insufficient or inadequate quality data upon which to base a recommendation for practice	*Chapter*
Basic care — Formal preconceptional care for all women	5
Fish oil supplementation to improve pregnancy outcome	6, 15
Prostaglandin precursors to improve pregnancy outcome	6, 15
Calcium supplementation to improve pregnancy outcome	6, 15, 24
Magnesium supplementation to improve pregnancy outcome	6, 15, 24
Zinc supplementation to improve pregnancy outcome	6
Antigen-avoidance diets to reduce risk of an atopic child	6
Screening and diagnosis — Placental grading by ultrasound to improve perinatal outcome	8, 12
Measuring placental proteins for pre-eclampsia	10
Doppler ultrasound of uterine artery for pre-eclampsia	10
Measuring hematocrit and platelets for following the course of pre-eclampsia	10
Fetal biophysical profile for fetal surveillance	12
Pregnancy problems — Acupressure for nausea and vomiting of pregnancy if simple measures are ineffective	13
Vitamin B6 for nausea and vomiting of pregnancy if simple measures are ineffective	13
Ginger for nausea and vomiting of pregnancy	13
Acid-suppressing drugs for heartburn	13
Rutosides for hemorrhoids	13
Rutosides for varicose veins	13
Exercise and education programs for backache	13
Increased salt intake for leg cramps	13
Oral magnesium for leg cramps	13
Progestogens for threatened miscarriage with a live fetus	14
Human Chorionic gonadotrophin (HCG) for threatened miscarriage with a live fetus	14
Steroids for women with auto-antibodies and recurrent miscarriage	14
Evacuation versus "wait and see" following spontaneous miscarriage	14
Medical versus surgical evacuation following spontaneous miscarriage	14
Hospitalization for women with pregnancy-induced hypertension	15
Bed-rest for women with pre-eclampsia	15
Antihypertensive drugs for mild to moderate hypertension	15
Antioxidant vitamins C and E to prevent pre-eclampsia	15
Magnesium sulphate for pre-eclampsia	15
Interventionist versus expectant management for severe early onset pre-eclampsia	15
Plasma volume expansion for pre-eclampsia	15
Hospitalization and bed-rest for impaired fetal growth	16
Abdominal decompression for impaired fetal growth	16
Betamimetics for impaired fetal growth	16
Oxygen treatment for impaired fetal growth	16
Hormone treatment for impaired fetal growth	16
Calcium channel blockers for impaired fetal growth	16
Plasma volume expanders for impaired fetal growth	16
Hospitalization and bed-rest for triplet and higher order pregnancy	17
Antiviral agents for women with a history of recurrent genital herpes	19
Prophylactic antibiotics for prelabor rupture of membranes at term or preterm	23

TABLE B-4   Forms of Care of Unknown Effectiveness (continued)

There are insufficient or inadequate quality data upon which to base a recommendation for practice		*Chapter*
Pregnancy problems (continued)	Postpartum prophylactic antibiotics after prelabor rupture of membranes	23
	Bed-rest to prevent preterm birth	24
	Progestogens to prevent preterm birth	24
	Calcium antagonists to stop preterm birth	24
	Antibiotic treatment in preterm labor	24
	Oxytocin antagonists to stop preterm labor	24
	Sweeping of the membranes to prevent post-term pregnancy	26, 40
	Nipple stimulation to prevent post-term pregnancy	26
Childbirth	Pre-admission assessment to determine if labor is in the active phase	29
	Routine amnioscopy to detect meconium-stained amniotic fluid in labor	30
	Routine artificial rupture of the membranes to detect meconium-stained amniotic fluid in labor	30
	Short periods of electronic fetal monitoring as a screening test on admission in labor	30
	Fetal stimulation tests for fetal assessment in labor	30
	Maternal oxygen administration for fetal distress in labor	30
	Institutional routines for repeating blood pressure measurements in labor	31
	Nipple stimulation to prevent postpartum hemorrhage	33
	Misoprostol in the third stage of labor to prevent postpartum hemorrhage	33
	Early versus late clamping of the umbilical cord at birth	33
	Methods of delivery of the placenta in the third stage of labor	33
	Injecting oxytocin in the umbilical vein in the third stage of labor	33
	Injecting oxytocin in the umbilical vein for retained placenta	33
Problems during childbirth	Abdominal decompression to relieve pain in labor	34
	Immersion in water to relieve pain in labor	34
	Acupuncture to relieve pain in labor	34
	Acupressure to relieve pain in labor	34
	Transcutaneous electrical nerve stimulation to relieve pain in labor	34
	Intradermal injection of sterile water to relieve pain in labor	34
	Aromatherapy to relieve pain in labor	34
	Hypnosis to relieve pain in labor	34
	Continuous infusion versus intermittent top-ups for epidural analgesia	34
	Free mobility during labor to augment slow labor	35
	Early use of oxytocin to augment slow or prolonged labor	35
	"Active management" of labor	35
	Cervical vibration for slow or prolonged labor	35
	Histoacryl tissue adhesive for perineal skin repair	36
	Cesarean section for very preterm delivery	37
	Cesarean section for preterm breech delivery	37
	Immediate versus delayed clamping of the umbilical cord of preterm infants	37
Techniques of induction and operative delivery	Oxytocin by automatic-infusion system versus "standard regiments" for induction of labor	40
	Misoprostol orally or vaginally for induction of labor	40
	Use of hemostatic stapler for the uterine incision at cesarean section	42
	Single- versus two-layer closure of the uterine incision at cesarean section	42
	Systemic versus intraperitoneal prophylactic antibiotics at cesarean section	43

TABLE B-4   Forms of Care of Unknown Effectiveness (continued)

There are insufficient or inadequate quality data upon which to base a recommendation for practice		*Chapter*
Care after childbirth	Tracheal suctioning for meconium in babies without respiratory depression	44
	Routine use of antiseptics on the umbilical cord stump	45
	Oral proteolytic enzymes for breast engorgement in breastfeeding mothers	46
	Cabbage leaves for breast engorgement in breastfeeding mothers	46
	Dopamine agonists to improve milk supply in breastfeeding mothers	46
	Oxytocin nasal spray to improve milk supply in breastfeeding mothers	46
	Oral proteolytic enzymes for perineal pain postpartum	47
	Ultrasound and pulsed electromagnetic energy for perineal pain	47
	Rubber rings and similar devices to prevent pressure for perineal pain	47
	Cabergoline versus physical methods of suppressing lactation	48

TABLE B-5   Forms of Care Unlikely to Be Beneficial

The evidence against these forms of care is not as firmly established as for those in Table 6		*Chapter*
Basic care	Reliance on expert opinion instead of on good evidence for decisions about care	2
	Routinely involving doctors in the care of all women during pregnancy and childbirth	3
	Routinely involving obstetricians in the care of all women during pregnancy and childbirth	3
	Not involving obstetricians in the care of women with serious risk factors	3
	Fragmentation of care during pregnancy and childbirth	3
	Social support for high-risk women to prevent preterm birth	3, 24
	Antenatal breast or nipple care for women who plan to breastfeed	46
	Advice to restrict sexual activity during pregnancy	5
	Prohibition of all alcohol intake during pregnancy	5
	Imposing dietary restrictions during pregnancy	6
	Routine vitamin supplementation in late pregnancy in well-nourished populations	6
	Routine hematinic supplementation in pregnancy in well-nourished populations	6
	High-protein dietary supplementation	6, 16
	Restriction of salt intake to prevent pre-eclampsia	6, 15
Screening and diagnosis	Routine use of ultrasound for fetal measurement in late pregnancy	8, 12
	Reliance on edema to screen for pre-eclampsia	10
	Angiontensin-sensitivity test to screen for pre-eclampsia	10
	Cold-pressor test to screen for pre-eclampsia	10
	Roll-over test to screen for pre-eclampsia	10
	Isometric exercise test to screen for pre-eclampsia	10
	Measuring uric acid as a diagnostic test for pre-eclampsia	10
	Screening for "gestational diabetes"	11
	Routine glucose challenge test during pregnancy	11
	Routine measurement of blood glucose during pregnancy	11
	Insulin plus diet treatment for "gestational diabetes"	11
	Routine fetal movement counting to improve perinatal outcome	12
	Routine use of Doppler ultrasound screening in all pregnancies	12
	Measurement of placental proteins or hormones (including estriol and human placental lactogen)	12
	Routine cervical assessment for prevention of preterm birth	24

TABLE B-5   Forms of Care Unlikely to Be Beneficial (continued)

The evidence against these forms of care is not as firmly established as for those in Table 6	*Chapter*
Pregnancy problems Calcium supplementation for leg cramps	13
Screening for, and treatment of, vaginal candidal colonization without symptoms	13
Screening for, and treatment of, vaginal trichomonas colonization without symptoms	13
Screening for, and treatment of, bacterial vaginosis without symptoms	13
Bed-rest for threatened miscarriage	14
Immunotherapy for recurrent miscarriage	14
Antithrombotic agents to prevent pre-eclampsia	15
Reducing salt intake to prevent pre-eclampsia	15
Diazoxide for pre-eclampsia or hypertension in pregnancy	15
Ketanserin for severe hypertension in pregnancy	15
Diuretics for pregnancy-induced hypertension	15
High protein dietary supplementation for impaired fetal growth	16
Hospitalization and bed-rest for uncomplicated twin pregnancy	17
Cervical cerclage for multiple pregnancy	17
Prophylactic betamimetics for multiple pregnancy	17
Routine cesarean section for multiple pregnancy	17
Routine screening for mycoplasmas during pregnancy	19
Screening for toxoplasmosis during pregnancy	19
Treatment for group B streptococcus colonization during pregnancy	19
Cesarean section for non-active herpes simplex before or at the onset of labor	19
Amniotomy in HIV-infected women	19, 35
Elective delivery before term in women with otherwise uncomplicated diabetes	20
Elective cesarean section for pregnant women with diabetes	20
Discouraging breastfeeding in women with diabetes	21
Vaginal or rectal examination when placenta previa is suspected	22
Postural techniques for turning breech into cephalic presentation	22
External cephalic version before term to avoid breech presentation at term	22
X-ray pelvimetry to diagnose cephalopelvic disproportion	22
Computer tomographic pelvimetry to predict cephalopelvic disproportion	22
Cesarean section for macrosomia without a trial of labor to prevent shoulder dystocia	22
Induction of labor to prevent cephalopelvic disproportion	22
Amniocentesis for prelabor rupture of the membranes preterm	23
Regular leucocyte counts for surveillance in prelabor rupture of the membranes	23
Home uterine activity monitoring for prevention of preterm birth	24
Magnesium sulphate to stop preterm labor	24
Betamimetics for preterm labor in women with heart disease or diabetes	24
Hydration to arrest preterm labor	24
Diazoxide to stop preterm labor	24
Adding thyrotrophin releasing hormone (TRH) to corticosteroids to promote fetal maturation	25
Childbirth Withholding food and drink from women in labor	29
Routine intravenous infusion in labor	29
Routine measurement of intrauterine pressure during oxytocin administration	31, 35
Wearing face masks during labor or for vaginal examinations	31
Frequent scheduled vaginal examinations in labor	31
Routine directed pushing during the second stage of labor	32
Pushing by sustained bearing down during the second stage of labor	32

TABLE B-5 Forms of Care Unlikely to Be Beneficial (continued)

The evidence against these forms of care is not as firmly established as for those in Table 6

Childbirth (continued)	Breath holding during the second stage of labor	32
	Early bearing down during the second stage of labor	32
	Arbitrary limitation of the duration of the second stage of labor	32
	"Ironing out" or massaging the perineum during the second stage of labor	32
	Routine manual exploration of the uterus after vaginal birth	32
	Injectable prostaglandins in the third stage of labor	33
	Encouraging early suckling to prevent postpartum hemorrhage	33
Problems during childbirth	Injecting saline into the umbilical vein for retained placenta	33
	Biofeedback to relieve pain in labor	34
	Sedatives and tranquilizers to relieve pain in labor	34
	Caudal block to prevent pain in labor	34
	Paracervical block to relieve pain in labor	35
	Intrapartum x-ray to diagnose cephalopelvic disproportion	35
	Diagnosing cephalopelvic disproportion without ensuring adequate uterine contractions	35
	Relaxin for slow or prolonged labor	35
	Hyaluronidase for slow or prolonged labor	35
	Vitamin K to the mother to prevent intraventricular hemorrhage in the very preterm infant	37
	Phenobarbitone to the mother to prevent intraventricular hemorrhage in the very preterm infant	37
	Delivery of a very preterm infant without adequate facilities to care for a very preterm baby	37
	Elective forceps delivery for preterm birth	37, 41
	Routine use of episiotomy for preterm birth	37
	Trial of labor after previous classical cesarean section	38
	Routine manual exploration of the uterus to assess a previous cesarean section scar	38
Techniques of induction and operative delivery	Relaxin for cervical ripening before induction of labor	39
	Nipple stimulation for cervical ripening before induction of labor	39
	Extra-amniotic instead of other prostaglandin regimens for cervical ripening	39
	Instrumental vaginal delivery to shorten the second stage of labor	41
	Routine exteriorization of the uterus for repair of the uterine incision at cesarean section	42
Care after childbirth	Silver nitrate to prevent eye infection in newborn babies	44
	Elective tracheal intubation for very low-birthweight infants who are not depressed	44
	Routine suctioning of newborn babies	44
	Medicated bathing of babies to reduce infection	45
	Wearing hospital gowns in newborn nurseries	45
	Restricting sibling visits to babies in hospitals	45
	Routine measurements of temperature, pulse, blood pressure, and fundal height postpartum	45
	Limiting use of women's own non-prescriptive drugs postpartum in hospital	45
	Administering non-prescription symptom-relieving drugs at regularly set intervals	45
	Prohibition of oral contraceptives for diabetic women	20
	Nipple shields for breastfeeding mothers	46
	Switching breasts before babies spontaneously terminate the feed	46
	Oxytocin for breast engorgement in breastfeeding mothers	46
	Antibiotics for localized breast engorgement (milk stasis)	46
	Discontinuing breastfeeding for localized breast engorgement (milk stasis)	46
	Combinations of local anesthetics and topical steroids for relief of perineal pain	47
	Relying on these tables without referring to the rest of the book	50

TABLE B-6   Forms of Care Likely to Be Ineffective or Harmful

Ineffectiveness or harm demonstrated by clear evidence		*Chapter*
Basic care	Dietary restriction to prevent pre-eclampsia	6, 15
Screening and diagnosis	Contraction stress cardiotocography to improve perinatal outcome	12
	Nipple-stimulation test cardiotocography to improve perinatal outcome	12
	Non-selective use of non-stress cardiotocography to improve perinatal outcome	12
Pregnancy problems	Adrenocorticotrophic hormone (ACTH) for severe vomiting of pregnancy	13
	Saline cathartics for constipation	13
	Lubricant oils for constipation	13
	Diethylstilbestrol during pregnancy	14
	Elective delivery for prelabor rupture of the membranes preterm	23
	Ethanol to stop preterm labor	24
	Progestogens to stop preterm labor	24
Childbirth	Routine enema in labor	29
	Routine pubic shaving in preparation for childbirth	29
	Electronic fetal monitoring without access to fetal scalp sampling during labor	30
	Prophylactic intrapartum amnio-infusion for oligohydramnios	30
	Rectal examinations to assess labor progress	31
	Requiring a supine (flat on back) position in the second stage of labor	32
	Routine use of the lithotomy position for the second stage of labor	32
	Routine or liberal episiotomy for birth	32
	Ergometrine instead of oxytocin prophylaxis in the third stage of labor	33
Problems in childbirth	Glycerol-impregnated catgut for perineal trauma	36
Techniques for induction and operative delivery	Oral prostaglandins for cervical ripening	39
	Estrogens for cervical ripening or for induction of labor	39
	Oxytocin for cervical ripening before induction of labor	39
Care after childbirth	Sodium bicarbonate for asphyxiated babies	44
	Routine restriction of mother-infant contact	45
	Routine nursery care for babies in hospital	45
	Antenatal Hoffman's exercises for inverted or flat nipples	46
	Antenatal breast shells for inverted or flat nipples	46
	Limitation of suckling time during breastfeeding	46
	Nipple creams or ointments for breastfeeding mothers	46
	Routine supplements of water or formula for breastfed babies	46
	Samples of formula for breastfeeding mothers	46
	Encouraging fluid intake beyond demands of thirst for breastfeeding mothers	46
	Combined estrogen-progesterone oral contraceptives for breastfeeding mothers	46
	Test weighing of breastfed infants	46
	Witch hazel for relief of perineal pain	47
	Adding salt to bath water for treating perineal pain	47
	Antiseptic solutions added to bath water for perineal pain	47
	Hormones for relief of breast symptoms in non-breastfeeding mothers	48
	Bromocriptine for relief of breast symptoms in non-breastfeeding mothers	48

Standards of Family-Centered Maternity Care

The following standards describe a competent level of performance in the professional nursing role. These standards include activities related to nursing practice, competencies, ethics, family health education and counseling, collaboration, and professional responsibility and accountability. All family-centered maternity care nurses are expected to engage in professional role activities appropriate to their education, position, and practice setting.

STANDARD 1—NURSING PRACTICE

The family-centered maternity care nurse provides direct nursing care in accordance with the family-centered mission and philosophy of the maternity service.

The FCMC nurse demonstrates competency in meeting the following objectives:

- On admission, completes a family assessment and history for use in individualizing care for mother and baby during the antepartum, intrapartum, and postpartum periods. In order to meet this objective, the nurse will describe:
  - Roles and functions of family members.
  - Patterns of interaction and communication among family members, verbal and nonverbal.
  - The mother's and family's understanding of pregnancy, lactation, involution, neonatal transition, and postpartum physiologic and developmental changes.
  - The childbearing family's ethnic, cultural, and religious heritage.
  - The childbearing family's health beliefs and health teaching needs.
  - The childbearing family's spiritual needs.
- In collaboration with the family and within 24 hours of each woman's admission, develops a family nursing care plan for the antepartal, intrapartal, or postpartal period. This plan includes the following:
  - Family-centered goals that identify and promote strengths in childbearing women and their families and facilitate independence and empowerment.
  - Valid, measurable, and time-bound outcome criteria for stated goals.
  - Interventions for ongoing diagnosis, treatment, and education to accomplish the goals.
  - Evaluation data that describe whether the outcome criteria have been met.
- Documents the plan of care and patient and family response to the nursing interventions daily.
- Implements the interventions identified in the family nursing care plan.
- Evaluates the outcomes of the care plan every eight hours, and updates and revises the family nursing care plan as appropriate.

STANDARD 2—NURSING COMPETENCIES

The family-centered maternity care nurse demonstrates nursing actions based on knowledge of normal and abnormal patterns of biophysical and psychosocial growth, development, adaptation, and functioning of the pregnant woman, fetus, newborn, and family in the following content areas:

- Anatomy and physiology of human reproduction, pregnancy, birth, and the puerperium.
- Maternal, fetal, and newborn physiological, psychological, and developmental changes during the trimesters of pregnancy and the puerperium.

- Psychosocial adaptation of the woman and family during pregnancy, puerperium, and the first year of life.

- Nutritional requirements of pregnancy, lactation, and puerperium.

- Indicators of high-risk status for mothers, infants, and childbearing families.

- Impact of environmental factors and/or hazards on the pregnancy, fetus, newborn, and family health status.

- Effects of substance abuse on the pregnancy, fetus, and childbearing family.

- Laboratory and diagnostic tests routinely used to screen the health status of the mother, fetus, and newborn during the antepartum, intrapartum, puerperium, and newborn periods.

- Local and regional resources for the provision of social and psychological healthcare needs and financial support for childbearing families.

- Principles of health education and counseling to implement family-centered maternity care.

STANDARD 3—ETHICS

The family-centered maternity care nurse's decisions and actions on behalf of families are determined in an ethical manner.

The FCMC nurse demonstrates competency in meeting the following objectives:

- Delivers care in a nonjudgmental and nondiscriminatory manner.

- Maintains a safe environment for patient care:

  - Functions competently with all equipment on the maternity unit, identifying how the equipment relates to each individual patient's care.

  - Responds to emergencies appropriately.

- Supports a woman's natural ability to give birth.

- Provides nursing care according to family-centered guidelines, policies, procedures, and protocols.

- Recognizes patient rights and responsibilities.

- Treats each family with respect and dignity.

- Maintains patient and family confidentiality and privacy.

- Explains all treatments and procedures to the woman and her family, or asks the physician or midwife to do so, as appropriate.

- Listens to the family with patience and understanding.

- Seeks available resources to help formulate ethical decisions.

- Provides support and supportive services to the family.

- Acts as an advocate for mother and newborn.

- Involves family members and close friends for social and emotional support of the new mother as much as she wishes.

STANDARD 4—FAMILY HEALTH EDUCATION AND COUNSELING

The family-centered maternity care nurse demonstrates a commitment to providing experiences that allow new mothers and their families to learn about their baby and their changing roles within the family structure.

The FCMC nurse demonstrates competency in meeting the following objectives:

- Assesses and identifies daily the educational needs and skills of the woman and her family.

- Listens to the mother's and family's perspectives and priorities.

- Teaches families using adult teaching and learning principles and guidelines for maternal and newborn care.

- Uses respectful and easily understood language.

- Uses available educational resources in the practice environment.

- Documents and evaluates the families' responses to teaching.

- When teaching parents basic infant care, includes information related to:

  - Infant states of consciousness.

  - Newborn sensory motor skills.

  - Newborn behaviors and individual differences and temperaments.

  - Parent–infant interactions and relationships.

  - Parents' perceptions of their newborn.

- Assists families in understanding and coping with normal developmental and common situational crises during the childbearing experience.

- Supports and teaches mothers to breastfeed.

STANDARD 5—COLLABORATION

The family-centered maternity care nurse collaborates with other healthcare team members to provide care to childbearing families.

The FCMC nurse demonstrates competency in meeting the following objectives:

- Researches the family assessment and history, nursing care plan, flow sheet, and chart prior to administering patient care.

- Gives and receives 1:1 report on families in care assignment.

- Consults with other healthcare providers, as needed.

- Assists colleagues in the care of families as needed.
- Refers families to community agencies, peer and support resources, and other resources as appropriate.
- As appropriate, uses federal, state, and county maternal-child health resources in providing care to families.
- Makes referrals, including provisions for continuity of care.
- Influences peers through positive role modeling.
- Communicates all pertinent information to all team members.
- Requests assistance from nursing leadership when necessary.

STANDARD 6—PROFESSIONAL RESPONSIBILITY AND ACCOUNTABILITY

The family-centered maternity care nurse maintains competencies and participates in activities that contribute to ongoing personal development and to development of other healthcare providers and the profession.

The FCMC nurse demonstrates competency in meeting the following objectives:

- Attends staff meetings and shares knowledge and skills with colleagues.
- Provides peers with constructive feedback regarding their practice.
- Maintains certification and recertification in standard hospital programs.
- Conforms to family-centered hospital, nursing, and division policies.
- Participates in ongoing educational activities and learning experiences to improve quality of care to families.
- Performs ongoing self-evaluation, identifying areas for practice development as well as areas of strength.
- Demonstrates a family-centered approach in caring for mothers, newborns, and families throughout the childbearing experience.
- Uses research findings in practice.
- Participates in research activities as appropriate.
- Demonstrates flexibility in response to change.
- Commits to lifelong learning.

An Overview of the Family-Centered Maternity Nursing Screening Tool

The Family-Centered Maternity Nursing Screening Tool is designed to select technical skills, critical thinking skills, and family-centered maternity care talents. Talent, as used in this tool, is more important than experience, skills, or intelligence. It is an aspect of one's experience; it is a pattern of thought, feeling, or behavior that can be productively applied.

This tool presents an objective method for assessing three dimensions of competent performance for nurses: critical thinking, interpersonal relations (attitudes), and technical skills.

TECHNICAL SKILLS

These skills measure experience and are assessed through a two-tiered process.

Step 1, the initial application process, provides an opportunity to review applications and to select interview candidates who appear to meet minimum criteria as established by the interviewers. During this phase of the process, the applicant completes core skills lists for mother–baby nursing and labor and delivery practice. The completed core skills lists are submitted with the completed application form.

Step 2 applies only to those candidates who are invited to attend an interview session following successful screening in Step 1. These applicants complete an advanced skills list and engage in a detailed discussion about family-centered care with the interviewer.

INTERPERSONAL RELATIONS SKILLS

These skills measure talent ("attitude") and are assessed through two 10-item sections of statements. Separate items are presented for labor and delivery and for mother–baby care. Questions are presented with two different response sets, one indicating a contemporary practitioner and one indicating a more traditional caregiver. Using a key that is provided with the instrument, applicants receive one point for each family-centered response and 0 points for non-family-centered responses. A perfect score would be +10 for the L&D questions and +10 for the M–B questions. The applicant should have a minimum score of +8 for each set of questions.

CRITICAL THINKING SKILLS

These skills measure behavior and are assessed through vignettes that present the applicant with a variety of typical situations. The candidate is required to provide a response as to what a family-centered nurse would do in each situation. There are five typical events and five that are specific to diverse cultural needs.

The Centering Pregnancy Program: A Model for Group Prenatal Care

The Centering Pregnancy Program is an innovative model for providing complete prenatal care within a group setting. Its overriding mission is to empower pregnant women by encouraging them to take responsibility for themselves and to interact positively with the healthcare system, while meeting their health and educational needs.

HISTORY

The first Centering pilot groups were conducted in 1993 in Waterbury, Connecticut. Centering's founder, Sharon Schindler Rising, MSN, CNM, FACNM, created the model based on her work at the University of Minnesota, where she developed the graduate nurse-midwifery educational program and the Childbearing Childrearing Center. The data from the initial 13 groups—3 of them teens—were encouraging. Visit compliance was as high as 92% in some groups and ER use was down. Most promising, however, was the patient satisfaction: 96% of the participating women stated that they preferred receiving their care in this way.

In 1998, Sharon began conducting two-day workshops throughout the United States to train providers in the Centering method of facilitative leadership and to assist in establishing a program in their facility. Additional support services were created to meet the increasing interest, including individual consultation, The Centering web site, and the newsletter *Centering Circuit*. Government and private research agencies also took note and began committing time and funds to evaluate and support the apparent benefits of Centering.

In 2001, as awareness of the model and the number of sites offering Centering group care steadily grew, the strength and size of the organization led its leaders to make the step of creating a new nonprofit corporation: Centering Pregnancy and Parenting Association.

The benefits of this structure are numerous. Most importantly, it reflects the mission of Centering—to change the paradigm of the care of the pregnant woman and family—and ensures that it will be accomplished exclusively for the benefit of pregnant women and their families and those involved in their care. Additionally, it opens up opportunities for membership and participation for interested individuals, institutions, and organizations that may or may not be directly conducting Centering groups.

Today, the Centering model is enthusiastically accepted in a variety of patient populations, from inner city teens to suburban private practices to large institutional services. And with the growing evidence of its strengths, the Centering network steadily increases.

Philosophy

The Centering Pregnancy model is based on the philosophy that pregnancy is a process of wellness, and a time when many women can be encouraged to take responsibility for their own health and learn to participate in self-care. It is also a time of introspection and transition for most women, and therefore an important opportunity for caregivers to assist maturation and effect behavioral change. The program is built on the premise that prenatal care is most effectively and efficiently provided to women in groups; that learning and support are enhanced by group resource, including the guidance of the professional care provider and an atmosphere that facilitates learning, encourages free exchange, and develops mutual support; and that this high quality of care can be difficult to achieve with the traditional structure of individual examination room visits.

Structure

Centering Pregnancy brings women out of the confines of the traditional exam room for the majority of their care by providing three components of prenatal care—assessment, support, and education—within a group setting under the facilitative leadership of a skilled practitioner. Groups of eight to twelve women of similar gestational age meet at regular intervals throughout pregnancy, beginning at approximately 14 weeks of pregnancy and ending one-month postpartum. During the 90- to 120-minute sessions the women receive their basic prenatal physical assessments and engage in self-care activities related to this process, socialize and get support from other women/couples, and gain knowledge and skills related to pregnancy, childbirth, and parenting. The issues addressed in the sessions include nutrition, common discomforts, relationships, labor and delivery, infant care, and postpartum, all of which are described in detail in the *Centering Pregnancy Handbook*.

THE HANDBOOK

The *Centering Pregnancy Handbook* contains the material needed to establish and conduct a Centering program. It is designed for any skilled group leader involved in delivering prenatal care: nurse-midwife, nurse practitioner, social worker, clinical nurse specialist, mental health clinician, or physician. The contents include instructions on how to develop a total program suitable for a variety of agencies. Learning objectives and detailed session outlines support the educational component of Centering, along with worksheets, handouts, and evaluation materials in English and Spanish.

BENEFITS

Configuring prenatal care into groups offers advantages over traditional prenatal care to the pregnant woman/couple, the practitioner, and the facility in which it is conducted. Group prenatal care provides substantially more contact with caregivers, provides support services, and is integrated to respond to the complex needs of pregnant women. More specifically, group care affords the opportunity to:

- Discuss the physical and psychosocial changes of pregnancy and the behavioral changes that may be required to maintain a healthy pregnancy.

- Cover a broader and deeper scope of topics than would be possible on an individual basis.

- Expose all women to information, including those who may be too embarrassed to discuss sensitive issues such as HIV/STDs, condom use, or interpersonal violence, during a one-to-one visit.

- Increase contact time with each woman dramatically, from approximately 90 minutes over the course of a pregnancy in the standard individual prenatal care, to 15 hours in the group setting.

- Include single pregnant women and couples.

- Create a "community" of support, that often continues beyond pregnancy, for women/couples who may be isolated or without family.

- Mirror concerns, thus normalizing the pregnancy experience.

- Create an environment that is stimulating and challenging to the practitioner/facilitator.

- Provide efficient use of time and space, freeing exam rooms for other activities.

- Ensure reimbursement through the usual systems of billing prenatal care; managed care companies should find this model attractive in its efficiency and scope.

CENTERING SITE SUPPORT SERVICES

Behind the Centering Pregnancy name is a great organization that can provide assistance in education, promotion, and program support. Here are the services that are offered:

Instructional workshops provide individuals and agencies with the skills and knowledge to successfully establish and run a Centering program. The attendees are those who are interested in the model and are seeking detailed information; those who have decided to set up a Centering Pregnancy program in their facility and require guidance; and those participating in an ongoing Centering program seeking advice on specific problems. Workshops are conducted for a group of individuals, or for one or more agencies, within a geographic area.

Professional consultation is available to individual clinic and private practice sites, as well as educational/preceptor programs. Services include assistance with assessment of current care delivery system, preparation of staff to conduct a group program, modification of the Centering program to your setting, and evaluation of outcomes. Speakers are available for presentations to students, faculty, and service personnel, and at formal roundtables and conferences. Daylong information workshops are also offered to acquaint individuals and agencies with the concept of group prenatal care delivered through Centering Pregnancy, and to provide an overview of Centering Pregnancy with the opportunity to explore patterns of implementation.

The Centering web site contains the background and a detailed description of the Centering Pregnancy model. You can also find the dates for upcoming workshops, read the latest news from the Centering network, and order handbooks. It can be viewed at www.centeringpregnancy.com.

Centering Circuit, the newsletter of Centering Pregnancy, gives the latest Centering happenings. It features news articles on Centering, announcements of upcoming workshops and speaking dates, updates on ongoing programs, and personal comments and advice on the Centering experience. It is published 2–4 times a year, and is available on request.

Urban Midwife Associates: The UMA Foundation

68 Glendale Street, Dorchester, MA 02125

15 Saxon Terrace, Newton, MA 02461

SUMMARY

Birth Sisters^SM is an intensive program of lay community-based social support for women across the childbearing cycle. The Birth Sisters^SM Model was developed in 1994 by Urban Midwife Associates (UMA), as part of its overall model program. The name Birth Sisters^SM is a registered Service Mark of Urban Midwife Associates and may not be used without permission.

DEFINITION OF THE BIRTH SISTERS^SM PROGRAM MODEL

Birth Sisters^SM are lay women from a particular community who are trained to provide social support across the childbearing cycle. The training and care must include the following essential components:

- Contact in the antepartum period between Birth Sister and client.

- Continuous intrapartum emotional support and physical presence and provision of "labor support" techniques as appropriate.

- Postpartum home visiting in the first two weeks after delivery, with direct services to include assistance in child care and household chores, breastfeeding support and teaching, and emotional caring and support.

- Provision of training to potential Birth Sisters^SM is eligible for DONA* certification.

- Birth Sisters^SM must be recruited from the neighborhoods and cultural groups served by the entity providing the program.

GOALS OF THE BIRTH SISTERS^SM PROGRAM MODEL

- Increased satisfaction with the childbearing experience and increased self-esteem on the part of the pregnant woman

- Increased incidence of breastfeeding, longer duration of breastfeeding and its associated medical benefits to the mother and the infant

- Decreased utilization of expensive obstetrical technology, i.e., fewer cesarean sections and operative deliveries

- Enhancement of supportive connections between women and the building of community, preservation of culturally specific social childbirth practices

HISTORY OF THE BIRTH SISTERS^SM MODEL

The Birth Sisters^SM Program was developed by Urban Midwife Associates in 1994 as part of its overall program of services, which includes:

- Comprehensive primary care midwifery

- Continuity of care and caregiver over time in the context of a personal relationship

- Community-based, community-building care

- Evidence-based care and appropriate use of technology

- Education for health promotion and prevention

- Culturally and linguistically sensitive care and social support

This program was targeted to women at high social risk of poor pregnancy outcome due to adolescence, homelessness, drug addiction, incarceration, HIV infection, physical or mental disability, immigrant status or language barrier, or residence in neighborhoods historically plagued by the effects of poverty, discrimination, and limited care options. The model was also intended to be beneficial for and made available to any woman who was interested in the kind of care offered, regardless of ability to pay.

The Birth Sisters^{SM} Program was initially funded in 1995 by the March of Dimes, under a grant written by Urban Midwife Associates. In 1998 Urban Midwife Associates donated the unused portion of that grant to Boston Medical Center to develop a Birth Sisters^{SM} Program using the model, making it available to all women delivering at that hospital.

USE OF THE BIRTH SISTERS^{SM} MODEL

Urban Midwife Associates will make the model available to any group that wishes to use it, as well as the name and the logo, without cost, provided that certain requirements are met. These include:

1. Each of the above components of the model must be fully included.

2. The name Birth Sisters^{SM} must always be written to include the Service Mark (SM) and the written notation "The name Birth Sisters^{SM} is a registered Service Mark of Urban Midwife Associates, Inc."

3. All written and nonwritten descriptions of the Birth Sisters^{SM} program in question must include the acknowledgement that the Birth Sisters^{SM} model was developed by Urban Midwife Associates.

4. All Birth Sisters^{SM} literature must include the notation "The name Birth Sisters^{SM} is a registered Service Mark of Urban Midwife Associates, Inc., and may not be used without permission."

5. Any entity requesting to use the model must agree to submit yearly reports to UMA verifying that it is continuing to provide the model as described, to submit yearly statistical information about its version of the program for research purposes, and any other requirements decided upon by Urban Midwife Associates in order to certify that the model is properly applied.

Telephone: 617/287-8707

Urban Midwife Associates Fax: 617/825-7585

UMA Foundation Fax: 617/244-3661

Resources for Information on Family-Centered Maternity Care

American Academy of Family Physicians (AAFP)
1140 Tomahawk Creek Parkway
Leawood, KS 66211-2672 USA
913/906-6000
www.aafp.org

American Academy of Husband-Coached Childbirth (AAHCC)
(The Bradley Method)
P.O. Box 5224
Sherman Oaks, CA 91413-5224 USA
818/788-6662
www.bradleybirth.com

American Academy of Pediatrics (AAP)
141 NW Point Boulevard
Elk Grove, IL 60007 USA
847/228-5005
www.aap.org

American College of Nurse-Midwives
818 Connecticut Ave. NW, Suite 900
Washington, DC 20006 USA
202/728-9860
Fax 202/728-9897
www.acnm.org

American College of Obstetricians and Gynecologists (ACOG)
409 12th St. SW
P.O. Box 96920
Washington, DC 20090-6920 USA
202/638-5577
www.acog.org

American Medical Association
515 North State St.
Chicago, IL 60610 USA
310/464-5000
or
1101 Vermont Ave. NW
Washington, DC 20005 USA
202/789-7400
www.ama-assn.org

American Nurses Association
600 Maryland Ave. SW, Suite 100 West
Washington, DC 20024 USA
800/600-2662
Fax 202/651-7001
www.ana.org

American Public Health Association (APHA)
800 I St. NW
Washington, DC 20001-3710 USA
202/777-2742
Fax 202/777-2532
www.apha.org

American Red Cross
National Headquarters
811 Gatehouse Road
Falls Church, VA 22042 USA
703/206-6000
www.redcross.org

Association of Labor Assistants and Childbirth Educators (ALACE)
(Formerly Informed Birth and Parenting)
P.O. Cambridge, MA 02238-2724 USA
617/441-2500
www.alace.org

Association of Women's Health, Obstetric and Neonatal Nurses (AWHONN)
2000 L. St. NW Suite 740
Washington, DC 20036
800/673-8499 USA
800/245-0231 Canada
www.awhonn.org

Brazelton Institute
1295 Boylston Street, Suite 320
Boston, MA 02115 USA
617/355-4959
Fax 617/859-7215
www.brazelton-institute/com

Breastfeeding Committee for Canada
Box 65114
Toronto, ON M4K 3Z2 Canada
Fax 416/465-8265
email: www.bfc@istar.ca

Canadian Institute of Child Health
384 Bank St., Suite 300
Ottawa, ON K2P 1Y4 Canada
613/230-8838
Fax 613/230-6654
www.cich.ca

Canadian Medical Association
1862 Alta Vista Dr.
Ottawa, ON K1G 3Y6 Canada
613/731-9331
Fax 613/236-8864
www.cma.ca

Canadian Nurses Association
50 Driveway
Ottawa, ON K2P 1E2 Canada
613/237-2133
800/361-8404
Fax 613/237-3520
www.cna-nurses.ca

Canadian Paediatric Society
2204 Walkley Rd.
Ottawa, ON K1G 4G8 Canada
613/526-9397
www.cps.ca

Centering Pregnancy and Parenting Association (CPPA)
50 Mountain Rd.
Cheshire, CT 06410 USA
www.centeringpregnancy.com

Childbirth and Postpartum Professional Association (CAPPA)
310 Sweet Ivy Lane
Lawrenceville, GA 30042 USA
888/548-3674
www.childbirthprofessional.com

Children's Medical Ventures, Inc.
541 Main Street
S. Weymouth, MA 02190 USA
800/377-3449
904/285-1613
email: info@childmed.com

Coalition for Improving Maternity Services (CIMS)
P.O. Box 2346
Ponte Vedra Beach, FL 32004 USA
888/282-CIMS
904/285-1613
Fax 904/285-2120
www.motherfriendly.org
email: info@motherfriendly.org

The Compassionate Friends, Inc.
P.O. Box 3696
Oak Brook, IL 60522-3696 USA
630/990-0010
www.compassionatefriends.org

Depression After Delivery
PO Box 278
Belle Mead, NJ 08502 USA
908/575-9121
www.depressionafterdelivery.com

Doulas of North America (DONA)
13513 North Grove Dr.
Alpine, UT 84004 USA
801/756-7331
Fax 801/763-1847
www.dona.org

Health Canada
A.L. 0913A
Ottawa, ON K1A 0K9 Canada
613/941-5366
Fax 613/957-2991
www.hc-sc.gc.ca

Hypnobirthing Institute
PO Box 810
Epsom, NH 03234 USA
603/798-3286
www.hypnobirthing.com

Institute for Family-Centered Care
7900 Wisconsin Avenue, Suite 405
Bethesda, MD 20814
301/652-0281
Fax 301/652-0186
www.familycenteredcare.org
email: ifcc@aol.com

I Am Your Child
www.iamyourchild.org

International Association of Infant Massage
1891 Goodyear Ave., Suite 622
Ventura, CA 93003 USA
805/644-8524
Fax 805/644-7699
www.health4all.com/infantmassage

International Cesarean Awareness Network, Inc. (ICAN)
1304 Kingsdale Ave.
Redondo Beach, CA 90278 USA
310/542-6400
Fax 310/542-5386
www.childbirth.org/section/ICAN.html

International Childbirth Education Association (ICEA)
P.O. Box 20048
Minneapolis, MN 55420 USA
952/854-8660
FAX 952/854-8772
www.icea.org
email: info@icea.org

International Lactation Consultant Association (ILCA)
1500 Sunday Drive, Suite 102
Raleigh, NC 27607 USA
919/787-5181
Fax 919/787-4916
www.ilca.org

Johnson & Johnson Pediatric Institute
1-877/565-5465
www.JJPI.com

La Leche League International (LLLI)
1400 N. Meacham Rd.
PO Box 4079
Schaumburg, IL 60173-4048 USA
874/519-7730
1-800/LA-LECHE
www.lalecheleague.org

Lamaze International
2025 M Street NW, Suite 800
Washington, DC 20036-3309 USA
202/367-1128
Fax 202/367-2128
www.lamaze-childbirth.com

March of Dimes Birth Defects Foundation
1275 Mamaronek Ave.
White Plains, NY 10605 USA
914/428-7100
www.modimes.org

Maternity Center Association
281 Park Ave.
New York, NY 10010 USA
212/777-5000
www.maternity.org

Midwives Alliance of North America
P.O. Box 175
Newton, KS 67114 USA
316/283-4543
www.mana.org

National Association of Childbearing Centers (NACC)
3123 Gottschall Rd.
Perkiomenville, PA 18074 USA
215/234-8068
www.birthcenters.org

National Association for Parents and Professionals for Safe Alternatives in Childbirth (NAPSAC)
Route 1, Box 646
Marble Hill, MO 63764 USA
314/238-2010

National Center for Complementary and Alternative Medicine
P.O. Box 8218
Silver Springs, MD 20907-8218
888/644-6226
http://altmed.od.nih.gov

National Center for Education in Maternal and Child Health
2000 15th St., Suite 701
Georgetown University
Arlington, VA 22201-2617 USA
703/524-7802
www.ncemch.org

National Council on Family Relations
3989 Central Avenue NE, Suite 550
Minneapolis, MN 55421 USA
612/781-9331
www.ncfr.org

National Healthy Mothers Healthy Babies Coalition
121 North Washington Street, Suite 300
Alexandria, VA 22314 USA
703/826-6610
Fax 703/836-3470
www.hmhb.org

National Organization of Mothers of Twins Clubs
877/540-2200
www.nomotc.org

National Perinatal Association (NPA)
University Professional Center, Suite 209
3500 E. Fletcher Ave.
Tampa, FL 33613-4707 USA
813/971-1008
888/971-3295
www.nationalperinatal.org

National Society of Genetic Counselors (NSGC)
233 Canterbury Dr.
Wallingford, PA 19086-6617
610/872-7608
www.nsgc.org

National Women's Health Network
514 10th St. NW, Suite 400
Washington, DC 20005 USA
202/347-1140
Fax 202/347-1168
www.womenshealthnetwork.org

Pampers Parenting Institute
www.pampers.com

Parents Without Partners
www.parentswithoutpartners.org

Postpartum Support International
927 Kellogg Ave.
Santa Barbara, CA 93111 USA
www.chss.iup.edu/postpartum

Sidelines National Support Network
This is a national nonprofit organization for women on pregnancy-related bed rest.
2805 Park Place
Laguna Beach, CA 92651 USA
714/497-2265
www.sidelines.org

UNICEF
UNICEF House
3 United Nations Plaza
New York, NY 10017 USA
www.unicef.org

U.S. Department of Agriculture (WIC)
Food and Consumer Service
Special Supplement Nutrition Program for Women, Infants and Children (WIC)
3101 Park Center Drive, Room 540
Alexandria, PA 22302 USA
www.theusda.gov/wic

U.S. Department of Labor Women's Bureau
200 Constitution Avenue, NW
Room S-3002
Washington, DC 20210
800/827-5335
Fax 202/219-5529
www.dol.gov/wb

World Health Organization
Avenue Appia 20
1211 Geneva 27 Switzerland
+004122 791-2111
Fax +004122 791-3111
www.who.int

Worldwide Fund for Mothers Injured in Childbirth
7200 Sears Tower
Chicago, IL 60606 USA
www.wfmic.org

Assessment Criteria for a Family Beginnings™ Maternity Program

This tool is designed to identify specific practices, policies, and procedures that demonstrate actual day-to-day implementation of the principles of family-centered maternity care. Completing this assessment tool aids in prioritizing and planning change to family-centered maternity care.

194

PHILOSOPHY OF CARE

	Yes	No

1. The maternity service has a written mission statement that conveys a commitment to family-centered maternity care (FCMC). ☐ ☐

2. The maternity service has a written philosophy of FCMC. ☐ ☐

3. The FCMC philosophy is discussed with applicants for employment in the hospital's Maternity Unit and/or antepartal clinic, and the applicant's response is noted in the interview record. ☐ ☐

4. During their orientation, all Maternity employees are given the following:

   a. A copy of the FCMC philosophy and mission. ☐ ☐

   b. In-service education about FCMC. ☐ ☐

   and this is so noted in their personnel file. ☐ ☐

5. All professionals with practice privileges in the Maternity Service are given a copy of the FCMC philosophy annually. ☐ ☐

6. The written FCMC philosophy is reviewed and reaffirmed annually by all maternity care providers employed by or affiliated with the hospital. ☐ ☐

   a. Position descriptions and performance appraisals evaluate family-centered practice. ☐ ☐

7. The FCMC philosophy includes a commitment to the following components:

   a. Providing the information and education needed for informed childbirth, early parenting, and decision making. ☐ ☐

   b. Continuity of care. ☐ ☐

   c. Individualized care based on the uniqueness of each woman and her family. ☐ ☐

   d. Each woman defines her "family" and identifies her support person(s). ☐ ☐

   e. Involving the woman and her family in assessing her and their needs. ☐ ☐

   f. Involving the woman and her family in program planning, implementation, and evaluation.

   g. Flexibility in providing birth choices and preferences. ☐ ☐

   h. Early and frequent contact between family members and their newborn. ☐ ☐

   i. Recognizing childbearing as a normal, natural process rather than a risk or an illness requiring medical intervention. ☐ ☐

   j. Recognizing childbearing as a normal life cycle event and developmental opportunity and a transition to parenting. ☐ ☐

   k. Recognizing the psychosocial, cultural, spiritual, economic, and educational needs of the woman and her family as well as their physical needs. ☐ ☐

8. A hospital committee exists to develop, implement, maintain, and evaluate family-centered maternity care in the hospital and the antepartal clinic. ☐ ☐

   a. The committee's composition is multidisciplinary, including representation of ancillary services that routinely interact with Maternity. ☐ ☐

   b. There are at least two consumer members on this committee. ☐ ☐

   c. At least every two years, the committee conducts a community survey to determine consumer preferences and feedback regarding maternity services. ☐ ☐

   d. The results of the community survey form one basis for committee recommendations for appropriate hospital, medical, and nursing administrators and committees. ☐ ☐

	Yes	**No**

e. The committee is responsible for consumer satisfaction questionnaires specific to maternity and newborn care.. ☐ ☐

    1) The committee annually reviews and revises the questionnaires as needed. .... ☐ ☐

    2) The committee reviews the questionnaire results quarterly. .... ☐ ☐

    3) The results of the consumer satisfaction questionnaires form one basis for committee recommendations for appropriate hospital, medical, and nursing administrators and committees.. ☐ ☐

    4) The hospital provides support services for the committee for:

        a) Reviewing responses.. ☐ ☐

        b) Secretarial services... ☐ ☐

        c) Written responses to consumer comments, compliments, or complaints. .... ☐ ☐

f. The committee is responsible for planning and implementing an annual continuing education conference on FCMC. .... ☐ ☐

g. The committee collaborates with the Family Advisory Council on quality improvement initiatives.. ☐ ☐

9. A Family Advisory Council exists to participate in designing, evaluating, and interpreting quality improvement initiatives. .... ☐ ☐

10. The FCMC philosophy is printed, framed, and displayed:

    a. On the Maternity Unit. .... ☐ ☐

    b. In the antepartal clinic. .... ☐ ☐

11. The FCMC philosophy is printed and distributed to all childbearing women on admission to the maternity service:

    a. In the hospital. .... ☐ ☐

    b. In the antepartal clinic. .... ☐ ☐

12. All staff introduce themselves to women, family members, and other support person(s) in all interactions.. ☐ ☐

13. There is evidence that values embodied in the mission and philosophy statements are lived throughout the organization and reflected in communication, treatment of employees, and decision making.. ☐ ☐

    a. Staff morale is high. .... ☐ ☐

    b. Staff attitudes are positive and reflect trust and respect for administration............................. ☐ ☐

    c. Staff demonstrates loyalty to the hospital .... ☐ ☐

ACCESS AND COMMUNICATION—CONTACT PRIOR TO ADMISSION

1. There is a designated hospital phone number for information regarding maternity services.......... ☐ ☐

2. The person answering this phone number has a warm phone manner, is courteous, and communicates interest and a desire to be helpful... ☐ ☐

3. The person answering this phone number is able to provide the following information and services as requested:

    a. Answer questions about the specific provisions for family-centered maternity care in the hospital... ☐ ☐

		Yes	No

b. Give the time, meeting place, contact person, and phone number for Maternity Unit tours .... ☐ ☐

c. Give the time, meeting place, contact person, and phone number for hospital-provided childbirth education classes. .... ☐ ☐

d. Send a list of the names and phone numbers of all childbirth educators in the catchment area. ☐ ☐

e. Give the hours and phone number of the outpatient antepartal clinic, if applicable. .... ☐ ☐

f. Send a list of names and phone numbers of all physicians and certified nurse-midwives with obstetrical practice privileges in the hospital. .... ☐ ☐

g. Answer questions about the cost and methods of payment for various aspects of hospitalization. .... ☐ ☐

h. Send preadmission forms. .... ☐ ☐

i. Answer questions about admission and visitor parking. .... ☐ ☐

j. Answer questions about what to bring to the hospital when admitted. .... ☐ ☐

k. Give directions to the Maternity Unit, outpatient antepartal clinic, ultrasonography, laboratories, and other relevant specialized areas. .... ☐ ☐

4. The hospital provides, at a minimum, the following preadmission maternity education classes:

   a. Orientation to the Maternity Unit, which includes: .... ☐ ☐

      1) Orientation to family-centered maternity care. .... ☐ ☐

      2) Giving each woman and her family a copy of the hospital's written FCMC philosophy. . ☐ ☐

      3) Giving each woman a reading list of recommended books and Internet sites on pregnancy, childbirth preparation, and parenting. .... ☐ ☐

      4) Discussion of available options for labor and birth. .... ☐ ☐

      5) Giving each woman and her family access to a copy of the hospital's policies and procedures as they pertain to the Maternity Unit. .... ☐ ☐

      6) A tour of the Maternity Unit. .... ☐ ☐

      7) Giving each woman and her family a list of the names and phone numbers of the Maternity nursing supervisors and head nurses, the medical chief of the obstetrical department, and the hospital's chief executive officer. .... ☐ ☐

   b. Maternity Unit orientation and tour for siblings. .... ☐ ☐

   c. Childbirth education individual sessions or group classes for hospitalized women with antepartal complications. .... ☐ ☐

5. The hospital provides the following classes as needed:

   a. Preconceptional. .... ☐ ☐

   b. Early pregnancy. .... ☐ ☐

   c. Cesarean birth. .... ☐ ☐

   d. Vaginal birth after Cesarean. .... ☐ ☐

   e. Preparation for birth:

      1) Focusing primarily on uncomplicated vaginal birth, emphasizing self-help strategies and support from others. .... ☐ ☐

      2) Including information about epidurals in areas where epidural anesthesia is an option.... ☐ ☐

   f. Sibling preparation. .... ☐ ☐

	Yes	No

g. Parenting and the transition to parenthood... ☐ ☐

h. Prenatal and postnatal exercises. .... ☐ ☐

i. Nutrition, emphasizing the importance of folic acid.................................. ☐ ☐

j. Breastfeeding. .... ☐ ☐

k. Grandparenting. .... ☐ ☐

l. Adolescent pregnancy.. ☐ ☐

6. To all who request it, the hospital provides a list of the names and phone numbers of all community educators providing the classes listed in #5 above. .... ☐ ☐

7. Women are encouraged to identify their preferences for their birth experiences and those of their families and support person(s) and to develop a written birth plan........................... ☐ ☐

8. Birth classes inform families orally and in writing of the risks, benefits, and alternatives to epidural anesthesia in an unbiased manner with evidence-based information. .... ☐ ☐

9. All classes emphasize informed consent and parent participation in decision making. .... ☐ ☐

10. All classes emphasize healthy behaviors and lifestyles. .... ☐ ☐

PARTNERSHIP BETWEEN PATIENT, FAMILY, AND CARE PROVIDERS—CHILDBIRTH AND PARENTING EDUCATION

1. Class schedules, a contact person and their phone number, and meeting places and times are publicized in catchment area newspapers, community calendars, radio and television public service announcements, and service advertisements. .... ☐ ☐

2. Class size enables the following optimal learning situations:

   a. Individualized attention and monitoring of exercises. .... ☐ ☐

   b. Time to respond to everyone's questions within the established timeframe. .... ☐ ☐

   c. Everyone can see and handle teaching aids. .... ☐ ☐

   d. Comfortable personal space, which is not cramped.................................. ☐ ☐

3. There are a sufficient number of class series and/or childbirth educators to enable the optimal class situation specified in #2 above. .... ☐ ☐

4. Childbirth educators are qualified, as determined by successfully completing a course or certification given by a recognized independent agency (e.g., ASPO/LAMAZE, ICEA, or Bradley); or by successfully completing a course or module in professional nursing, nurse-midwifery, or medical education. .... ☐ ☐

5. Statistics are kept on the number of class series offered and how many people attend each series. ... ☐ ☐

6. Written childbirth education goals reflect the hospital's FCMC philosophy. .... ☐ ☐

7. There are written objectives and an outline for each class. .... ☐ ☐

8. The objectives and outline for each class reflect the following:

   a. Written goals for the hospital's childbirth education program.......................... ☐ ☐

   b. The principles of adult learning. .... ☐ ☐

   c. Engagement of the learner in their learning process..................................... ☐ ☐

   d. A variety of teaching techniques and strategies. .... ☐ ☐

   e. Use of a variety of teaching tools.. ☐ ☐

	Yes	No

f. Division of the class into two parts:

   1) Information sharing, group process, and theoretical content. .... ☐ ☐

   2) Self-help tools and exercises. .... ☐ ☐

g. An emphasis on self-empowerment. .... ☐ ☐

9. The content of the classes includes the following:

a. Physiological processes of childbearing throughout the maternity cycle. .... ☐ ☐

b. Physical adjustments throughout the maternity cycle, including:

   1) Personal hygiene. .... ☐ ☐

   2) Sexual. .... ☐ ☐

   3) Discomforts and comfort measures. .... ☐ ☐

c. Psychosocial adjustments throughout the maternity cycle for:

   1) Mother. .... ☐ ☐

   2) Family members. .... ☐ ☐

d. Basic reproductive anatomy. .... ☐ ☐

e. Nutrition during pregnancy and lactation. .... ☐ ☐

f. Effects of smoking, alcohol, and drugs. .... ☐ ☐

g. Participatory decision-making skills. .... ☐ ☐

h. Options and choices in childbirth. .... ☐ ☐

i. Possible medical and nursing interventions, rationale, and technology used for:

   1) Mother. .... ☐ ☐

   2) Newborn. .... ☐ ☐

j. The principles of informed consent and family-centered maternity care. .... ☐ ☐

k. Cesarean birth. .... ☐ ☐

l. Self-help tools and coping techniques. .... ☐ ☐

m. Pain control using body conditioning, relaxation, positioning, and breathing exercises as well as medication (IV/PO) and regional analgesia and anesthesia. .... ☐ ☐

n. Characteristics of the normal newborn. .... ☐ ☐

o. Newborn care, safety, and feeding. .... ☐ ☐

p. Family planning. .... ☐ ☐

q. Parenting. .... ☐ ☐

r. Breastfeeding. .... ☐ ☐

s. Bonding and attachment. .... ☐ ☐

t. The value of mother–baby nursing. .... ☐ ☐

u. Infant security. .... ☐ ☐

10. Written evaluations of each class series are obtained from the participants, reviewed, and used as the basis for change. .... ☐ ☐

11. Class series are held at times and locations convenient to women and their families. .... ☐ ☐

ANTEPARTAL CARE

	Yes	No

Education and Communication

1. Childbirth education classes are provided as part of the antepartal plan of care............................ ☐ ☐

2. Printed instructional materials are available and are appropriate for the population served:

   a. In English.. ☐ ☐

   b. In languages other than English if there are non–English-speaking populations. .... ☐ ☐

3. Audiotapes and/or audiovisual materials are available and are appropriate for the population served:

   a. In English.. ☐ ☐

   b. In languages other than English if there are non–English-speaking populations. .... ☐ ☐

4. Informational posters are displayed on the walls and are appropriate for the population served:

   a. In English.. ☐ ☐

   b. In languages other than English if there are non–English-speaking populations. .... ☐ ☐

5. A recommended list of books, videos, CDs, and Internet sites on pregnancy, childbirth preparation, and parenting books is given to each woman. .... ☐ ☐

6. A lending library of pregnancy, childbirth, and parenting books is available in the Antepartal Clinic and is appropriate for the population served:

   a. In English.. ☐ ☐

   b. In languages other than English if there are non–English-speaking populations. .... ☐ ☐

7. Each woman is given a list of community resources for childbirth education, support groups, parenting, breastfeeding, and child care with the name and phone number of a contact person for each resource. .... ☐ ☐

8. Translation services are available if there are non–English-speaking populations......................... ☐ ☐

9. Interpreters are available for hearing-impaired women. .... ☐ ☐

10. The person answering the phone and scheduling appointments has a warm phone manner, is courteous, and communicates interest and a desire to be helpful. .... ☐ ☐

11. A record of information and education given during appointments is included as part of the medical record. .... ☐ ☐

12. Each woman and her family is informed of available birth options:

   a. An explanation of each option is given... ☐ ☐

   b. The woman's birth preferences and plan, including method of infant feeding, becomes part of her medical record, which is available to the in-hospital Maternity Unit upon admission. ...... ☐ ☐

13. Each woman and her family receives information about breastfeeding and its value so she can make an informed decision early in pregnancy.. ☐ ☐

Care Practices

1. The initial appointment is scheduled within one week of initial contact....................................... ☐ ☐

2. The woman is encouraged to bring family members with her to her appointments by:

   a. The person scheduling the appointment... ☐ ☐

   b. Nursing staff. .... ☐ ☐

   c. The primary care provider.. ☐ ☐

	Yes	No

3. The woman first meets her primary care provider at each visit while still dressed. .... ☐ ☐

4. Family members and care providers are all introduced to each other upon meeting. .... ☐ ☐

5. Prior to implementing or administering examinations, procedures, treatments, or medications:

    a. Explanations are routinely given. .... ☐ ☐

    b. Patient consent is obtained. .... ☐ ☐

6. In addition to assessing and evaluating the physical well-being of mother and baby, each visit includes the following:

    a. Opportunity to express concerns. .... ☐ ☐

    b. Opportunity to ask questions. .... ☐ ☐

    c. Anticipatory guidance:

        1) Appropriate to physical findings and gestational age. .... ☐ ☐

        2) Emphasizing health promotion. .... ☐ ☐

        3) Emphasizing self-care and self-help. .... ☐ ☐

    d. Information and education appropriate to gestational age regarding:

        1) Fetal growth and development. .... ☐ ☐

        2) Maternal physiological changes. .... ☐ ☐

        3) Personal hygiene. .... ☐ ☐

        4) Discomforts and comfort measures. .... ☐ ☐

    e. Assessment and evaluation of:

        1) Maternal psychological and psychosexual well being. .... ☐ ☐

        2) Family functioning. .... ☐ ☐

        3) Family reactions, responses, and questions. .... ☐ ☐

        4) Socioeconomic factors requiring referrals. .... ☐ ☐

7. The woman and her family members are encouraged to participate in the conduct of the visit. ...... ☐ ☐

8. A woman's birth preferences and plan, including method of infant feeding, is developed and recorded during her pregnancy in collaboration with those whom she wishes to involve. .... ☐ ☐

9. Each woman is given a list of the names and phone numbers of:

    a. The Antepartal Clinic nursing supervisor and head nurse, medical chief, and executive officer. .... ☐ ☐

    b. Places she can call any hour of the day or night with questions, for information, in the event of an emergency, or when she thinks she is in labor. .... ☐ ☐

10. The appointment system is flexible and accommodates working women and family members. ...... ☐ ☐

11. The woman's chart is accessible to her for reading. .... ☐ ☐

12. Prenatal care is coordinated with and referrals made to community services and programs as appropriate. .... ☐ ☐

Environment and Design

1. Walls are clean and attractive. .... ☐ ☐

2. Rooms and furnishings are clean. .... ☐ ☐

	Yes	No

3. There is a play area for children. .... ☐ ☐

4. Picture books, audiovisuals, and toys designed for helping children understand pregnancy, fetal development, birth, and sibling relationships are available. .... ☐ ☐

5. The Antepartal Clinic is well lit. .... ☐ ☐

6. There are windows in the:

   a. Common areas. .... ☐ ☐

   b. Examining rooms. .... ☐ ☐

7. Seating is comfortable:

   a. The chairs are comfortable. .... ☐ ☐

   b. There is sufficient personal space. .... ☐ ☐

8. Nourishing snacks are available in the area. .... ☐ ☐

9. There is sufficient space to accommodate support person(s) and children in the:

   a. Waiting room. .... ☐ ☐

   b. Examining rooms. .... ☐ ☐

   c. Consultation rooms. .... ☐ ☐

10. Space meets practice and family needs and supports nonseparation. .... ☐ ☐

IN-HOSPITAL

Education and Communication

1. Signs directing women and their families and visitors to the maternity area are clearly placed, easy to read, and in the language(s) of the population served. .... ☐ ☐

2. There is a sign at the entrance to the Maternity Unit that specifically welcomes family members and support persons. .... ☐ ☐

3. Signs within the maternity area are worded to reflect the hospital's FCMC philosophy. .... ☐ ☐

4. Translation services are available if there are non–English-speaking populations. .... ☐ ☐

5. Interpreters are available for hearing-impaired women. .... ☐ ☐

6. The person(s) answering the phone(s) has a warm phone manner, is courteous, and communicates interest and a desire to be helpful. .... ☐ ☐

7. Printed instructional materials are available and routinely distributed as needed to all women and are appropriate for the population served:

   a. In English. .... ☐ ☐

   b. In languages other than English if there are non–English-speaking populations .... ☐ ☐

   which supplement individual and group teaching on:

   a. Hospital practices and policies. .... ☐ ☐

   b. The process and progress of labor. .... ☐ ☐

   c. Labor and delivery options, risks, and benefits. .... ☐ ☐

   d. Adjusting the birthing and postpartum bed to various positions for comfort as well as physiologic positioning. .... ☐ ☐

		Yes	No
e.	Self-help tools and coping techniques during labor.	☐	☐
f.	Postpartum self-care:		
	1) In hospital.	☐	☐
	2) At home.	☐	☐
g.	Infant care:		
	1) In hospital.	☐	☐
	2) At home.	☐	☐
h.	Breastfeeding.	☐	☐
i.	Bottle feeding.	☐	☐
j.	Infant behavior and cues.	☐	☐
k.	Circumcision.	☐	☐
l.	Personal adaptations and adjustments during the postpartum period.	☐	☐
m.	Family adaptations and adjustments during the postpartum period.	☐	☐
n.	Early parenting.	☐	☐
o.	Family planning and fertility awareness.	☐	☐

8. The following teaching methods are available for use during the maternity stay:

		Yes	No
a.	Individual one-to-one instruction.	☐	☐
b.	Group instruction.	☐	☐
c.	Return demonstration.	☐	☐
d.	Routine nursing care activities are used as opportunities to teach.	☐	☐

9. Teaching includes:

		Yes	No
a.	Hospital practices and policies.	☐	☐
b.	The process and progress of labor.	☐	☐
c.	Delivery options.	☐	☐
d.	Adjusting the birthing and postpartum bed to various positions for comfort.	☐	☐
e.	Self-help tools and coping techniques during labor.	☐	☐
f.	Postpartum self-care:		
	1) In hospital.	☐	☐
	2) At home.	☐	☐
g.	Infant care:		
	1) In hospital.	☐	☐
	2) At home.	☐	☐
h.	Breastfeeding.	☐	☐
i.	Bottle feeding.	☐	☐
j.	Infant behavior and cues.	☐	☐
k.	Circumcision.	☐	☐

	Yes	No

l.   Personal adaptations and adjustments during the postpartum period. .... ☐ ☐

m. Family adaptations and adjustments during the postpartum period......................... ☐ ☐

n.   Early parenting. .... ☐ ☐

o.   Family planning and fertility awareness. .... ☐ ☐

10. Audiotapes and/or audiovisual materials are available and appropriate to the population served:

    a.   In English.. ☐ ☐

    b.   In languages other than English if there are non–English-speaking populations. .... ☐ ☐

11. A lending library is available with postpartum, infant care, and parenting books that are appropriate to the population served:

    a.   In English.. ☐ ☐

    b.   In languages other than English if there are non–English-speaking populations. .... ☐ ☐

12. Up-to-date professional references are available on the unit, including:

    a.   Textbooks:

        1) Midwifery. .... ☐ ☐

        2) Nursing .... ☐ ☐

        3) Medical. .... ☐ ☐

    b.   Journals:

        1) Midwifery. .... ☐ ☐

        2) Nursing .... ☐ ☐

        3) Medical. .... ☐ ☐

    c.   Professional standards and guidelines for maternity care (AAP, ACNM, ACOG, ANA, JCAH, AWHONN). .... ☐ ☐

13. Documentation of information and education given during the hospital stay is included as part of the permanent medical record... ☐ ☐

14. Support persons are oriented to:

    a.   The Maternity Unit.. ☐ ☐

    b.   The location of the bathroom. .... ☐ ☐

    c.   The location of nourishment.. ☐ ☐

    d.   Ways they can help the mother.. ☐ ☐

Antepartal and Intrapartal Care Practices

1.   Personnel provide the following continuity of care:

    a.   Admitting, labor, delivery, recovery, postpartum, and newborn personnel are the same......... ☐ ☐

    b.   Admitting, labor, delivery, and recovery personnel are the same................................. ☐ ☐

    c.   Admitting, labor, and delivery personnel are the same... ☐ ☐

    d.   Labor and delivery personnel are the same... ☐ ☐

    e.   Postpartum and newborn personnel are the same. .... ☐ ☐

		Yes	No
f.	A single nurse cares for both mother and baby wherever they are during:		
	1) Day shift.	☐	☐
	2) Evening shift.	☐	☐
	3) Night shift.	☐	☐
g.	Family and community paraprofessionals (doulas) are available to support women during labor and birth.	☐	☐
2.	A woman is admitted directly to the Maternity Unit.	☐	☐
3.	A birthing woman's support person does not have to leave her to complete admission procedures in the Business or Admitting Office.	☐	☐
4.	Privacy is provided for families to answer questions during the admission process.	☐	☐
5.	The woman and her family's preferences for the birth experience are reviewed or ascertained during the admitting process.	☐	☐
6.	The woman's birth plan is shared and respected by:		
a.	Antepartal staff.	☐	☐
b.	Labor and delivery staff.	☐	☐
c.	Physicians.	☐	☐
d.	Postpartum staff.	☐	☐
7.	Prior to implementing or administering examinations, procedures, treatments, or medications:		
a.	Explanations are routinely given.	☐	☐
b.	Patient consent is obtained.	☐	☐
8.	Maternity policies and procedures.		
a.	Reflect the hospital's written FCMC philosophy.	☐	☐
b.	Are consumer sensitive in their language.	☐	☐
c.	Do not use words such as "permit" or "allow."	☐	☐
9.	The use of LDRs or LDRPs is routine.	☐	☐

Intrapartum Care Practices

		Yes	No
1.	The woman's support person(s) are encouraged to be present:		
a.	During procedures.	☐	☐
b.	During a birth.	☐	☐
	regardless of:		
a.	The pregnancy's risk status.	☐	☐
b.	The mode of delivery.	☐	☐
c.	Prior attendance at a preparatory class.	☐	☐
2.	Nourishment is available for support persons during labor.	☐	☐
3.	Labor and birth staff and primary care professionals provide support and manage labor to minimize the technologic and pathologic aspects of pregnancy in low-risk situations:		
a.	According to normal physiological principles.	☐	☐
b.	Without unnecessary interference.	☐	☐

	Yes	No
c. With attention to psychosocial needs.	☐	☐
d. While encouraging self-help.	☐	☐
e. While encouraging questions and self-knowledge.	☐	☐
f. Maintaining a sustaining human presence (possibly a doula).	☐	☐
g. With acceptance of attitudes and behavior.	☐	☐
h. With adaptations for cultural variations.	☐	☐

4. The woman and her support person(s) are assisted in the specific relaxation and breathing techniques they have learned and are encouraged to use them. .... ☐ ☐

5. Women without any childbirth education are:

	Yes	No
a. Taught self-help measures as needed.	☐	☐
b. Given appropriate explanations of labor process and progress.	☐	☐
c. Assisted by their support person(s) who are:		
1) Taught helping measures.	☐	☐
2) Involved in the woman's care.	☐	☐

6. The following procedures are not done "routinely":

	Yes	No
a. Perineal shave or mini-prep.	☐	☐
b. Enema.	☐	☐
c. Intravenous infusion.	☐	☐
d. Amniotomy.	☐	☐
e. Hourly or every other hour vaginal examinations.	☐	☐
f. Continuous electronic fetal monitoring:		
1) External.	☐	☐
2) Internal.	☐	☐
g. IV or PO analgesia.	☐	☐
h. Epidural anesthesia or analgesia.	☐	☐
i. Saddle blocks or spinal anesthesia.	☐	☐
j. Pitocin augmentation.	☐	☐
k. Episiotomy.	☐	☐
l. Lithotomy position or stirrups for delivery.	☐	☐

7. Women with normal pregnancies in normal labor are encouraged to:

	Yes	No
a. Change positions often.	☐	☐
b. Ambulate.	☐	☐
c. Bathe (shower, tub, Jacuzzi).	☐	☐
d. Drink fluids.	☐	☐
e. Use birthing balls.	☐	☐

	Yes	No

8. Structured intermittent monitoring is used to assure fetal well-being:

    a. Maternal mobility. ☐ ☐

    b. Improved comfort. ☐ ☐

9. Siblings are welcome:

    a. As determined by the parents. ☐ ☐

    b. Without age restriction. ☐ ☐

    c. If they have been prepared and been given a tour. ☐ ☐

    d. If they are accompanied by a responsible adult other than the woman's primary support person. ☐ ☐

and are welcome to be present during:

    a. Labor. ☐ ☐

    b. Birth. ☐ ☐

    c. Recovery. ☐ ☐

    d. Postpartum. ☐ ☐

10. There are no arbitrary restrictions on the number of family members and/or support people who may be present for a birth. ☐ ☐

11. The following options are available at the time of birth:

    a. Position of the woman's choice.

        1) Lateral Simms. ☐ ☐

        2) Squatting. ☐ ☐

    b. Dimming of lights. ☐ ☐

    c. Music of the woman and her partner's choice. ☐ ☐

    d. Intermittent monitoring. ☐ ☐

    e. Ironing and massage of the perineum. ☐ ☐

    f. Audiotaping, video recording, and photographing. ☐ ☐

    g. Skin-to-skin contact with baby upon delivery. ☐ ☐

    h. Delay of ophthalmic eye ointment or drops. ☐ ☐

    i. Eye prophylaxis other than silver nitrate. ☐ ☐

12. Women having a Cesarean birth are routinely given the option of conduction anesthesia in order to be awake for the delivery. ☐ ☐

Postpartum Care Practices

1. There is no separation of the baby from the mother unless medically indicated or desired by the mother:

    a. After vaginal birth. ☐ ☐

    b. After Cesarean birth. ☐ ☐

2. Women having Cesarean birth may see and touch and hold their babies immediately after birth if warranted by the physical condition of both mother and baby. ☐ ☐

	Yes	No

3. Family members and support persons are not separated from mother and baby during the recovery period:

   a. After vaginal birth. .... ☐ ☐

   b. After Cesarean birth. .... ☐ ☐

4. Breastfeeding mothers are encouraged to initiate breastfeeding immediately after birth if warranted by the physical condition of both mother and baby:

   a. After vaginal birth. .... ☐ ☐

   b. After Cesarean birth. .... ☐ ☐

5. Assistance with feeding is routinely provided to those who are:

   a. Breastfeeding. .... ☐ ☐

   b. Bottle feeding. .... ☐ ☐

6. Breastfeeding babies are not fed:

   a. Glucose water. .... ☐ ☐

   b. Formula. .... ☐ ☐

7. Breastfeeding mothers are not given formula gift packs.......................... ☐ ☐

8. Routine procedures on the baby are done in full view of the mother or while the baby is in her arms, including:

   a. Weighing. .... ☐ ☐

   b. Foot printing. .... ☐ ☐

   c. Banding. .... ☐ ☐

   d. Physical examination. .... ☐ ☐

   e. Gestational age assessment. .... ☐ ☐

   f. Instillation of eye prophylaxis. .... ☐ ☐

   g. Injections. .... ☐ ☐

9. Mother–baby nursing practice is the standard of care, including:

   a. Nonseparation of mother and baby... ☐ ☐

   b. Infant teaching and examination at the mother's bedside by:

      1) The nurse. .... ☐ ☐

      2) The physician. .... ☐ ☐

10. Parents, appropriately identified and attired, may enter the normal newborn nursery to move their baby to the mother's room... ☐ ☐

11. The mother is assessed prior to discharge for:

   a. Necessary infant care skills. .... ☐ ☐

   b. Satisfactory initiation of breastfeeding, if applicable........................ ☐ ☐

12. Referral to appropriate support groups is given for:

   a. Breastfeeding. .... ☐ ☐

   b. Cesarean birth. .... ☐ ☐

   c. Parenting. .... ☐ ☐

	Yes	No

13. Postpartum support options include:

    a. Follow-up phone calls. .... ☐ ☐

    b. Home visiting. .... ☐ ☐

    c. After birth classes. .... ☐ ☐

    d. Mother–baby return visits.. ☐ ☐

    e. Postpartum support groups. .... ☐ ☐

14. Referrals are made to appropriate community agencies as needed........................ ☐ ☐

15. The mother's chart is accessible to her for reading... ☐ ☐

16. The infant's chart is accessible to the mother for reading.................................. ☐ ☐

17. A screening tool, which is:

    a. Written. .... ☐ ☐

    b. Culturally sensitive. .... ☐ ☐

    is used by the nursing staff to individually assess:

    a. Mother–infant interaction and bonding.. ☐ ☐

    b. Family relationships. .... ☐ ☐

    c. Maternal self-care skills. .... ☐ ☐

    d. Infant care skills. .... ☐ ☐

18. Visiting hours facilitate FCMC.. ☐ ☐

19. If the baby is in the Newborn Intensive Care Unit:

    a. Techniques are used to personalize the baby.................................. ☐ ☐

    b. Parents are encouraged to visit at any time.................................... ☐ ☐

    c. Siblings and grandparents are encouraged to visit.......................... ☐ ☐

    d. Parents are encouraged to participate in:

        1) Their infant's daily care. .... ☐ ☐

        2) Decision making regarding their child's care. .... ☐ ☐

    e. The professionals giving care to the baby provide continuity. .... ☐ ☐

    f. Mothers are assisted in obtaining, storing, delivering, and feeding their breast milk. .... ☐ ☐

    g. Mothers are encouraged to verbalize their fears, guilt, doubts, grief, and learning needs. .... ☐ ☐

    h. The woman and her family are referred to support groups....................... ☐ ☐

    i. The woman and her family are offered social services............................. ☐ ☐

    j. Assistance is given in locating affordable overnight accommodations when parents are coming from a distance. .... ☐ ☐

    k. Prior to discharge:

        1) A home assessment is done, if needed. .... ☐ ☐

        2) In-hospital "nesting rooms" and teaching are made available for learning necessary caretaking skills.................................... ☐ ☐

        3) Parents are comfortable with necessary caretaking skills............... ☐ ☐

	Yes	No

20. If the baby is transferred to another hospital:

    a. The mother and her partner are encouraged to see and touch the baby before being separated. ... ☐ ☐

    b. A family member is encouraged to accompany the infant, if possible. ☐ ☐

    c. A picture is taken of the infant before transfer and given to the mother and her partner. ☐ ☐

    d. The mother and her family are given a phone number at the transfer hospital that will connect them with information, support, and education. ☐ ☐

21. Women who relinquish their babies are:

    a. Encouraged to see and hold their baby. ☐ ☐

    b. Assisted with their plans:

        1) For the baby. ☐ ☐

        2) For themselves. ☐ ☐

    c. Assisted in their grief process. ☐ ☐

22. If the baby is stillborn or dies while in the hospital:

    a. Opportunity is provided for: ☐ ☐

        1) Privacy for the woman and her family to:

            a) Hold their baby while he or she dies. ☐ ☐

            b) Grieve. ☐ ☐

        2) Seeing, holding, and touching their baby. ☐ ☐

        3) Taking pictures of their baby. ☐ ☐

        4) Having their baby's identification items and other keepsakes and mementos. ☐ ☐

        5) Explanations of their baby's birth and death. ☐ ☐

        6) The mother and father or support person to be together day and night, as desired. ☐ ☐

    b. The woman is given her choice of remaining on the Maternity Unit or being moved to another unit. ☐ ☐

    c. Help is provided regarding:

        1) Naming their baby. ☐ ☐

        2) Baptism or other religious rite. ☐ ☐

        3) Autopsy. ☐ ☐

        4) Cremation or burial. ☐ ☐

        5) Funeral or memorial service. ☐ ☐

        6) Grief process. ☐ ☐

    d. Referral to grief support groups is offered to the woman and her family. ☐ ☐

    e. Autopsy permits and cremation forms are worded sensitively. ☐ ☐

23. Annual statistics are kept as shown in the Appendix A. ☐ ☐

Environment and Design

		Yes	No
1.	There is adequate and safe parking.	☐	☐
2.	The architecture and interior design create a supporting, welcoming atmosphere for families.	☐	☐
3.	Walls are clean and attractive.	☐	☐
4.	Women can be checked for diagnosis of labor or evaluation of pregnancy problems without being formally admitted to the hospital.	☐	☐

5. There is an early labor lounge, which has:

		Yes	No
a.	A television.	☐	☐
b.	A radio.	☐	☐
c.	A stereo with tape deck.	☐	☐
d.	Windows.	☐	☐
e.	Pleasant décor.	☐	☐
f.	Comfortable furnishings.	☐	☐
g.	A telephone.	☐	☐
h.	Reading material	☐	☐
i.	Games.	☐	☐
j.	A mini-kitchen for nourishing snacks.	☐	☐

		Yes	No
6.	There is a children's play area.	☐	☐
7.	Space is provided for family members, including siblings, and support persons to have relaxation breaks away from the laboring woman.	☐	☐

8. The following room(s):

   a. LDR.

   b. LDRP.

   c. Private postpartum.

   have: (Write number of room[s] in Yes or No column.)

		Yes	No
a.	A door to knock on for permission to enter.	☐	☐
b.	A private toilet.	☐	☐
c.	A private shower or bath.	☐	☐
d.	Sufficient space to accommodate:		
	1) Family and support person(s).	☐	☐
	2) Comfortable furnishings.	☐	☐
	3) Personal possessions.	☐	☐
	4) An infant crib and supplies.	☐	☐
	5) A sofa that makes into a bed for overnights.	☐	☐
	6) Equipment and professional personnel, as needed.	☐	☐
e.	A portable mirror.	☐	☐
f.	An outside mirror.	☐	☐
g.	A telephone.	☐	☐

	Yes	No

h. Individual control of the amount of light in the room. .... ☐ ☐

i. Attractive décor that deemphasizes the hospital environment. .... ☐ ☐

j. Equipment and supplies for obstetrical or medical emergencies:

    1) Stored out of sight. .... ☐ ☐

    2) Readily accessible. .... ☐ ☐

9. Rooms and furnishings are clean. .... ☐ ☐

10. The number of LDR rooms is adequate to serve all women with vaginal births. .... ☐ ☐

11. All women have a private room in which to labor and birth. .... ☐ ☐

12. The temperature of all patient care rooms can be individually adjusted. .... ☐ ☐

13. Space is provided on the Maternity Unit for group infant care and parenting classes. .... ☐ ☐

14. Space is provided for families to eat together during the postpartum stay. .... ☐ ☐

15. There is adequate education space for prenatal classes. .... ☐ ☐

16. There is a lactation center. .... ☐ ☐

17. There are private breastfeeding rooms for mothers of babies in the NICU. .... ☐ ☐

HOME FOLLOW-UP AND PARENTING SUPPORT—CONTACT AFTER DISCHARGE

1. The mother is given the telephone numbers of her and her baby's primary care providers and/or a hospital number where they can call any hour of the day with self-care or infant-care questions or concerns. .... ☐ ☐

2. An RN from the Maternity Unit is assigned to make a follow-up phone call within one week of discharge. .... ☐ ☐

3. A written form documenting this phone call is included in the medical record. .... ☐ ☐

4. An RN from the Maternity Unit is assigned to make a home visit within 48 hours of discharge for those mothers and babies who are identified to be at risk. .... ☐ ☐

5. Doulas are available to provide postpartum support at home. .... ☐ ☐

6. A written form documenting this home visit is included in the medical record. .... ☐ ☐

7. The nurse makes referrals as indicated to the primary care providers. .... ☐ ☐

8. There is a written, planned, family-centered follow-up program for mothers whose:

    a. Baby died in the hospital or was stillborn. .... ☐ ☐

    b. Baby was in the Newborn Intensive Care Unit. .... ☐ ☐

    c. Baby was transferred to another hospital. .... ☐ ☐

    d. Baby was born with congenital anomalies. .... ☐ ☐

    e. In-hospital assessment revealed risk for maternal neglect or child abuse. .... ☐ ☐

9. The hospital's consumer satisfaction questionnaire specific to maternity care is mailed within 24 hours of the mother's discharge. .... ☐ ☐

10. The hospital's consumer satisfaction questionnaire specific to newborn care is mailed within 24 hours of the baby's discharge. .... ☐ ☐

ANNUAL STATISTICS

Approximate Percentage of All Deliveries That:

	0–10%	11–25%	26–40%	41–55%	56–70%	71–85%	86–100%
1. Were with women who took a childbirth education series.	___	___	___	___	___	___	___
2. Were Cesarean births.	___	___	___	___	___	___	___
3. Took place in a:							
a. LDR	___	___	___	___	___	___	___
b. LDRP	___	___	___	___	___	___	___
4. Were inductions.	___	___	___	___	___	___	___
5. Were women who experienced mother–baby nursing day and night.	___	___	___	___	___	___	___
6. Were women who breastfed.	___	___	___	___	___	___	___
7. Were women who did not use epidural analgesia.	___	___	___	___	___	___	___
8. Were of infants who were admitted to a Neonatal Intensive Care Unit (in this hospital or another hospital).							
a. For observation	___	___	___	___	___	___	___
b. For care greater than 48 hours in duration	___	___	___	___	___	___	___
9. Were of women who ambulated during labor.	___	___	___	___	___	___	___
10. Took place in the following positions:							
a. Lithotomy	___	___	___	___	___	___	___
b. Dorsal (no stirrups)	___	___	___	___	___	___	___
c. Lateral	___	___	___	___	___	___	___
d. Squatting	___	___	___	___	___	___	___
e. Knee–chest	___	___	___	___	___	___	___
f. Other	___	___	___	___	___	___	___

ANNUAL STATISTICS (continued)

Approximate Percent of All Deliveries That:

	0–10%	11–25%	26–40%	41–55%	56–70%	71–85%	86–100%
11. Were women who had:							
a. A perineal shave or mini-prep	___	___	___	___	___	___	___
b. An enema	___	___	___	___	___	___	___
c. An intravenous infusion	___	___	___	___	___	___	___
d. External continuous fetal monitoring	___	___	___	___	___	___	___
e. Internal continuous fetal monitoring	___	___	___	___	___	___	___
f. An episiotomy	___	___	___	___	___	___	___
g. Labor augmentation with Pitocin	___	___	___	___	___	___	___
12. Were women who had:							
a. Analgesia	___	___	___	___	___	___	___
b. Epidural anesthesia	___	___	___	___	___	___	___
c. Saddle blocks or spinal anesthesia	___	___	___	___	___	___	___
d. Pudendal or local anesthesia	___	___	___	___	___	___	___
13. Were attended by:							
a. A significant other support person(s)	___	___	___	___	___	___	___
b. Siblings	___	___	___	___	___	___	___

Competency-Based Skills Checklist for Mother–Baby Nursing

MOTHER–BABY UNIT

Please complete this checklist to demonstrate that you understand how a mother–baby unit functions.

Mother–Baby Unit Checklist

Performance Objective	Yes	No
1. Competency: Demonstrate understanding of hospital and unit functioning.		
Verbally summarize the unit mission and philosophy, identifying major points:		
• Unit standards of care for the postpartum mother, baby, and family..........................	☐	☐
Identify unit communication mechanisms:		
• Shift report...	☐	☐
• Unit CE announcements..	☐	☐
• In-house publications from various departments...	☐	☐
• Occurrence reports and incidence reports..	☐	☐
• Reporting broken and damaged equipment...	☐	☐
• Staff and department meetings...	☐	☐
• In-unit communications..	☐	☐
• Employee accident and injury report...	☐	☐
• Requisitions: lab, X-ray, etc.	☐	☐
• Unit and hospital computer functions..	☐	☐
Locate unit reference materials:		
• Disaster plan..	☐	☐
• Documentation (charting and forms manual)...	☐	☐

Completed

	Completed	
	Yes	**No**
• Equipment manual	☐	☐
• Emergency procedures/safety	☐	☐
• Hospital and unit policies and procedures manuals	☐	☐
• Infection control and isolation manual	☐	☐
• Laboratory manual	☐	☐
• Nursing diagnosis and care plans	☐	☐
• Planning references	☐	☐
• Nursing reference texts	☐	☐
• Physician Desk Reference and hospital formulary	☐	☐

Transport specimens for analysis according to procedure:

• Arterial blood gases and scalp pH samples	☐	☐
• Cord gases	☐	☐
• Sputum	☐	☐
• Stool	☐	☐
• Throat	☐	☐
• Urine		
• UA	☐	☐
• C & S	☐	☐
• Other	☐	☐

Locate unit rooms, equipment, and supplies, including:

• Emergency keys	☐	☐
• IV supplies	☐	☐
• IV pumps and PCA pumps	☐	☐
• CS supplies	☐	☐
• Linen	☐	☐
• Clean utility	☐	☐
• Equipment storage	☐	☐
• Kitchen and ice	☐	☐
• Soiled utility	☐	☐
• Lockers	☐	☐
• Lounge	☐	☐
• Restrooms for staff	☐	☐
• Waiting rooms for visitors	☐	☐
• Public restrooms	☐	☐

	Completed	
	Yes	**No**
• Items stored in various cupboards, etc.	☐	☐
• Stock meds	☐	☐
• Narcotics	☐	☐
• Sterile equipment and supplies	☐	☐
• Code cart	☐	☐
• Scales	☐	☐
• Thermometers	☐	☐
• Cleaning equipment	☐	☐

Demonstrate proper use of equipment and supplies in the patient's room:

	Yes	No
• Patient protective equipment (gloves, masks, goggles, etc.)	☐	☐
• Bed and room numbering	☐	☐
• Operation of bed	☐	☐
• Lights	☐	☐
• Telephone	☐	☐
• Television	☐	☐
• VCR	☐	☐
• Temperature control	☐	☐
• Call light, canceling, and intercom	☐	☐
• Bathroom call light	☐	☐
• Toilet and hopper	☐	☐
• Shower	☐	☐
• Tub	☐	☐
• Emergency alarm	☐	☐
• CPR masks	☐	☐
• Oxygen	☐	☐
• Suction	☐	☐
• Sharps disposal	☐	☐
• Other	☐	☐

Charge for items used, including:

	Yes	No
• General supplies	☐	☐
• IV therapy	☐	☐
• Medications	☐	☐
• Other	☐	☐

218

SELF-ASSESSMENT

Read through the performance objectives, and complete the first column ("Self-assess") using the following key:

3 = Can perform without review
* = Needs review
0 = Never done

Mother–Baby Nursing Self-Assessment

	Self-assess	Read P&P	Discuss and observe	Perform with assistance	Perform inde-pendently	No opportunity
2. Competency: Maintain a safe environment.						
Comply with unit safety policy.	___	___	___	___	___	___
Demonstrate principles of body mechanics in mobilizing patients and/or objects.	___	___	___	___	___	___
Practice electrical safety:						
• Verbally explain actions to take when equipment malfunctions or frayed electrical cords are found:	___	___	___	___	___	___
• Remove equipment from use.	___	___	___	___	___	___
• Label with the problem.	___	___	___	___	___	___
• Report to the appropriate department.	___	___	___	___	___	___
Explain actions to take when a patient's personal equipment is brought from home.	___	___	___	___	___	___
Incorporate principles of infection control into nursing practice, including:						
• Location of gloves, masks, gowns, and goggles on the unit.	___	___	___	___	___	___
• Universal precautions appropriate to each situation.	___	___	___	___	___	___
• Isolation techniques when indicated.	___	___	___	___	___	___
• Safe disposal of sharps.	___	___	___	___	___	___
3. Competency: Manage selected emergency situations.						
Locate fire equipment on the unit including alarm boxes, fire extinguishers, and fire hoses.	___	___	___	___	___	___
Verbally explain nursing responsibilities in the event of an actual, suspected, or practice fire.	___	___	___	___	___	___
Verbally explain nursing responsibilities in the event of an external disaster.	___	___	___	___	___	___
Verbally explain nursing responsibilities in the event of a power failure.	___	___	___	___	___	___
Be prepared for a cardiac or respiratory arrest in an adult and a newborn:						
• Locate emergency equipment on the unit:						
• Resuscitation masks	___	___	___	___	___	___
• Code carts	___	___	___	___	___	___
• Verbally explain the process for activating a Code Team response.	___	___	___	___	___	___

	Self-assess	Read P&P	Discuss and observe	Perform with assistance	Perform independently	No opportunity
• Verbally explain the procedure for initiating stat calls for a physician, respiratory therapy, anesthesia, and others as needed.	___	___	___	___	___	___
• Check emergency equipment and supplies; document the checks.	___	___	___	___	___	___
• Replace items from the code cart and unit stock meds.	___	___	___	___	___	___
• Explain hospital policy for no code status.	___	___	___	___	___	___

4. Competency: Demonstrate professional responsibility in the RN licensed nurse role.

	Self-assess	Read P&P	Discuss and observe	Perform with assistance	Perform independently	No opportunity
Comply with personnel policies for actions and appearance.	___	___	___	___	___	___
Delegate nursing activities appropriately.	___	___	___	___	___	___
Change behavior based on feedback regarding performance.	___	___	___	___	___	___
Evaluate achievement of orientation objectives.	___	___	___	___	___	___
Identify own learning needs.	___	___	___	___	___	___
Take responsibility for meeting own learning needs.	___	___	___	___	___	___
Document attendance at CE programs on own CE Record.	___	___	___	___	___	___
Maintain confidentiality when interacting with patients, families, personnel, and the public.	___	___	___	___	___	___

5. Competency: Organize nursing care for a group of patients.

	Self-assess	Read P&P	Discuss and observe	Perform with assistance	Perform independently	No opportunity
Establish priorities and rationales for patient care activities.	___	___	___	___	___	___
Revise patient care priorities as needed.	___	___	___	___	___	___
Adapt to unexpected events on the unit, such as patient admits and emergencies.	___	___	___	___	___	___
Complete assignments within allotted time frames.	___	___	___	___	___	___
Develop a mechanism for being organized in the delivery of patient care.	___	___	___	___	___	___

6. Competency: Communicate relevant patient information.

Regularly report changes in patient status in a timely fashion as appropriate to:

	Self-assess	Read P&P	Discuss and observe	Perform with assistance	Perform independently	No opportunity
• Physician or resident or nurse midwife	___	___	___	___	___	___
• Charge nurse	___	___	___	___	___	___
• Coworkers	___	___	___	___	___	___
• Other health team members	___	___	___	___	___	___

Document nursing care consistent with the charting system in use:

	Self-assess	Read P&P	Discuss and observe	Perform with assistance	Perform independently	No opportunity
• Admission assessment	___	___	___	___	___	___
• Special records (if applicable)	___	___	___	___	___	___
• Clinical record	___	___	___	___	___	___

	Self-assess	Read P&P	Discuss and observe	Perform with assistance	Perform inde- pendently	No opportunity
• Blood admin record	____	____	____	____	____	____
• Diabetic record	____	____	____	____	____	____
• PIH record	____	____	____	____	____	____
• Nutritional support form	____	____	____	____	____	____
• Medication record						
• Routine	____	____	____	____	____	____
• PRN, stat, one-time dose	____	____	____	____	____	____
• Nursing care plan and/or care path	____	____	____	____	____	____
• Nursing flowsheet and nurse's notes	____	____	____	____	____	____
• Parental fluid record	____	____	____	____	____	____
• Patient and family teaching record	____	____	____	____	____	____
• Referral forms	____	____	____	____	____	____
• Other	____	____	____	____	____	____
Receive physician's orders; communicate and document appropriately.	____	____	____	____	____	____
Orient patients and their families to the hospital environment.	____	____	____	____	____	____

7. **Competency: In collaboration with the mother, family, and healthcare team members, conduct an initial and ongoing assessment to gather data and implement appropriate plans of care for the new mother.**

Recognize antepartal and intrapartal events significant for the postpartum period:

	Self-assess	Read P&P	Discuss and observe	Perform with assistance	Perform inde- pendently	No opportunity
• Evaluate the maternal history.	____	____	____	____	____	____
• Recognize significant data and events from the maternal history.	____	____	____	____	____	____
• Implement nursing interventions that reflect history.	____	____	____	____	____	____

Screen for signs and symptoms of obstetrical and medical complications, including:

	Self-assess	Read P&P	Discuss and observe	Perform with assistance	Perform inde- pendently	No opportunity
• Puerperal infection, shock, sepsis	____	____	____	____	____	____
• Thrombophlebitis	____	____	____	____	____	____
• Pulmonary embolism	____	____	____	____	____	____
• Postpartum hemorrhage	____	____	____	____	____	____
• Pelvic hematoma	____	____	____	____	____	____
• Urinary tract infections	____	____	____	____	____	____
• Mastitis	____	____	____	____	____	____
• PIH	____	____	____	____	____	____
• Herpes	____	____	____	____	____	____

	Self-assess	Read P&P	Discuss and observe	Perform with assistance	Perform inde- pendently	No opportunity
• STDs	⎯	⎯	⎯	⎯	⎯	⎯
• Hepatitis	⎯	⎯	⎯	⎯	⎯	⎯
• HIV	⎯	⎯	⎯	⎯	⎯	⎯

Assess maternal physical status:

- Assess for physiologic changes resulting from childbirth

  - Uterine involution

	Self-assess	Read P&P	Discuss and observe	Perform with assistance	Perform inde- pendently	No opportunity
• Fundus height and position	⎯	⎯	⎯	⎯	⎯	⎯
• Firmness	⎯	⎯	⎯	⎯	⎯	⎯

  - Lochia

	Self-assess	Read P&P	Discuss and observe	Perform with assistance	Perform inde- pendently	No opportunity
• Type	⎯	⎯	⎯	⎯	⎯	⎯
• Amount	⎯	⎯	⎯	⎯	⎯	⎯
• Color	⎯	⎯	⎯	⎯	⎯	⎯
• Clots	⎯	⎯	⎯	⎯	⎯	⎯
• Bladder function	⎯	⎯	⎯	⎯	⎯	⎯
• Hematoma development and treatment	⎯	⎯	⎯	⎯	⎯	⎯
• Symptoms of infection or hemorrhage	⎯	⎯	⎯	⎯	⎯	⎯
• Postpartum anemia	⎯	⎯	⎯	⎯	⎯	⎯
• Hemorrhoid care	⎯	⎯	⎯	⎯	⎯	⎯
• Neurological assessment (DTRs, clonus)	⎯	⎯	⎯	⎯	⎯	⎯
• Homans' signs	⎯	⎯	⎯	⎯	⎯	⎯
• Calf circumference measurements	⎯	⎯	⎯	⎯	⎯	⎯

- Perform and instruct new mother concerning perineal care

  - Peri hygiene

	Self-assess	Read P&P	Discuss and observe	Perform with assistance	Perform inde- pendently	No opportunity
• Wash and wipe front to back	⎯	⎯	⎯	⎯	⎯	⎯
• Sprays, ointments, and compresses	⎯	⎯	⎯	⎯	⎯	⎯
• Sitz baths or whirlpool	⎯	⎯	⎯	⎯	⎯	⎯
• Hand washing	⎯	⎯	⎯	⎯	⎯	⎯
• Care of postpartum epidural patient	⎯	⎯	⎯	⎯	⎯	⎯
• Instruct patient about and assist with resumption of activity	⎯	⎯	⎯	⎯	⎯	⎯

- Assess nutrition and hydration status

	Self-assess	Read P&P	Discuss and observe	Perform with assistance	Perform inde- pendently	No opportunity
• State indications for NPO status	⎯	⎯	⎯	⎯	⎯	⎯
• Clear liquids	⎯	⎯	⎯	⎯	⎯	⎯
• Discuss implementation of progressive diet	⎯	⎯	⎯	⎯	⎯	⎯
• Measure and record intake and output	⎯	⎯	⎯	⎯	⎯	⎯

	Self-assess	Read P&P	Discuss and observe	Perform with assistance	Perform inde-pendently	No opportunity
• Weigh patient and record weight; understand the significance of increase	___	___	___	___	___	___
• Assess elimination status						
• Bladder size, emptying	___	___	___	___	___	___
• State indications for catheterization	___	___	___	___	___	___
• Insert straight catheter	___	___	___	___	___	___
• Insert Foley catheter	___	___	___	___	___	___
• Administer enemas	___	___	___	___	___	___
• State indication and use for enemas for postpartum patient	___	___	___	___	___	___
• Give SS enema	___	___	___	___	___	___
• Give Fleets enema	___	___	___	___	___	___
• Demonstrate knowledge and understanding of postpartum hemorrhage:						
• State predisposing factors	___	___	___	___	___	___
• Describe causes	___	___	___	___	___	___
• Describe interventions and possible treatments	___	___	___	___	___	___
• Medications	___	___	___	___	___	___
• Lab	___	___	___	___	___	___
Demonstrate knowledge and understanding of physiology relating to surgical repair of cesarean-delivered mother:						
• Assess hydration status	___	___	___	___	___	___
• Assess for restoration of bowel and bladder function						
• Bowel sounds and abdominal distention	___	___	___	___	___	___
• Bladder palpation	___	___	___	___	___	___
• Flatus	___	___	___	___	___	___
• Demonstrate turning and positioning, coughing, and deep breathing	___	___	___	___	___	___
• Ambulating	___	___	___	___	___	___
• Patient teaching—rest and hygiene	___	___	___	___	___	___
• Wound checking: incision and drainage	___	___	___	___	___	___
• Catheterization						
• Straight	___	___	___	___	___	___
• Foley	___	___	___	___	___	___
• Demonstrate knowledge of and care for:						
• Hemovac drain	___	___	___	___	___	___
• Levine tube	___	___	___	___	___	___

	Self-assess	Read P&P	Discuss and observe	Perform with assistance	Perform independently	No opportunity
• Jackson Pratt drain	___	___	___	___	___	___
• Penrose drain	___	___	___	___	___	___
• Suprapubic catheter	___	___	___	___	___	___

• Appropriately use and instruct patient about binders and support aids

	Self-assess	Read P&P	Discuss and observe	Perform with assistance	Perform independently	No opportunity
• Scultetus binder	___	___	___	___	___	___
• Abdominal binder	___	___	___	___	___	___
• Compression stockings	___	___	___	___	___	___
• Application of ace bandages	___	___	___	___	___	___

• Demonstrate knowledge of:

	Self-assess	Read P&P	Discuss and observe	Perform with assistance	Perform independently	No opportunity
• Sterile hot and cold compresses	___	___	___	___	___	___
• Moist compresses	___	___	___	___	___	___
• Operative site assessment	___	___	___	___	___	___
• Perform dressing change using clean technique	___	___	___	___	___	___

Perform procedures and document according to hospital procedure manual, including:

	Self-assess	Read P&P	Discuss and observe	Perform with assistance	Perform independently	No opportunity
• Vaginal exam	___	___	___	___	___	___
• Rectal exam	___	___	___	___	___	___
• Suture removal	___	___	___	___	___	___
• Staple removal	___	___	___	___	___	___
• Vaginal pack removal	___	___	___	___	___	___
• Suprapubic catheter removal	___	___	___	___	___	___
• RhoGAM administration	___	___	___	___	___	___
• Rubella vaccine administration	___	___	___	___	___	___
• Venipuncture and label for specimen	___	___	___	___	___	___
• Insertion of IV cannula	___	___	___	___	___	___
• Set up and label peripheral and piggyback IV bottles	___	___	___	___	___	___
• Infusion pumps	___	___	___	___	___	___

Treatments:

• Thermal

	Self-assess	Read P&P	Discuss and observe	Perform with assistance	Perform independently	No opportunity
• K-pad	___	___	___	___	___	___
• Ice pack to perineum	___	___	___	___	___	___
• Ice packs to breast	___	___	___	___	___	___

• Inhalation

	Self-assess	Read P&P	Discuss and observe	Perform with assistance	Perform independently	No opportunity
• Wall oxygen	___	___	___	___	___	___
• Mask	___	___	___	___	___	___

	Self-assess	Read P&P	Discuss and observe	Perform with assistance	Perform independently	No opportunity
• Cannula	___	___	___	___	___	___
• Aerosol	___	___	___	___	___	___
• IPPB	___	___	___	___	___	___
• Catheter	___	___	___	___	___	___
• Douche	___	___	___	___	___	___
• Oral-nasal suctioning	___	___	___	___	___	___

Assess psychosocial needs, including:

	Self-assess	Read P&P	Discuss and observe	Perform with assistance	Perform independently	No opportunity
• Taking-in and taking-hold stages	___		___	___	___	___
• Mother–baby acquaintance process	___	___	___	___	___	___
• Parent–infant attachment	___	___	___	___	___	___
• Family interaction and social situation	___	___	___	___	___	___
• Knowledge of blues versus depression as grieving	___	___	___	___	___	___
• Coping skills	___	___	___	___	___	___
• Identify criteria and demonstrate referral to:						
• Social worker	___	___	___	___	___	___
• Home health	___	___	___	___	___	___
• Chaplain	___	___	___	___	___	___
• Identify maladaptive mother–baby attachment	___	___	___	___	___	___

Assess educational needs of mother, infant, and partner, including:

Infant care

	Self-assess	Read P&P	Discuss and observe	Perform with assistance	Perform independently	No opportunity
• Infant nutrition—breast- and formula-feeding	___	___	___	___	___	___
• Infant states, state-related behaviors, and individual differences	___	___	___	___	___	___
• Infant stimulation	___	___	___	___	___	___
• Infant growth and development	___	___	___	___	___	___
• Parenting	___	___	___	___	___	___
• Birth control and family planning	___	___	___	___	___	___
• Diabetes	___	___	___	___	___	___
• Pre- and post-op care	___	___	___	___	___	___

Demonstrate knowledge and understanding of administration of blood:

	Self-assess	Read P&P	Discuss and observe	Perform with assistance	Perform independently	No opportunity
• Describe indications for blood administration	___	___	___	___	___	___
• Perform the procedure according to policies	___	___	___	___	___	___
• State interventions for suspected or actual transfusion reaction	___	___	___	___	___	___

	Self-assess	Read P&P	Discuss and observe	Perform with assistance	Perform inde-pendently	No opportunity
• Document blood transfusion	————	————	————	————	————	————

Demonstrate nursing interventions for patients with:

	Self-assess	Read P&P	Discuss and observe	Perform with assistance	Perform inde-pendently	No opportunity
• Uterine atony and subinvolution	————	————	————	————	————	————
• Retained placental tissue	————	————	————	————	————	————
• Unrepaired birth canal laceration	————	————	————	————	————	————
• Birth canal hematoma	————	————	————	————	————	————
• Spinal headache	————	————	————	————	————	————
• Pre-eclampsia or eclampsia	————	————	————	————	————	————
• Diabetes						
• Classification	————	————	————	————	————	————
• Signs						
• Insulin shock	————	————	————	————	————	————
• Diabetic coma	————	————	————	————	————	————
• Insulin administration						
• Sliding scale	————	————	————	————	————	————
• Continuous infusion	————	————	————	————	————	————
• Lab tests						
• FBS/RBS	————	————	————	————	————	————
• Chem BG	————	————	————	————	————	————
• Normal values	————	————	————	————	————	————
• Postpartum anemia	————	————	————	————	————	————
• Postpartum infection	————	————	————	————	————	————

Demonstrate knowledge of commonly used medications:

	Self-assess	Read P&P	Discuss and observe	Perform with assistance	Perform inde-pendently	No opportunity
• Codeine	————	————	————	————	————	————
• RhoGAM	————	————	————	————	————	————
• PPD	————	————	————	————	————	————
• Rubella	————	————	————	————	————	————
• Pitocin	————	————	————	————	————	————
• Methergine/Ergotrate	————	————	————	————	————	————
• Insulin	————	————	————	————	————	————
• FeSO4	————	————	————	————	————	————
• MgSO4	————	————	————	————	————	————
• Colace	————	————	————	————	————	————
• Antibiotics	————	————	————	————	————	————
• Tylenol	————	————	————	————	————	————

	Self-assess	Read P&P	Discuss and observe	Perform with assistance	Perform inde-pendently	No opportunity
• Motrin	___	___	___	___	___	___
• Hepatitis B vaccine	___	___	___	___	___	___

Determine the patient's response to the environment, including:

• Degree of orientation	___	___	___	___	___	___
• Level of anxiety	___	___	___	___	___	___
• Quality of communication	___	___	___	___	___	___
• Sleep patterns	___	___	___	___	___	___

Assess patients for pain:

• Describe pain in the patient's terms	___	___	___	___	___	___
• Elicit information from the patient regarding onset, duration, and relief of pain	___	___	___	___	___	___

Assess for mother–baby bonding	___	___	___	___	___	___

Provide emotional support to the mother and family, including:

• Grief or loss program	___	___	___	___	___	___
• When infant is sick	___	___	___	___	___	___
• Normal birth	___	___	___	___	___	___

Explain hospital policies and procedures to new mothers and families	___	___	___	___	___	___

Control the patient environment in relation to:

• Sleep	___	___	___	___	___	___
• Privacy	___	___	___	___	___	___
• Visitors	___	___	___	___	___	___
• Noise	___	___	___	___	___	___
• Other staff	___	___	___	___	___	___

Provide care and comfort measures for the new mother:

• Promote a return to normalization of physical and emotional status	___	___	___	___	___	___

• Promote rapid healing of tissue trauma following pregnancy and birth by implementing appropriate comfort measures:

• Apply cold or heat to the perineum	___	___	___	___	___	___
• Care of hemorrhoids	___	___	___	___	___	___
• Perineal care	___	___	___	___	___	___
• Know use of abdominal binder and how to apply	___	___	___	___	___	___
• State epidural duromorph care	___	___	___	___	___	___

	Self-assess	Read P&P	Discuss and observe	Perform with assistance	Perform independently	No opportunity
• Assist the mother with suppressing lactation with minimal discomfort						
• Tight-fitting bra	___	___	___	___	___	___
• Breast care and ice	___	___	___	___	___	___
• Teach comfort measures	___	___	___	___	___	___
• Avoid stimulating the nipple or breast	___	___	___	___	___	___
• Care for mothers in pain						
• Determine strategies to relieve pain and modify nursing care plan	___	___	___	___	___	___
• Administer pain medication as prescribed	___	___	___	___	___	___
Promote successful breastfeeding						
• Assist the new mother with nipple and breast care	___	___	___	___	___	___
• Know types of breast pumps and how to store breast milk	___	___	___	___	___	___
• Assist mother with breastfeeding						
• Properly position infant at breast	___	___	___	___	___	___
• Identify signs of correct infant latch-on	___	___	___	___	___	___
• Describe frequency, duration, and establishment of milk supply	___	___	___	___	___	___
• Alert mother to infant's feeding cues	___	___	___	___	___	___
• Assess infant's hydration status	___	___	___	___	___	___
• Perform LATCH scoring (See "Explanation of the LATCH System" on page 236)	___	___	___	___	___	___
Refer to lactation specialist or community resources in non-threatening way as needed	___	___	___	___	___	___
Identify breastfeeding problems and take appropriate nursing actions:						
• Breast refusal (infant sleepy or fussy)	___	___	___	___	___	___
• Incorrect suck	___	___	___	___	___	___
• Breaks in nipple integrity	___	___	___	___	___	___
• Engorgement	___	___	___	___	___	___
Teach mother and infant care that will promote family wellness and successful parenting						
• Assess learning needs through observation and questioning	___	___	___	___	___	___
• Plan and implement teaching to provide learning experiences	___	___	___	___	___	___
Support a woman's decision to bottle feed her newborn.	___	___	___	___	___	___

	Self-assess	Read P&P	Discuss and observe	Perform with assistance	Perform independently	No opportunity
Demonstrate and explain to mother formula preparation and storage	___	___	___	___	___	___

8. Competency: In collaboration with the mother, family, and healthcare team members, conduct an initial and ongoing assessment to gather data and to implement the appropriate plans of care for the new baby.

	Self-assess	Read P&P	Discuss and observe	Perform with assistance	Perform independently	No opportunity
Review the maternal–fetal and neonatal history, identifying significant data to individualize nursing care	___	___	___	___	___	

Assess the neonate's physical status, including vital signs, recognizing abnormal findings and intervening to meet the neonate's needs:

- Assess the head and neck:

	Self-assess	Read P&P	Discuss and observe	Perform with assistance	Perform independently	No opportunity
• Observe and palpate the neonate's head for symmetry, noting absence or presence of caput succedaneum and presence of cephalohematoma	___	___	___	___	___	___
• Palpate the fontanels and sutures for fullness, depression, overriding, and shape	___	___	___	___	___	___
• Measure the head's circumference	___	___	___	___	___	___
• Evaluate the face's symmetry	___	___	___	___	___	___
• Observe the eyes for shape, position, size, appearance of pupils, and presence of hemorrhage	___	___	___	___	___	___
• Evaluate the mouth for clefts and teeth	___	___	___	___	___	___
• Note the neck's length, its relationship to the body, mobility, presence of webbing and/or fat pad	___	___	___	___	___	___
• Observe skin color for presence of duskiness, cyanosis, jaundice, bruising, or edema	___	___	___	___	___	___
• Note and record presence of any skin breaks, abrasions and/or contusions on the head, face, or neck	___	___	___	___	___	___
• Observe the nose for symmetry, septum, flaring, and patency	___	___	___	___	___	___

- Assess the body:

	Self-assess	Read P&P	Discuss and observe	Perform with assistance	Perform independently	No opportunity
• Palpate clavicles for masses and intactness	___	___	___	___	___	___
• Inspect the size, symmetry, and shape of the thorax, and any retracting	___	___	___	___	___	___
• Auscultate breath and heart sounds	___	___	___	___	___	___
• Count respiratory and heart rates	___	___	___	___	___	___
• Describe any murmurs (location, loudness, and intensity)	___	___	___	___	___	___

- Abdomen:

	Self-assess	Read P&P	Discuss and observe	Perform with assistance	Perform independently	No opportunity
• Inspect the abdomen's shape	___	___	___	___	___	___
• Observe the cord for the number of vessels	___	___	___	___	___	___

	Self-assess	Read P&P	Discuss and observe	Perform with assistance	Perform inde- pendently	No opportunity
• Palpate femoral pulses	____	____	____	____	____	____

• Genitals

• Observe for appropriateness of visible genitals per the neonate's stated sex	____	____	____	____	____	____
• Observe female neonates for the labia's maturation and for vaginal discharge	____	____	____	____	____	____
• Observe male neonates for the urethral opening's position, the presence of testes, and the scrotum's maturation................................	____	____	____	____	____	____
• Note elimination of urine and stool color, amount, and number................................	____	____	____	____	____	____

• Posterior

• Determine the anus's patency	____	____	____	____	____	____
• Observe for pilonidal dimple	____	____	____	____	____	____
• Palpate and inspect the spinal column for masses and for vertebrae symmetry	____	____	____	____	____	____

• Extremities

• Note the symmetry and the neonate's ability to move all extremities	____	____	____	____	____	____
• Count the digits on hands and feet................................	____	____	____	____	____	____
• Observe the digits for polydactylia and/or syndactylia	____	____	____	____	____	____
• Evaluate the rotation of hips by abducting the thighs to the bed, rotating the hips through a full range of motion, and observing the symmetry of leg creases....	____	____	____	____	____	____
• Evaluate peripheral pulses and compare the upper pulse with the lower for strength	____	____	____	____	____	____

• Assess reflexes

• Elicit and evaluate rooting and sucking responses	____	____	____	____	____	____
• Elicit and evaluate the grasp response in both hands ..	____	____	____	____	____	____
• Elicit and evaluate the ability to be pulled to a sitting position, noting head and arm positions	____	____	____	____	____	____
• Elicit and evaluate a Moro response	____	____	____	____	____	____
• Observe and evaluate tone, tremulousness, jitteriness, etc.	____	____	____	____	____	____

Assess the neonate's neurological, behavioral, and maturational status:

• Perform and document a Ballard exam at the appropriate time	____	____	____	____	____	____
• Intervene appropriately if the infant is LGA or SGA	____	____	____	____	____	____

	Self-assess	Read P&P	Discuss and observe	Perform with assistance	Perform independently	No opportunity

- Identify the three stages of activity immediately following birth (term infant):

	Self-assess	Read P&P	Discuss and observe	Perform with assistance	Perform independently	No opportunity
• Alert/active phase (Stage I)	___	___	___	___	___	___
• Quiet phase (Stage II)	___	___	___	___	___	___
• Alert/active phase (Stage III)	___	___	___	___	___	___

- Identify sleeping and waking states:
  - Sleep states:

	Self-assess	Read P&P	Discuss and observe	Perform with assistance	Perform independently	No opportunity
• Quiet	___	___	___	___	___	___
• Deep	___	___	___	___	___	___

  - Wake states:

	Self-assess	Read P&P	Discuss and observe	Perform with assistance	Perform independently	No opportunity
• Drowsiness	___	___	___	___	___	___
• Active alert	___	___	___	___	___	___
• Quiet alert	___	___	___	___	___	___
• Crying	___	___	___	___	___	___

Identify the infant at risk and intervene appropriately for:

	Self-assess	Read P&P	Discuss and observe	Perform with assistance	Perform independently	No opportunity
• Well, at risk, and sick newborns	___	___	___	___	___	___
• Congenital abnormality	___	___	___	___	___	___
• SGA/LGA status	___	___	___	___	___	___
• IDM	___	___	___	___	___	___
• Risk factors of postterm infants	___	___	___	___	___	___
• Risk factors of preterm infants	___	___	___	___	___	___
• Infants with FAS/drug dependency	___	___	___	___	___	___
• Congenital heart defects	___	___	___	___	___	___
• Hypoglycemia	___	___	___	___	___	___
• Neonatal sepsis	___	___	___	___	___	___
• Hyperbilirubinemia	___	___	___	___	___	___
• Strep B	___	___	___	___	___	___
• Hepatitis	___	___	___	___	___	___
• HIV	___	___	___	___	___	___
• Hypothermia	___	___	___	___	___	___
• Respiratory distress	___	___	___	___	___	___

9. **Competency: In collaboration with the mother, family, and healthcare team members, implement plans of care for neonates when care deviates from normal.**

In hyperviscosity, state normal lab values:

	Self-assess	Read P&P	Discuss and observe	Perform with assistance	Perform independently	No opportunity
• Hct	___	___	___	___	___	___
• Bilirubin	___	___	___	___	___	___

	Self-assess	Read P&P	Discuss and observe	Perform with assistance	Perform independently	No opportunity
• Ca						
• CBC						

For prevention of hypoglycemia, demonstrate:

	Self-assess	Read P&P	Discuss and observe	Perform with assistance	Perform independently	No opportunity
• Site selection and techniques for dextrostix						
• Chemstrips						
• Use of D10w—formula						
• Use of dextrometer						
• Interpretation of lab values						

Detect and treat hyperbilirubinemia:

	Self-assess	Read P&P	Discuss and observe	Perform with assistance	Perform independently	No opportunity
• Assess for jaundice according to protocol						
• Interpret lab results appropriately						
• Perform phototherapy per orders:						
• Eye protection						
• Thermal regulation						
• Bilimeter						
• Positioning						
• Feeding						
• Fluids						

Recognize a distressed versus a normal infant, including:

	Self-assess	Read P&P	Discuss and observe	Perform with assistance	Perform independently	No opportunity
• Anomalies						
• Abnormal vital signs						
• Neurological deficits such as lethargy or jitteriness						
• Color changes						
• Neonatal sepsis						
• Hypothermia						
• Respiratory distress						

Perform suctioning:

	Self-assess	Read P&P	Discuss and observe	Perform with assistance	Perform independently	No opportunity
• Bulb syringe						
• Delee suction						
• Wall units						
• Assist with insertion of chest tubes						
• Documentation						

Perform specimen collection and obtain cultures:

	Self-assess	Read P&P	Discuss and observe	Perform with assistance	Perform independently	No opportunity
• U-bags						
• Supra-pubic aspiration						

	Self-assess	Read P&P	Discuss and observe	Perform with assistance	Perform independently	No opportunity
• Cultures						
• Gastric aspirate	___	___	___	___	___	___
• Ear, nose, and throat	___	___	___	___	___	___
• Skin	___	___	___	___	___	___
• Stool	___	___	___	___	___	___
• Heel sticks for glucose levels	___	___	___	___	___	___
• Urine specific gravity	___	___	___	___	___	___
• Assist with special procedures, including:						
• Intubation	___	___	___	___	___	___
• Insertion of umbilical catheter	___	___	___	___	___	___
• Lumbar puncture	___	___	___	___	___	___
• Exchange transfusion	___	___	___	___	___	___
• Physician exam	___	___	___	___	___	___
• Circumcision	___	___	___	___	___	___
• Notify the health department and infection control nurse	___	___	___	___	___	___
• PKU, T4 testing	___	___	___	___	___	___
• IVs	___	___	___	___	___	___
• Care of IDM	___	___	___	___	___	___
• Blood gases	___	___	___	___	___	___

Correctly and accurately perform nursing care and procedures on the newborn, including:

	Self-assess	Read P&P	Discuss and observe	Perform with assistance	Perform independently	No opportunity
• Post-circumcision care	___	___	___	___	___	___
• Umbilical cord care	___	___	___	___	___	___
• Phototherapy care	___	___	___	___	___	___
• Gastric lavage	___	___	___	___	___	___
• Maintenance of adequate respiratory status	___	___	___	___	___	___
• Maintenance of a neutral thermal environment	___	___	___	___	___	___
• Perform all aspects of care for SGA and preterm infants	___	___	___	___	___	___
• Administer Hepatitis B vaccine	___	___	___	___	___	___
• Perform capillary blood sampling for MDT and supplemental screening	___	___	___	___	___	___
• Assess suck, swallow, and breathing coordination during bottle feedings	___	___	___	___	___	___
• Assess and promote mother–baby bonding	___	___	___	___	___	___

Identify infants in need of resuscitation and the appropriate method of resuscitation.

	Self-assess	Read P&P	Discuss and observe	Perform with assistance	Perform independently	No opportunity
	___	___	___	___	___	___

	Self-assess	Read P&P	Discuss and observe	Perform with assistance	Perform inde-pendently	No opportunity
• Identify and care for "sick" infants:						
• Draw warmed heel gases	___	___	___	___	___	___
• Demonstrate basic knowledge of gases	___	___	___	___	___	___
• Recognize the signs of infant distress	___	___	___	___	___	___
• Correctly assess cardiopulmonary status	___	___	___	___	___	___
• Perform infant CPR correctly	___	___	___	___	___	___
• Use a bag mask correctly	___	___	___	___	___	___
• Apply O_2 when appropriate	___	___	___	___	___	___
• Verbalize understanding of the newborn transitional period	___	___	___	___	___	___
• Demonstrate neonatal resuscitation	___	___	___	___	___	___

Identify the needs of and provide nursing support for families in crisis:

	Self-assess	Read P&P	Discuss and observe	Perform with assistance	Perform inde-pendently	No opportunity
• Describe the therapeutic aspects of crisis counseling	___	___	___	___	___	___
• Discuss the nurse's role in assisting the family that experiences a loss	___	___	___	___	___	___
• Complete all documentation according to the Perinatal Loss Policy	___	___	___	___	___	___
• Discuss the needs of and provide nursing support for a family whose baby is in the SCN or has been transported to the NICU	___	___	___	___	___	___
• Identify the assessments and nursing care for families with attachment problems	___	___	___	___	___	___
• Discuss nursing care of the mother who is relinquishing her baby	___	___	___	___	___	___
• Complete all documentation according to the Adoption and Abandonment Policy	___	___	___	___	___	___
• Identify the signs of a family at risk for child abuse	___	___	___	___	___	___
• Discuss the nursing care for a single parent family	___	___	___	___	___	___

10. Competency: In collaboration with the mother, family, and healthcare team members, identify nursing diagnoses for selected patients.

	Self-assess	Read P&P	Discuss and observe	Perform with assistance	Perform inde-pendently	No opportunity
Identify nursing diagnoses based on patient assessment data	___	___	___	___	___	___
Formulate an etiology for each diagnosis	___	___	___	___	___	___

11. Competency: In collaboration with the mother, family, and healthcare team members, develop nursing care plans for selected patients.

Identify expected outcomes for each nursing diagnosis:

	Self-assess	Read P&P	Discuss and observe	Perform with assistance	Perform inde-pendently	No opportunity
• Develop realistic, measurable, and achievable outcomes for specific patient needs	___	___	___	___	___	___

	Self-assess	Read P&P	Discuss and observe	Perform with assistance	Perform inde-pendently	No opportunity
Plan nursing interventions to achieve each desired outcome:						
• Achieve culturally appropriate interventions	___	___	___	___	___	___
• Collaborate with other healthcare team members	___	___	___	___	___	___
• Integrate other patient care activities into the patient's care	___	___	___	___	___	___
Prioritize patient care activities appropriately	___	___	___	___	___	___
Document discharge planning on the nursing care plan:						
• Incorporate patient teaching	___	___	___	___	___	___
• Make referrals for postdischarge needs	___	___	___	___	___	___
• Address unresolved problems in discharge teaching	___	___	___	___	___	___

12. Competency: In collaboration with the mother, family, and healthcare team members, evaluate the outcomes of nursing care.

	Self-assess	Read P&P	Discuss and observe	Perform with assistance	Perform inde-pendently	No opportunity
Compare patient's responses to desired outcomes	___	___	___	___	___	___
Modify and/or revise the nursing care plan as needed	___	___	___	___	___	___

13. Competency: In collaboration with the mother, family, and healthcare team members, plan and provide maternal and newborn education.

	Self-assess	Read P&P	Discuss and observe	Perform with assistance	Perform inde-pendently	No opportunity
Discuss maternal self-care, including:						
• Perineal care	___	___	___	___	___	___
• Hemorrhoids	___	___	___	___	___	___
• Breasts and nipples	___	___	___	___	___	___
• Activity limitations	___	___	___	___	___	___
• Nutrition	___	___	___	___	___	___
• Need for balance of exercise and rest	___	___	___	___	___	___
• Sexuality and contraception	___	___	___	___	___	___
• Psychosocial aspects of postpartum period	___	___	___	___	___	___
• Signs and symptoms of complications to report to the healthcare provider	___	___	___	___	___	___
Discuss newborn care, including:						
• Nutritional needs	___	___	___	___	___	___
• Growth and development	___	___	___	___	___	___
• Cord care	___	___	___	___	___	___
• Circumcision care, if indicated	___	___	___	___	___	___
• Bathing	___	___	___	___	___	___
• Diapering	___	___	___	___	___	___
• Taking a temperature	___	___	___	___	___	___

	Self-assess	Read P&P	Discuss and observe	Perform with assistance	Perform inde-pendently	No opportunity
• Signs and symptoms to report to the healthcare provider...	___	___	___	___	___	___
• Environmental safety...	___	___	___	___	___	___
• Infant states of consciousness	___	___	___	___	___	___
• Infant temperament..	___	___	___	___	___	___

Discuss support person(s) and family adaptation, including:

	Self-assess	Read P&P	Discuss and observe	Perform with assistance	Perform inde-pendently	No opportunity
• Transition to new roles......................................	___	___	___	___	___	___
• Communication among the mother, support person(s), and family—expectations versus reality	___	___	___	___	___	___
• Siblings						
• Possible age-appropriate regression............................	___	___	___	___	___	___
• Strategies for meeting sibling needs	___	___	___	___	___	___

	Self-assess	Read P&P	Discuss and observe	Perform with assistance	Perform inde-pendently	No opportunity
Provide community resource information for short- and long-term maternal and newborn follow-up.	___	___	___	___	___	___

EXPLANATION OF THE LATCH SYSTEM

The LATCH system is a documentation tool for breastfeeding charting and assessment. The LATCH tool was modeled on the Apgar scoring system. A composite score of 0–10 is possible, depending upon the identified criteria met in each of the key areas of breastfeeding (see the table at the end of this section). It is not a judgement of the breastfeeding dyad or staff member helping; rather, it is a method to identify interventions needed and to facilitate charting.

Each letter of the acronym LATCH denotes a key component of breastfeeding. *L* is the infant's ability to latch onto the breast. *A* is for the presence of audible swallowing of the infant at the breast. *T* is for the mother's nipple type. *C* is for the mother's sense of comfort. *H* is for the holding, or the breastfeeding position, used by the mother, and the amount of help the mother requires in holding the infant (see the following table).

The *L* Assessment

The importance of assessing the infant's ability to latch correctly onto the breast during breastfeeding is well documented. The *L* assessment is scored as a 2 if the infant's gum line is placed well over the mother's lactiferous sinuses, the tongue is positioned under the areola, and both lips are flanged outward. Jaw movement should be visible at the temple area and adequate suction demonstrated by full cheeks without dimpling. There also should be a sustained latch with rhythmic sucking outbursts of 6–7 compressions every 10 seconds. A score of 1 is given if these criteria are met only after repeated attempts or if the staff must hold the nipple in the infant's mouth and repeatedly stimulate the infant to suck. If the infant takes only the nipple tip and is unable to compress the lactiferous sinuses, the assessment score also is a 1. An infant who is too sleepy or reluctant to nurse and, therefore, does not latch on receives an assessment score of 0.

The *A* Assessment

The audible swallowing of the infant at the breast is assessed next. Swallowing at the breast is an indicator of milk intake and is a necessary component of breastfeeding. The observation of swallowing also provides the mother with encouragement and reinforcement that she is providing milk for her infant. The *A* assessment is scored as a 2 if swallowing is heard as a short, forceful expiration of air. During the first 24–48 hours, several bursts of sucking may precede the swallowing sound. At 3–4 days after birth, the frequency of swallowing should increase. If swallowing is heard infrequently and usually only with stimulation, the assessment score is 1. If no audible swallowing is noted, the assessment score is 0.

The *T* Assessment

The shape, size, and texture of the nipple is an important factor in the ability of the infant to latch onto the breast and maintain a sucking effort. *T* is for the mother's nipple type. The nipple type is an important indicator of the amount and kind of intervention that may be required. If the nipple is everted and projects outward at rest or after stimulation, the assessment score is 2. A nipple that is flat or projects forward minimally receives an assessment score of 1. Inverted nipples receive an assessment score of 0.

The *C* Assessment

The mother's comfort is an important factor in the continued breastfeeding of her infant. Pain in the breast or nipple area influences not only the let-down reflex, but also the mother's willingness to continue to breastfeed and her feelings of competence. The assessment of the mother's comfort includes both breast and nipple areas. The assessment score is 2 if the breast tissue is soft and elastic and the nipples have no visible signs of redness, bruising, blistering, bleeding, or cracking. When asked, the mother also must state that she is comfortable. If the mother indicates that she is experiencing mild to moderate tenderness, if she is experiencing a decrease in tissue elasticity when her breasts fill, or if her nipples are reddened with small blisters, the assessment score is 1. Mothers who indicate severe discomfort and have breasts that are engorged, firm, tender with nonelastic tissue, and nipples that are cracked, bleeding, very reddened, or have large blisters or bruises receive an assessment score of 0.

The *H* Assessment

The final component of the LATCH assessment considers the breastfeeding position the mother uses and the amount of help she requires from the staff to hold the infant. Many positions can be used for breastfeeding depending upon the mother's preference and the infant's needs. The *H* assessment area is an important indicator of the mother's need for further teaching before discharge or referral to a lactation consultant. This assessment area also serves as documentation of the amount of assistance required by the breastfeeding dyad experiencing a problem. The breastfeeding infant's body should be flexed and should exhibit no muscular rigidity. The head should be aligned with the trunk, facing the breast and not turned laterally or hyperextended. The mother should support her breast with a cupped hand. Pillows are used to support the infant's body at breast level. The assessment score is 2 if the mother is able to position the infant at the breast (in a cradle, football, or side-lying hold), as described above, without assistance from the nursing staff. If the mother needs assistance from the nursing staff with positioning and attaching the infant at the first breast, but is able independently to achieve the infant's latch-on at the second breast, the assessment score is 1. If the mother needs the nursing staff's full assistance to attach and hold the infant at the breast for the entire feeding, the assessment score is 0.

TABLE I-1   The LATCH System

	0	1	2
L *Latch*	• Too sleepy or reluctant • No latch achieved	• Repeated attempts • Hold nipple in mouth • Stimulate to suck	• Grasps breast • Tongue down • Lips flanged • Rhythmic sucking
A *Audible Swallowing*	• None	• A few with stimulation	• Spontaneous and intermittent <24 hours old • Spontaneous and frequent >24 hours old
T *Type of Nipple*	• Inverted	• Flat	• Everted (after stimulation)
C *Comfort (Breast and Nipple)*	• Engorged • Cracked, bleeding, large blisters, or bruises	• Filling • Reddened, small blisters or bruises • Mild or moderate discomfort	• Soft • Tender
H *Hold (Positioning)*	• Full assist (staff holds infant at the breast)	• Minimal assist (i.e., elevates head of bed, place pillows for support) • Teach one side; mother does other. Staff holds and then mother takes over	• No assist from staff • Mother able to position and hold infant

Sample Policies, Procedures, and Patient Handouts for Family-Centered Maternity Care

BILL OF RIGHTS AND RESPONSIBILITIES FOR A PREGNANT PATIENT
Policy and Procedure

Procedure

Provide care for all antepartum and postpartum patients according to The Pregnant Patient's Bill of Rights and The Pregnant Patient's Responsibilities.

Policy

Staff will ensure that all antepartum and postpartum patients are encouraged to participate in decisions affecting their well-being and that of their unborn children.

Equipment

1. The Pregnant Patient's Bill of Rights (attached).
2. The Pregnant Patient's Responsibilities (attached).

Implementation

I. Follow the guidelines of The Pregnant Patient's Bill of Rights and The Pregnant Patient's Responsibilities when providing care to the antepartum or postpartum patient.

II. Assist the mother in understanding her rights and responsibilities.

_____

VP Nursing

_____

Department Chair

(continued)

(continued)

The Pregnant Patient's Bill of Rights

I. The pregnant woman has the right to:

   A. Be informed, prior to the administration of any drug or procedure, by the health professional caring for her of any potential direct or indirect effects, risks, or hazards to herself or her unborn or newborn infant that may result from the use of a drug or procedure prescribed for or administered to her during pregnancy, labor, birth, or lactation.

   B. Be informed, prior to the proposed therapy, not only of the benefits, risks, and hazards of the proposed therapy, but also of known alternative therapy.

   C. Be informed, prior to the administration of any drug, by the health professional who is prescribing or administering the drug to her that any drug which she receives during pregnancy, labor, or birth, no matter how or when the drug is taken or administered, may adversely affect her unborn baby, directly or indirectly, and that there is no drug or chemical that has been proven safe for the unborn child.

   D. Be informed, if Cesarean section is anticipated, prior to the administration of any drug, and preferably prior to her hospitalization, that minimizing her intake and, in turn, her baby's intake of nonessential preoperative medication will benefit her baby.

   E. Be informed, prior to the administration of a drug or procedure, if there is no properly controlled follow-up research that has established the safety of the drug or procedure regarding its direct and/or indirect effects on the physiologic, mental, and neurologic development of the child exposed, via the mother, to the drug or procedure during pregnancy, labor, birth, or lactation.

   F. Be informed, prior to the administration of any drug, of the brand name and generic name of the drug so she may advise the health professional of any past adverse reaction to the drug.

   G. Determine for herself, without pressure from her attendant, whether she will accept the risks inherent in the proposed therapy or refuse a drug or procedure.

   H. Know the name and qualifications of the individual administering a medication or procedure to her during labor or birth.

   I. Be informed, prior to the administration of any procedure, as to whether that procedure is being administered to her for her or her baby's benefit (medically indicated) or as an elective procedure (for convenience or teaching purposes).

   J. Be accompanied during the stress of labor and birth by someone she cares for and to whom she looks for emotional comfort and encouragement.

   K. Choose a position, after appropriate medical consultation, for labor and for birth which is least stressful to her baby and herself, and promotes her comfort and the physiologic progress of her labor.

II. The new mother has the right to:

   A. Have her baby cared for at her bedside if her baby is normal, and to feed her baby according to her baby's needs rather than according to hospital regimen.

   B. Be informed in writing of the name of the person who actually delivered her baby and that person's professional qualifications. This information should also be on the birth certificate.

   C. Be informed if there is any known or indicated aspect of her or her baby's care or condition that may cause her or her baby later difficulty or problems.

   D. Have her and her baby's hospital medical records complete, accurate, and legible, and to have the hospital retain these records, including nurses' notes, until the child reaches at least the age of majority or, alternatively, to have the records offered to her before they are destroyed.

   E. Have access, both during and after her hospital stay, to her complete medical records, and to receive a copy upon payment of a reasonable fee and without incurring the expense of an attorney.

It is the obstetric patient and her baby, not the health professional, who must sustain any trauma or injury resulting from the use of a drug or obstetric procedure. Observing the rights listed above will not only permit the obstetric patient to participate in decisions involving her and her baby's health care, but will help to protect the health professional and the hospital against litigation arising from resentment or misunderstanding on the mother's part.

Prepared by: Doris Haire, Chair, Committee on Health Law and Regulation, International Childbirth Education Association.

(continued)

(continued)

The Pregnant Patient's Responsibilities

In addition to understanding her rights, the pregnant woman should also understand that she too has certain responsibilities.

I. The pregnant woman is responsible for:

   A. Learning about the physical and psychological process of labor, birth, and postpartum recovery. The better informed expectant parents are, the better they will be able to participate in decisions concerning the planning of their care.

   B. Learning what comprises good prenatal and intranatal care and for making an effort to obtain the best care possible.

   C. Knowing about those hospital policies and regulations that will affect their birth and postpartum experience.

   D. Arranging for a companion or support person (husband, mother, sister, friend, etc.) who will share in her plans for birth and who will accompany her during her labor and birth experience.

   E. Making her preferences known clearly to the health professionals involved in her care in a courteous and cooperative manner and for making mutually agreed-upon arrangements regarding maternity care alternatives with her physician and hospital in advance of labor.

   F. Listening to their chosen physician or midwife with an open mind, just as they expect him or her to listen openly to them.

   G. Seeing, to the best of their ability, that their program, once the have agreed to a course of health care, is carried out in consultation with others with whom they have made the agreement.

   H. Obtaining information in advance regarding the approximate cost of her obstetric and hospital care.

   I. Notifying all concerned, when intending to change her physician or hospital, well in advance of the birth if possible, and for informing both of her reasons for changing.

   J. Learning, during her hospital stay, about her baby's continuing care after discharge from the hospital.

II. The parents are responsible for:

   A. Behaving toward those caring for them, in all their interactions with medical and nursing personnel, with the same respect and consideration they would like.

   B. Writing, after birth, constructive comments and feelings of satisfaction and/or dissatisfaction with the care (nursing, medical, and personal) they received. Good service to families in the future will be facilitated by those parents who take the time and responsibility to write letters expressing their feelings about the maternity care they received.

All the previous statements assume a normal birth and postpartum experience. Expectant parents should realize that if complications develop in their cases, there will be an increased need to trust the expertise of the physician and hospital staff they have chosen. However, if problems occur, the childbearing woman still retains her responsibility for making informed decisions about her care or treatment and that of her baby. If she is incapable of assuming that responsibility because of her physical condition, her previously authorized companion or support person should assume responsibility for making informed decisions on her behalf.

Prepared by members of the International Childbirth Education Association.

BIRTH PLAN
Gaston Memorial Hospital, Gastonia, North Carolina

The Birthplace
Gaston Memorial Hospital
Birth Plan

Welcome to The Birthplace! Our goal is to make your birth experience positive and unique, personal and private.

Name_____ **Date of Admission**_____

Support person(s)_____

Please check the options below <u>in the shaded boxes</u> which you would like to try (your nurse can describe them if needed):

Comfort Measures	Yes	No	Used by pt.	Stage of Labor/RN Comments
Jacuzzi				
Birthing Ball				
Walking				
Rocking Chair				
Labor Massage				
Relaxation/Breathing				
Visualization				
Position Changes				
Counter Pressure				
Knee Press				
Pain Medication				
Epidural				
Following Delivery:				
Labor partner to cut umbilical cord?				
Baby to be placed on Mom's abdomen?				
Pediatrician to check baby in Mom's room?				
I plan to: Breastfeed				
Bottle-feed				

Special Requests _____

_____

BONDING BETWEEN PARENT AND INFANT
Policy and Procedure

Procedure

Promote healthy attachment between parent(s) and infant attachment through careful interventions.

Policy

All unit staff will promote parent and infant bonding, a component of family-centered maternity care, at all times.

Equipment

Radiant warmer or warming light for the newborn.

Patient Education

Encourage questions and provide parenting education during the newborn assessment.

Implementation

I.   Encourage skin to skin contact with the mother immediately after the newborn's birth.

II. Encourage support persons to interact with the newborn by touching, holding, and talking.

III. Delay administering prophylactic eye medication until the initial bonding process has begun.

IV. Encourage breastfeeding during the immediate recovery period as early feedings are optimal for breastfeeding success.

V.   Use the newborn admission assessment, dressing, and infant bathing as teaching opportunities. Explain all findings to the new parents.

VI. Support the mother's caretaking efforts.

VII. Provide mother–baby care for cesarean mothers at the bedside or returning with the newborn from the holding nursery for frequent visits.

VIII. Assess bonding and document findings. Report potential maladaption to the charge nurse and infant care provider.

_____

VP Nursing

_____

Department Chair

BREAST CARE FOR BREASTFEEDING MOTHERS
Policy and Procedure

Procedure

Support and educate the breastfeeding mother to help ensure that the newborn has an adequate supply of breast milk and that the risk of bacterial contamination is reduced.

Policy

Staff will provide all breastfeeding postpartum mothers with information on breast care, including information on the electric and/or manual breast pump, breast milk expression, and storage

Equipment

1. Non-toxic nipple cream (preferably containing lanolin), if ordered.
2. Electric breast pump and/or manual pump.
3. Warm compresses.
4. Ice packs.
5. Discharge teaching checklist.

Patient Education

Provide breastfeeding education and nursing support. Encourage and answer all questions. Document teaching on the discharge checklist.

Implementation

I. General breast care.

   A. Instruct the mother to wear a supportive bra immediately after delivery.

   B. Offer nipple cream with instructions on its use. Apply cream to the nipples and areolas after feeding and wipe off with a tissue before feeding (if toxic or infant refuses to nurse). Use sparingly.

   C. Instruct the mother to wash her breasts with warm water only. Avoid soaps or perfumes on the nipples to prevent cracking.

   D. Allow breasts to air-dry completely after feeding. Apply dry bra pads.

   E. Instruct the mother to apply warm compresses if her breasts become engorged. Massage her breasts prior to feeding. This will assist with milk expression and emptying.

II. Support needs.

   A. Initiate breastfeeding early.

   B. Assist the mother in correctly positioning the infant at her breast.

   C. Encourage a demand-feeding schedule.

   D. Do not offer the infant supplemental feedings unless medically indicated and/or ordered by the infant care provider.

   E. Teach the mother to use techniques to stimulate milk letdown: deep breaths, visualizing the infant, sensory stimulation such as baby items or baby smells. The nurse of the mother's partner may massage the mother's shoulders to enhance relaxation.

   F. Offer psychological support.

VP Nursing

Department Chair

FATHERS OR DESIGNATED SIGNIFICANT OTHERS AT BIRTH
Policy and Procedure

Procedure

Provide support, lessen the mother's anxiety, and promote a family atmosphere. Facilitate the involvement of the father or support person(s) in a safe and supervised environment for birth.

Policy

Staff will welcome the father or support person(s) into the maternity unit during labor, birth, and the recovery period.

Patient Education

Explain procedures and define designated sterile areas to avoid contamination. Instruct the father and support person(s) on proper hand washing and the prevention and spreading of communicable infections.

Implementation

I.   Instruct the father (or support persons) to wash his hands thoroughly.

II.   A scrub suit, shoe covers, mask, and hair cover must be worn for Cesarean births.

III. Encourage the father to observe and participate during the infant's initial assessment and care.

IV.   Encourage and answer all questions.

_____
VP Nursing

_____
Department Chair

HYDROTHERAPY FOR LABOR AND POSTPARTUM PAIN RELIEF
Policy and Procedure

Procedure

Use hydrotherapy as an effective source of pain relief in labor and the postpartum period.

Policy

Upon order of the provider, the maternity unit staff will initiate and maintain hydrotherapy while continuing observation and assessment of the laboring or postpartum woman.

Equipment

1. Hydrotherapy tub.
2. Doppler and aquasonic gel.
3. Thermometer.
4. Nonslip bath mat, towels, and washcloths.
5. Bath skimmer.
6. Nonabrasive cleaner.

Patient Education

Explain the procedure to the woman, orient her to the room, the tub, and the emergency call system.

Hydrotherapy includes the following benefits:

1. Effective in providing pain relief in labor.
2. Effective in relieving postpartum cramping, episiotomy pain, muscle aches associated with labor and pushing, and breast tenderness.
3. Beneficial in facilitating breast stimulation for milk production and relieving engorgement by assisting relaxation and let-down reflex.

Implementation

I.   Hydrotherapy may be initiated when:

    A. Maternal vital signs are within normal limits.

    B. Fetal well-being has been established.

    C. Status of membranes has been documented. Membranes may be ruptured or intact. May use hydrotherapy if fluid is clear or is lightly meconium stained.

    D. During cervical priming with any type of prostaglandin product. (Should be used no sooner than two hours following application.)

    E. The patient has an IV.

II. Contraindications for using hydrotherapy include but are not limited to the following:

    A. Patients in which tocolysis is desired.

    B. Patients with heavy bleeding (more than usual bloody show or heavy lochia flow).

    C. Patients with a history of precipitous or rapid labor.

    D. Patients who are dilated more than 6 cm.

    E. Patients with epidural catheter in place.

    F. Patients with internal scalp electrode or needing close observation of fetal well-being.

    G. Patients whose labors are being augmented or stimulated with oxytocin and therefore need constant fetal monitoring.

III. Preparing the patient.

    A. Obtain baseline data, including vital signs and a minimum of 20 minutes reactive fetal monitor strip. Take vital signs as follows:

        1. Check and record maternal temperature every hour while the woman is laboring in the tub.

        2. Check blood pressure hourly or any time the mother expresses light-headedness. If her blood pressure is low, immediately remove the mother from the tub. If her blood pressure remains stable, the mother may return to the tub.

        3. Assess fetal heart rate according to ACOG guidelines for the low-risk patient (every 30 minutes in active phase of labor, every 15 minutes during second stage). If fetal tachycardia is present, cool the water or assist the mother out of the tub to cool down. If tachycardia persists, the mother must not return to tub, but needs continuous fetal monitoring.

(continued)

(continued)

    B. Obtain an order for hydrotherapy from the primary healthcare provider.

IV. Using hydrotherapy during labor.

    A. Maintain the water temperature to not exceed 100 degrees Fahrenheit.

    B. Primip mothers may remain in the tub up to four hours and multip mothers up to three hours, then reassess them out of the tub. The mother may use the jet tub during labor as long as both mother and fetus tolerate the procedure. Encourage the mother to ambulate if the labor begins to slow down.

    C. Provide hydration for the mother with cold drinks (preferably apple juice or Gatorade-type replacement fluids).

    D. Never leave the mother alone during hydrotherapy. Designated support persons may stay with the patient during the procedure if the nurse or provider is not present. Instruct attending support persons on using the emergency call system.

    E. For greatest benefit, completely undress and submerge the mother with her breasts underwater and the jets directed so that the agitation facilitates nipple stimulation, thereby facilitating the release of oxytocin. If the patient is modest, place a towel over her during hydrotherapy.

    F. Check and record the water temperature hourly. Add warm water as needed to maintain water temperature. Skim the water as needed to remove particulate matter.

V. Using hydrotherapy during birth.

    A. Have the mother assume a comfortable position for pushing. This may be sitting, squatting, or being held by her partner.

    B. Provide perineum support as needed.

    C. Lift the infant's head out of the water as soon as the infant is born. The infant's body may remain underwater.

    D. Perform bulb suctioning and cord clamping in the usual fashion.

    E. Suction the infant immediately after exiting the water. Standby suction should be available in case of unexpected meconium.

    F. The infant should be submerged except for face or removed from the tub, dried and wrapped for optimal thermoregulation.

    G. Complete infant admission procedure.

    H. Have the mother exit the tub prior to delivering the placenta. Assist her to the bed or have her sit on the side of the tub.

    Note: Mother must sign designated permit.

VI. Using hydrotherapy postpartum.

    A. Maintain the water temperature between 102–104 degrees Fahrenheit.

    B. The mother must have completed the initial recovery period (one to four hours). Vital signs should be stable with no known postpartal complications existing.

    C. The mother may use the jet tub as long as she tolerates the procedure. Ask her to discontinue usage at any time deemed necessary.

    D. Do not leave the woman alone during hydrotherapy. Designated support persons may observe the woman during the procedure if a nurse or provider is not present. Instruct on using the emergency call system.

    E. Check and record water temperature every hour. Add warm water as needed to maintain the temperature. Skim the water as needed to remove particulate matter.

VII. Tub cleaning and sanitation.

    A. Clean the tub after each use even when being used by the same woman.

    B. Refill the emptied tub until the jets are covered.

    C. Add a hospital-approved cleaning agent and turn the jets on. Skim any visible matter and leave the skimmer in the tub for disinfection.

    D. Circulate the water through the system for ten minutes. Drain the tub. Refill the tub with plain water and run the jets for five to ten minutes.

    E. Drain the tub and clean the surface with a nonabrasive cleaner.

    F. Rinse thoroughly.

_____

VP Nursing

_____

Department Chair

KANGAROO CARE
Policy and Procedure

Policy

To facilitate parent/infant closeness by promoting increased physical contact, to ease psychological burdens imposed by a premature birth, and to aid parents to feel more confident in responding to their infant's needs.

The procedure of skin-to-skin Kangaroo care (KC) will be used in the SCN.

Implementation

1. Receive or verify provider's orders to initiate KC.

2. Place rocking chair with pillows for support in draft-free private area.

3. Instruct parent to wear a medium weight blouse that can zip or button over the infant's back or have mother undress to waist and wear a cover gown. The infant's back is then covered with a warmed receiving blanket folded in fourths.

4. Place a hat on the infant's head, remove all other clothing except the diaper.

5. After explaining all procedures to the mother, have her sit in the rocking chair, position pillows for comfort, and place the baby upright onto her chest, between her breasts, from under the bottom of the blouse (so the leads, cords, and wires do not obstruct the view of the baby). Adjust oxygen if used. (The baby may need less oxygen flow under the mom's blouse as it acts like an oxygen "hood").

6. Obtain baseline vital signs (axillary, T, RR, HR, O_2 saturation) on the infant and take them again 20–30 minutes after KC initiated. Some infants warm up to an individual threshold at which they begin to squirm. If this happens, take the infant's temperature. Repeat vital signs checks when infant returned to incubator.

7. Give mother as much support as she needs. Emphasize that she is not hurting the baby. Stay close to the isolette during Kangaroo care for the first few days, until she tells you that she can be left with other nurses monitoring the baby.

8. Teach the mother how to hold, handle, breastfeed, and care for her baby, as well as to recognize and respond to behavioral cues. For example, teach the mother that if the infant shows such signs as finger splaying, extended limbs, tongue extension, or averted gaze, then she should withdraw some stimulation, such as rocking, singing, or talking, and offer such activities one at a time. As Kangaroo care progresses over weeks, encourage the mother to take control over care-taking activities.

9. If temperature is ± 37°, unfold the blanket covering the infant's back so only 2 folds are against the infant. Reassess the temperature in another 10 minutes.

10. If the infant is bottle feeding, offer the bottle when the infant begins to move his/her head from side-to-side.

11. Encourage the mother to take breaks as needed, usually at least every 2 hours. The mother can participate in Kangaroo care for as long or as briefly as she wishes, but the level of satisfaction and knowledge about the baby seem to be improved as more time is spent with baby.

12. If infant shows signs of unrest (not attributable to hunger, burping, and/or elimination) that persists for more than 5 minutes or if infant is in physiologic compromise (sustained desaturating, color changes, respiratory distress, HR instability, irritability), remove from KC.

13. Document initiation of, use of, and modifications to this policy.

14. Document start and stop times, vital signs, topics discussed, parental concerns, infant's behavioral and physiological responses to Kangaroo care.

Additional Information

Supportive Data

1. Breastfeeding mothers who give Kangaroo Care (KC) are inclined to produce more milk.

2. Infants given KC have adequate oxygenation.

3. Infants are warmer when being held in KC than when in open air cribs, so heat loss is not a real concern.

4. There is no rationale to support policies limiting and dictating incremental increases in the amount of time spent in KC. In many European sites, 4–5 hours per KC session is recommended to allow maximum benefit from KC.

5. Infants are shown to have fewer episodes of periodic breathing and apnea.

6. Infants receiving KC have had earlier hospital discharges.

7. Dressing/undressing and movement from crib to mother and back can be physiologically stressful to preterm infants. *At least one hour of KC at a time is recommended.*

ASSISTING THE NICU BREASTFEEDING MOTHER
Policy and Procedure

Policy

Assistance and instruction will be offered to staff and parents in providing the best possible nutrition and the best method of feeding the preterm infant.

Procedure

1. The mother will be supported in her personal goals regarding breastfeeding her infant.

2. Parents will be encouraged to provide Kangaroo Care when ordered. The physical contact with the baby is also important to the mother as it helps to increase her milk supply and improve the milk let-down.

3. Non-nutritive sucking will be encouraged to provide comfort, promote neurobehavioral organization, and increase oral-facial muscle tone and strength. Non-nutritive sucking helps increase ability to provide good intra-oral pressure for effective breastfeeding.

4. If supplementation is offered by bottle, use a firmer, standard size or NUK nipples when possible, to slow the flow of liquid. Red, premie nipples are not recommended.

5. Only appropriate size and type pacifiers should be used. Bottle nipples should not be used as pacifiers.

6. Mothers should be referred to lactation services for breastfeeding following discharge.

7. See NICU Breastfeeding Unit guide for specific suggestions regarding establishing breastfeeding for the NICU infant.

8. Milk should be thawed slowly to room temperature before feeding to infant. Microwave thawing is not allowed nor high temperatures of water as valuable nutrients are destroyed in the process.

9. It is recommended that milk refrigerators or freezers accessible to the public should have locks to protect against sabotage.

10. To avoid using the wrong milk, the container should be checked as when giving meds to verify correct patient identification.

11. The integrity of the container will be confirmed before feeding stored breastmilk to infants.

12. When possible, use colostrum or breastmilk for the first feedings.

Courtesy of Barbara Ford, RN, IBCLC.

NURSING CARE OF A MOTHER AND NEWBORN
Policy and Procedure Memorial Hospital, Fairfield, Ohio

POLICY & PROCEDURE

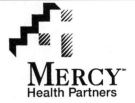

A general principle or plan that outlines expectations of a person or group in a defined situation, including a series of steps or a course of action used to complete the process and achieve an expected outcome.

MERCY
Health Partners

START DATE:	5/96		
REVIEW DATE:	10/04	**REVISED DATE:**	10/01
OWNERS:	Women's and Children's Services		
SCOPE OF CARE:	Women's and Children's Services		

TITLE: Mother Baby Care

PURPOSE: To provide standards for mother=baby nursing care from birth through discharge.

POLICY: Mother=baby couplet care is provided by the perinatal staff at the Mercy Family Birth Centers in accordance with national standards and within the framework of family=centered care.

PROCEDURE (steps/flowchart/decision algorithm)

I. Recovery period/Transition: when possible, care is provided with minimal interruption of family bonding.

   A. Maternal recovery—Recovery is complete when vital signs and assessments indicate the mother is stable

   1. Reassemble bed, place in low position with side rails up and call light within reach.

   2. Maternal vital signs and assessments are done every 15 minutes X 4, then 1 hour later.

      a. Vital signs include: pulse, respirations, blood pressure, with a temperature X 1 during recovery. Vital signs are taken more frequently as indicated.

      b. Fundus, lochia, and perineal status are assessed q 15 min. Also included during the recovery period are assessments of pain/comfort level, maternal infant attachment process, safety measures, IV, bladder, and effects of anesthesia.

   3. Encourage every opportunity for parent-infant interaction and support early breastfeeding as appropriate.

   4. Provide comfort/treatment measures as appropriate including warm blankets, ice to perineum, pain medication or medication for bleeding, bladder catheterization and the offering of food/fluids when patient is stable.

   B. Newborn transition:

   1. A TPR and assessment will be done at least 3 times with in the first 2 hours of life. This assessment will be done more frequently as indicated.

   2. Complete newborn assessment. Complete gestational age assessment if there is a question of mom's dates, no prenatalcare, or dates inconsitent with general newborn assessment.

   3. Verify notification of newborn physician's office of birth, presence of risk factors and any abnormal findings.

   4. Thermoregulation may be maintained by skin to skin contact, swaddling with warm blankets, or radiant warmer.

      a. If radiant warmer is used: apply servo-control probe to the infant's abdomen, but not over liver.

Courtesy of Mercy Hospital, Fairfield, Ohio. Reproduced with permission.

(continued)

(continued)

Cover the tip of the probe with a temperature probe cover. Care must be taken to keep the thermometer probe in constant contact with the infant's skin.

b.   Take axillary temperature when placing under the warmer and prior to removing from the warmer. Verify temperature rectally if axillary temperature is <97.6 or >99.6.

c.   If the infant has a low temperature, set the servo-control to 36.5 (97.8). Axillary temperatures should be monitored frequently until temperature is normal.

d.   The plexigalss sides of the bed should remain upright.

e.   If the infant is repositioned, the temperature probe should be in direct line with the heat source.

f.   Initial bath with soap may be given when infant's condition has stabilized and the axillary temperature is above 98.4.

   1)   Make every effort to minimize heat loss by giving the bath quickly and drying the infant thoroughly.

   2)   Assess temperature 30-60 minutes after the bath.

5.   Glucose screen and Hematocrit screen per policy.

6.   Newborn transitional period is complete when vital signs and assessments indicate newborn has stabilized.

II.   Continued Care of Mother-Baby Couplet. ALL women receive THE BABYKIND GUIDE BOOKLET and this is used as a reference for specific teaching.

A.   Maternal care following vaginal delivery (for care following Cesarean Delivery see Perioperative Care for Cesarean Patients policy)

1.   After mother's condition has stabilized, nursing assessments and vital signs are done every 8 hours for duration of hospitalization. Assessments are done more frequently as indicated.

2.   Educate the patient about good handwashing techiniques and the importance of handwashing after pericare, before caring for her infant, and after each infant's diaper change.

3.   Perineal care

a.   Instruct patient in appropriate perineal care and the use of a peribottle.

b.   Methods of perineal pain reduction include cold packs, witch hazel pads, hydrocortisone cream, Epifoam and sitz baths. These methods may be used singularly or in combination to provide needed pain relief as ordered by physician/CNM.

c.   Administer pain medication as needed.

4.   Breast care

a.   Breasts should be washed with water and a clean cloth daily during shower. No soap is necessary.

b.   Breastfeeding mothers will be assessed for nipple irritation or breakdown and will be taught how to examine and care for her breasts during lactation (Refer to "Breastfeeding", and "Use and Cleaning of Breast Pumps" policies).

c.   Educate non-lactating mothers on decreasing any stimulation of the breasts.

d.   Discuss the engorgement process with patient.

5.   Voiding

a.   Assess the bladder frequently for distention along with assessment of fundus deviation

b.   Offer bedpan if patient is unable to ambulate. When effects of anesthesia have worn off,

(continued)

encourage ambulation to bathroom with assistance.

   c. Educate patient on methods to promote voiding such as running water, pouring water over the vulva, or the use of sitz baths.

   d. Encourage patient's comfort level and administer pain medication (i.e. Ibuprofen) if patient has difficulty in voiding

   e. If patient remains unable to void, catheterize as ordered.

6. Rest

   a. Care including comfort measures, assessments and feedings.should be clustered when mother is awake

   b. Maternal rest should be encouraged and quiet periods protected.

7. Pain management continued as in recovery period.

B. Infant care

1. Nursing assessment and vital signs (TPR) are to be done every 4 hours X 24 hours and then every 8 hours thereafter.

2. Heat loss is minimized by dressing the infant with a hat, t-shirt and 2 blankets.

   a. If the infant's temperature is less than 97.6 with no extrinsic reason, methods to warm baby include wrapping in warm blankets, skin to skin contact or placing uncer radiant warmer. Reevaluate temperature hourly until above 98.

   b. If the infant"s temperature is above 99.6 wrap the infant loosely and reevaluate temperature hourly until 98.6. Evaluate maternal temperature.

   c. Notify physician of infants with a sustained decreased or elevated temperature.

3. Bathing: after the initial bath, an infant may be bathed with warm water every other day.

4. Weigh daily

5. Umbilical cord is to remain clean and dry. Remove cord clamp when cord is dry.

6. Infant feeding

   a. Breast feeding: place infant to breast as soon as possible after birth and then feed on demand (8-12 times in 24 hours). Refer to "Breastfeeding" Policy.

   b. Bottlefeeding: feed with preferred formula as soon as possible after birth and then feed on demand every 3-4 hours.

7. Infant identification

   a. Every infant should have two identification bands on.

   b. If for any reason the infant is taken out of the mother's room, her identification band and the infant's will be compared upon return of the infant to the room. (Refer to Safety, Identification and Security Policy)

8. If infant is to be circumcised refer to Circumcision policy.

9. Newborn Screening Test

   a. Infants discharged after 24 hours of age will have blood drawn prior to discharge.

   b. Infants discharged prior to 24 hours of age will have the initial Newborn Screen drawn before discharge and an additional Newborn Screen kit will be sent home with the parents. Instruct the parents to have the test repeated before the infant is two weeks of age.

10. Complete High Risk Hearing Questionnaire and make referrals as indicated.

(continued)

(continued)

11. Assess infant for jaundice before discharge and draw specimen for bilirubin test if baby is jaundiced. Notify physician of results of test prior to discharge.

III. Discharge of Mother-Baby Couplet

   A. Educational assessment

      1. Have mother complete discharge instruction sheet and review the topics with her that she has identified.

      2. Complete teaching sheet on mother and infant.

      3. When possible include family members/significant others in teaching.

      4. Have mother sign teaching sheet.

   B. Verify before discharge:

      1. Mother has "BabyKind Guide Booklet" and a copy of signed teaching sheet.

      2. Mother has prescriptions.

      3. Birth certificate Information sheet complete.

      4. Photos are taken of baby.

      5. Baby has voided and stooled.

      6. Cord clamp has been removed if appropriate

      7. Discharge orders are written for both mother and infant.

      7. RhoGam has been given if candidate.

      8. Rubella has been given as indicated.

      9. Hearing Screening Questionnaire has been completed.

     10. Second Newborn Screening form is provide if indicated.

     11. Mother verifies understanding to have or make appointments with both her and infant's health care providers.

     12. Mother's numbered band and one of Infant's matching bands removed and attached to baby's chart.

   C. Each mother is discharged per wheelchair with infant in her arms.

      1. The mother is wheeled tocar by hospital personnel.

      2. Parents place the infant(s) in the car seat(s). (See Car Seat policy)

   D. A discharge note is made on the mother's and infant's records which includes: time/date of discharge, how they were discharged, with whom they were discharged, and their condition upon discharge.

IV. Mother Discharged Prior to Infant:

   A. Instruct mother to keep her infant identification band on.

   B. Give the mother the nursery phone number and encourage parents to call and/or visit frequently.

   C. Teaching sheet is placed on infant's chart for completion prior to infant's discharge.

V. Infant Discharge Separate From Mother:

   A. Complete Social Service, Mother/baby home visit, and Public Health Referrals if indicated.

(continued)

(continued)

   B. Validate that educational assessment are complete (refer to teaching sheet). Have mother or other primary care giver sign the teaching sheet. Give copy of teaching sheet to care giver.

   C. Verify identification of the person to whom the infant is:

      1. Infant discharged to mother:

         a. Mother has identification bands: compare identifying information on both mother and infant; cut mother's numbered band, and a matching one from infant and attach to infant's chart.

         b. Mother does not have identification bands: verify identification of the mother with a picture ID; obtain driver's license number from the mother and document number in designated area; cut one band from infant and attach to the infant's chart.

      2. Infant discharged to person other than mother:

         a. Have mother sign the Consent to Release Child Form (obtained from the Social Service Department)

         b. Verify identification of person infant being discharged to with a picture ID; obtain the driver's license number from the person and document in infant's chart.

         c. Hospital personnel will transport the infant from the unit to the outside front door.

VI. Mothers wishing to dismiss their infants against medical advice must sign release form. Every effort will be made to discourage this action. The Shift Lead, mother and infant health care providers, and Social Service/Discharge Planning Department. will be notified of parents considering this.

VII. **Documentation will include assessments, nursing interventions, and evaluation of care given.**

- **DESIRED OUTCOME:** Mothers and infants will receive comprehensive physical and psychological care with optimal opportunity for family bonding and attachment and will be appropriately discharged in stable condition.

- **PERSONNEL:** Physician, CNM, NNP, RN, PCA.

- **EXCEPTIONS:** Critical situations involving mother or neonate may not allow continuous mother-baby couplet care.

- **ADAPTATIONS:** This policy contains information previously held in Intrapartum Nusing Policy and replaces Infant Discharge Separate from Maternal Discharge Policy.

- **REFERENCES:**

American Academy of Pediatrics and American College of Obstetricians and Gynecologists (Eds.). (1997). *Guidelines for Perinatal Care*, 4th Edition.

Egbert, Robin, and Peggy Foster, (2001). *The BabyKind Guide to Caring for You and Your Newborn Baby*, 2nd Edition. Cincinnati: Mercy Health Partners Greater Cincinnati.

Olds, Sally B., Marcia London, and Patricia Ladewig. (1999). *Maternal Newborn Nursing, A Family and Community Based Approach*, 6th Edition. New Jersey: Prentice-Hall Health.

Pilliterri, Adele. (1999). *Maternal and Child Health Nursing, Care of the Childbearing and Childrearing Family*, 3rd Edition. Philadelphia: Lippincott.

Simpson, Kathleen Rice, and Patricia A. Creehan. (2001). *Perinatal Nursing*, 2nd Edition AWHONN. Philadelphia: Lippincott.

- **DEFINITION OF TERMS: None**

USE OF THE BIRTHING BALL
Policy and Procedure   *The Good Samaritan Hospital, Lebanon, Pennsylvania*

Section: Maternal Care

Title: Use of the Birthing Ball

POLICY
It is the policy of the Maternity Unit to provide for the safe use of the birthing ball for low-risk women in labor.

PURPOSE
To outline the safe use of the birthing ball in the Maternity Unit.

EQUIPMENT
Birthing Ball

PROCEDURE
1. The staff member is responsible to explain the safe use of the birthing ball as a labor support mechanism. These include:

    a. Support person with patient at all times during use.

    b. Actual demonstration in use of the ball with a support mechanism in place for stabilization of patient (i.e., siderail, chair).

    c. Rocking motion to be utilized—not bouncing.

    d. Patient should have bare feet flat on floor to promote stabilization.

2. The nurse should observe patient utilizing ball and subsequently document return demonstration.

3. The labor ball is cleaned using the same solutions with which all other equipment is cleaned.

4. The labor ball should be approximately 65 cm in diameter when inflated.

5. Women over 280 pounds should not use the birthing ball.

Reproduced here with permission of Good Samaritan Hospital, Lebanon, Pennsylvania.

VISITING IN THE HOLDING NURSERY
Policy and Procedure

Procedure
Provide an opportunity for visitation with the infant in a safe and supervised environment.

Policy
Maternity nursing staff will ensure that parents or designated significant others may visit the newborn in the holding nursery anytime.

Implementation
1. Have the mother approve all visitors.

2. Screen visitors for communicable disease and exposure prior to the visit (e.g., upper respiratory, chicken pox, or influenza). Instruct visitors to wash their hands thoroughly with a hospital-approved soap.

3. Encourage and answer all questions.

4. Promote quiet time for visitors with the infant.

5. Plan on no more than 2 visitors at one time due to the need to maintain a restful environment in the holding nursery.

_____

VP Nursing

_____

Department Chair

POSTCESAREAN BIRTH RECOVERY CARE
Policy and Procedure

Procedure
Provide safe, effective care of new mothers immediately following cesarean birth.

Policy
An RN shall recover the cesarean mother for a minimum of one hour or until vital signs are stable and the course of recovery is normalized.

Equipment
1. Blood pressure monitoring equipment.
2. Thermometer.
3. Stethoscope.
4. Pulse oximeter.
5. Heart rate monitor.
6. Respiration monitor.
7. IV pole, fluids, and supplies.
8. Suction and catheters.
9. Oxygen and nasal cannula or mask.
10. Warm blankets.
11. Washcloths and towels.
12. Sanitary pads and belt.
A. Waterproof under-buttocks pads.
B. Crash cart.

Education
Explain the procedure to the woman and her family and answer their questions prior to the cesarean. Reassure and inform the new mother and her family during the recovery period. Limit visitors only if the mother requests.

Implementation
I. Observations and documentation.

   A. On the woman's arrival from the OB/OR suite, observe and chart the following:

      1. Vital signs.

      2. Level of consciousness.

      3. Subjective experience of pain.

      4. IV fluids:

         a. Type and number of bottles.

         b. Added medications.

         c. IV site and condition.

         d. Amount absorbed.

      5. Operative site:

         a. Cesarean and/or episiotomy site.

         b. Dressing—dry and intact.

         c. Drainage—(lochia) amount, type, and color.

      6. Drainage tubes:

         a. Type.

         b. Location.

(continued)

(continued)

    c. Amount of drainage.

    d. Type and color of drainage.

  7. Type of anesthesia administered.

  8. Medications and fluids used in the OR.

  9. Physician's orders checked and completed.

  10. Fundus:

    a. Location.

    b. Condition—firm, boggy, firm with massage.

B. Check and record every 15 minutes x 1 hour or until stable. Notify the physician of any abnormal findings. (After one hour or when the woman is stabilized, see Postsurgical Recovery Assessment, or follow the physician's orders.)

  1. Vital signs.

  2. Fundus:

    a. Location relative to umbilicus.

    b. Condition—firm, boggy, firm with massage, etc.

  3. Lochia—amount, appearance of episiotomy, if applicable, for swelling, hematoma.

  4. Condition of dressing.

  5. Mobility and sensation.

C. Check for bladder distention. Assess the catheter for patency if urine is less than 30cc per hour. Document the procedure, amount, and color. Pink- or blood-tinged urine may indicate bladder trauma. Notify the physician if urine output is less than 30cc per hour.

D. Give peri and catheter care as needed.

E. Check and record the new mother's temperature. Notify the physician if her temperature is above 100.4°F. Document notification and any orders received.

II. Special care required to maintain an airway after receiving a general anesthetic.

A. Using an oral airway.

  1. Stay at the bedside of a woman with an oral airway.

  2. Observe respirations for quality.

  3. Observe color—oxygen may be started if ordered.

  4. Suction PRN. Deep suction may cause bleeding.

  5. Airway removal:

    a. Wait until the woman either gags slightly or makes an effort to remove the oral airway herself.

    b. Never remove an oral airway forcefully; doing so may break her teeth.

    c. Never attempt to remove an oral airway if it is loose and she does not respond. Use nasal airways for women with caps or without an oral airway whose respirations are inadequate.

B. Administering oxygen.

  1. Regulate the oxygen flow rate and concentration to maintain the SaO_2 greater than 90 percent or as ordered by anesthesia. If unable to maintain SaO_2 greater than 90 percent, notify the anesthesiologist.

  2. Oxygen may be discontinued as ordered by anesthesia personnel.

  3. Have suction equipment set up and available. The woman may become nauseated and vomit. Suction as needed.

C. All women who receive general anesthesia will have their SaO_2 monitored with a pulse oximeter. Monitoring with a pulse oximeter may be discontinued as ordered by anesthesia personnel.

_____

VP Nursing

_____

Department Chair

POST CESAREAN RECOVERY ASSESSMENT
Policy and Procedure

Procedure
Prevent postoperative complications. Provide adequate postpartum care. Promote family attachment.

Policy
An RN will assess the new mother and maintain proper care and management after a cesarean birth.

Equipment
1. Cardiac monitor.
2. Pulse oximeter.
3. Blood pressure monitor.
4. Thermometer.
5. OB recovery assessment sheet.
6. Postpartum supply pack.
7. IV pole or infusion pump.
8. Basin.
9. Nurse call button.

Implementation
I.   Admission assessment.
    A. Check the woman's vital signs.
    B. Assess each body system, with particular attention to:
        1. Respiration—quality, frequency, and regularity.
        2. Circulation—the amount of bleeding from incision and lochia.
        3. Cardiac function—pulse, blood pressure, and rhythm strip.
        4. Urinary and genital—quantity of output and color.
        5. Fundal assessment—tone. Administer oxytocin, if prescribed.
        6. GI system—intake, abdominal distention, and bowel sounds.
II. Provide comfort measures for the new mother.
    A. Provide analgesics as ordered by physician
    B. Position for comfort.
    C. Explain splinting of the incision.
III. Begin postpartum and postoperative instructions. Document.
IV. Promote early interaction between the mother, father, and their infant. Document.
V.   Reunite the family in the recovery as soon as possible.
VI. If the baby must go to the nursery for special care, keep the mother informed of the status of the baby.
VII. Include siblings according to the family's wishes.

VP Nursing

Department Chair

PROVIDING BREAST MILK FOR THE NICU INFANT
Policy and Procedure

Policy

Assistance and instruction will be offered to the mother of the NICU infant to provide expressed breastmilk, assuring that the infant will receive the optimum immunological and nutritional benefits of mother's milk.

Procedure

1. Mothers will be assisted by staff to begin pumping as soon as possible after delivery or when the baby is admitted to the NICU. Preferably this will occur within 6 hours if mother is medically stable.

2. It is crucial to stimulate the breasts early and often to establish an adequate milk supply and a bond when separated from the infant.

3. Mothers will be instructed in the proper collection of breastmilk for the NICU infant.

4. Mothers will be instructed in the proper storage and transportation of breastmilk for their NICU infant. Mothers will be provided with written instructions to take home regarding pumping, collection, and storage procedures.

5. Hospital pumps in the NICU area used by multiple mothers should be cleaned daily using a hospital-approved germicide. See infection control guidelines.

6. Staff will only accept milk that is properly labeled.

7. Freezers and refrigerators that store human milk should be plugged into the hospital emergency power supply (red plugs). If a red plug is not available the temperature will be checked when the power is restored.

8. Milk is to be stored at 40 degrees F. and the refrigerator shall have a thermometer contained inside and easily visible.

9. Milk should be thawed slowly to room temperature before feeding to infant. Microwave thawing is not allowed nor high temperatures of water as valuable nutrients are destroyed in the process.

10. It is recommended that milk refrigerators or freezers accessible to the public should have locks to protect against sabotage.

11. To avoid using the wrong milk, the container should be checked as when giving meds to verify correct patient identification.

12. The integrity of the container will be confirmed before feeding stored breastmilk to infants.

13. When possible, use colostrums or breastmilk for the first feedings.

Courtesy of Barbara Ford, RN, IBCLC.

SAMPLE OF A WELCOME LETTER THAT CAN BE DISTRIBUTED TO VISITORS

Dear friends of the new family:

Welcome! Your visit reflects a loving community of support, which is important to every new family. We would like to offer some ideas on ways that you can help the new family.

At the hospital:

- Consider keeping your visit brief, about 15 minutes. This has several benefits: new parents will be less exhausted, nurses can spend more time teaching infant care, and babies can be fed when hungry. Feeding is a learning experience for both baby and mother and can be difficult in a room full of people.

- Ask the new family how you can help when they return home. Parents have told us that the following things really helped them in the first month:

  - Bring over a few meals that can go from freezer to oven.

  - Offer to drop by to do a few household tasks, such as laundry, grocery shopping, lawn mowing, or housecleaning.

  - If there are other children in the family, offer to take care of the other children for a few hours.

  - After a few weeks, offer to come over to watch the baby for an hour or two while the new parents go out.

At home, when you call or visit:

- Ask how the parents are doing, as well as how the new baby is doing.

- Offer lots of words of praise for the good job they are doing. All new parents need support in the hard work of taking care of their baby.

- Stress to parents that this is their special time to "be taken care of" by others; they should not have to care for anyone but the baby.

- It is usually best to offer advice only when asked for advice. New parents get so much advice they often feel overwhelmed. Support them as they learn about their role and this new and unique baby. They will really appreciate knowing you support their decisions about how they care for their baby.

- If concerns are expressed about the health of mom or baby, encourage the parents to call their doctor or midwife for guidance.

We hope these suggestions have been helpful to you. We are glad you came to visit! All new parents need to know others care about their new family.

The Staff

Adapted from Fairview Riverside Medical Center, Minneapolis, Minnesota.

PERINATAL LOSS
Policy and Procedure *The Good Samaritan Hospital, Lebanon, Pennsylvania*

Policy
It is the policy of The Maternity Unity to provide care to the family experiencing perinatal loss.

Procedure
It is the responsibility of all Nursing personnel to assist the family in the grief process. Nursing and Social Services must work closely in order to meet the requests of the family. If Social Services is not available, all concerns of the family are the responsibility of the nursing staff. Pronouncement of the death is the responsibility of the physician.

1. Initiate a Perinatal Loss Checklist as soon as it is evident that a fetal or neonatal death is imminent.

2. Begin a Perinatal Loss Admission folder providing complete chart including forms, death, and memorial certificates needed. Also found in folder, "When Hello Means Good Bye" should be given shortly after arrival on unit. Pink rose should be placed on patient door at this time. Place sympathy card in chart pocket. Nurses caring for the family may personally sign the nursing unit sympathy card. Address and place card in outgoing mail upon patient discharge.

3. Notify Social Service and/or Nursing Supervisor regarding the situation.

4. One-on-one nursing care prior to and in the initial hours following delivery should be followed whenever possible. The same nurse should be assigned to the patient whenever possible if her stay extends past 24 hours.

5. Select a Memento Memorial Box from bereavement supplies and place items to be used in photos in the box; i.e., baby ring, stuffed animal, baby block, and outfit.

6. Parents should be encouraged to see and hold their baby. The opportunity to have their baby remain in the crib at their bedside or held continually while family members visit is helpful in the grieving process. If they desire the baby to be removed from the room the body can be taken to the morgue or placed wrapped, on ice, and held in the soiled utility room until the family wants the body to hold again. In that case the body can be heated under an infant warmer for a few minutes to remove the ice/chilled feel of the body. Body must be picked up by the funeral home within 24 hours after delivery. Special attention should be given to not rush the family in their short time with their baby.

7. Offer parents the opportunity to bathe the baby or assist staff with the bathing and dressing of their baby. This can be done right on the mother's bed or bedside table to make it physically easier for her. Vaseline on a small piece of cotton or gauze can be placed in mouth and in nostrils if fluid is leaking from body.

8. Encourage parents to name their babies. Staff should refer to the baby by name whenever possible, i.e., "Would you like to help me bathe Michael?" Memorial Certificate should be completed and given to the patient before discharge from hospital.

9. Babies are to be dressed in an outfit provided by the family or by the hospital. Photos are to be taken by staff using a roll of film from the bereavement supply cabinet. In addition, a First Photo Bereavement Consent is obtained and First Photos are taken according to the directions.

   a. A consent is obtained—explain the package is free of charge and will arrive in approximately 3 weeks. White copy placed in package—yellow copy is placed on bulletin board in Assistant Clinical Manager's office—take care to include phone number on the yellow copy for follow-up.

   b. A new role of First Photo Film is used—up to 8 photos taken—enclose film and consent in preprinted package and place orange bereavement sticker on outer package.

   c. Mail same day.

   d. In the event a parent does not want the photos they are to be kept on file on the nursing unit for parents at a future date. While the First Photos require a consent—staff can take a roll of film for the family to later have access to. Family will be told the photos will be here for them if they desire them in the future.

Courtesy of Good Samaritan Hospital, Lebanon, Pennsylvania. Reproduced with permission.

(continued)

(continued)

10. Using film from the bereavement supplies closet, take photos of family members holding the baby and of the baby alone: dressed and at least two naked photos.

    a. Give special detail to using mementos that the family can later have to touch in remembrance of their baby i.e., stuffed animal, baby ring provided, baby block, door rose, offer to use wedding rings, religious medals or cross from mother. Return all items used in photos, including clothing and blanket to the mother's memorial/memento box.

    b. Take family photos that capture emotion.

    c. Refer to bereavement photo album for examples of how to take meaningful photos and what to avoid. There are instructions in the book.

11. Footprints:

    a. Plaster of paris and shells for an indented footprint: supplies in bereavement cabinet. Follow directions on plaster of paris container.

    b. When plaster print complete, place ink footprints on the identification certificate, the memorial certificate and inside the "memorial ring card" if it fits. (If having difficulty with the ink application on smooth feet, use the ink pad provided with the bereavement supplies—always do inking after the plaster print.

    c. Hand print can be alternative when necessary.

12. Lock of hair may be obtained if the parent desires some taken. Offer option to cut the hair themselves.

13. Infant ID bracelet: One on the body, one on the body wrap, and mother's on the foot print ID with baby footprints placed on permanent chart. Mother's signature obtained on Hollister ID. Mother may request infant ID from the funeral home.

14. Baptism of infant may be done by nurse, family, or minister/priest. See policy on Infant Baptism. Shell may be used to hold the water—holy water is in the bereavement supply cabinet. If a shell is used for water, place the shell in their memento box as a keepsake.

15. SHARE pamphlet should be given by staff in event Social Services is not available. This is in admission folder. Ask if SHARE may send them newsletters. If they say yes—check that their name may be placed on the mailing list on the perinatal loss check list.

    Ask if they would like a SHARE parent to contact them. Explain what SHARE is: a local group of parents who have experienced loss and support one another. Check appropriate space on perinatal loss check list and contact SHARE parent whose number is listed in the rolodex under SHARE parents.

16. Funeral arrangements must be made for every infant over 16 weeks gestation. The parents should select the funeral home. Suggest they ask older relatives for assistance with this task if having difficulty with a decision. Information about "Baby Land" located in Annville where the burial plot is at no cost to parents is also available in bereavement notebook.

    a. Some families desire to build their own casket. By Pennsylvania Law the body must first be treated with a chemical. Families can provide their own casket but the body will need to be treated and the death certificate filed by a funeral home. See Bereavement notebook on this topic.

17. Physician is responsible to discuss the option of autopsy and genetic studies with the family. Do not place infant and placenta in formalin if autopsy requested. Autopsy permits are on file in the nurse's station. If under 16 weeks a consent does not need to be signed; send placenta with the fetus and a pathology slip and notify the pathology lab. If greater than 16 weeks, send the fetus, the placenta, and lab slip and consent to the lab together. Also complete laboratory slips for chromosome analysis. Specimens for the chromosome analysis are to be obtained by the physician and placed in Hanks solution (found in OB med room refrigerator). Contact lab if no solution on unit prior to delivery. It is the responsibility of the lab pathologist to notify the funeral director when the autopsy is completed. The death certificate must accompany any fetus (16 weeks or greater) when sent for autopsy.

18. Patient is given option to transfer off the maternity unit. Pink rose placed on door again at time of transfer. May hold baby again on med-surg if she transfers. Refer to #5.

19. Provide family with as much privacy as possible. Unlimited visiting for family members as the parents desire. Encourage spouse to spend the night with patient. Family may have baby with them as long as they desire during the 24 hours period prior to leaving for funeral home.

(continued)

(continued)

20. A green fetal death certificate is completed on all stillborns of 16 weeks gestation or greater. Copy placed on mother's chart. A regular Death Certificate is completed if the infant is born alive in addition to a birth certificate. See policy on Fetal Death Certificates. A copy is placed on the infant chart and the original accompanies the body to the morgue and funeral home.

21. The Delaware Transplant Program must be notified of every stillborn and infant death. This can be done by the unit co-ordinator or the supervisor. Notify coroner's office in accordance with Pennsylvania Law.

22. All mementos are given to parent to take home. If parents do not desire to take the mementos, they are kept in storage on the maternity unit and offered again at a later date. Mementos are kept indefinitely.

23. Infant measurements—weight, length, head, and chest circumference—should be obtained and recorded on the delivery record. If an infant death occurs after 24 hours of age these measurements should be redone at that time and recorded on infant chart.

24. Preparing for the morgue: Undress baby and return the clothing to the parents. Baby should have ID bracelet on arm or leg. Wrap baby in a hospital baby blanket and then a blue Denison wrap. Affix label with baby name to the outside wrap. Use addressograph with mother's name if none available for baby. Mark label with mother's name, date, and sex of baby if known. Tape second ID bracelet to outer wrap securely.

25. Notify Security to meet you at the morgue. Log the baby name in the morgue log book. Security will assist you with this task. Place body in the cold closet along with the death certificate. Call funeral home to notify them the body is now in the morgue ready for release. Do not call funeral home for release if the parents are planning to hold the baby again before discharge.

26. Review discharge instructions found in perinatal loss admission folder with parent prior to discharge. DO NOT give the standard "New Beginnings" DC booklet.

27. Document all pertinent information regarding the infant's death in Nurses' Notes.

    a. Date and time that heart rate and respirations ceased.

    b. Date and time that physician was notified of same if not present.

    c. Date and time that physician pronounced infant death.

    d. Disposition of body:

        1. Date and time to morgue or lab.

        2. Date, time, and name of funeral home if pick-up time known.

    e. Infant care given prior to disposition.

    f. Parent contact, interventions, and outcome.

28. Return any personal items belonging to parents and document the same, i.e., cross necklace used for photos.

29. All portions of the Perinatal Loss Checklist should be as complete as possible. Perinatal Loss Checklist should remain on the mother's chart so communication of all interventions is clear to all staff members in regard to interventions complete and those still needing completion. Information documented on the checklist does not need to be documented a second time in the nurses' notes. Include additional information not placed on checklist in nurses' notes.

    a. Copy of Perinatal Loss Checklist to be placed in the Bereavement Notebook.

    b. Copy of Perinatal Loss Checklist is to be sent to Social Services: "attention Ginger" on inter-hospital mail envelope.

30. Maternity Phone Call follow-up sheet should be placed in bereavement follow-up notebook for staff person assigned to grief follow-up to use to call patient after discharge from hospital. When call is completed, white copy is sent to medical record for permanent chart, pink copy to physician's office, yellow copy remains in bereavement book.

Index